Reproducing Race

Reproducing Race

AN ETHNOGRAPHY OF PREGNANCY
AS A SITE OF RACIALIZATION

Khiara M. Bridges

UNIVERSITY OF CALIFORNIA PRESS
BERKELEY LOS ANGELES LONDON

University of California Press, one of the most distinguished university presses in the United States, enriches lives around the world by advancing scholarship in the humanities, social sciences, and natural sciences. Its activities are supported by the UC Press Foundation and by philanthropic contributions from individuals and institutions. For more information, visit www.ucpress.edu.

University of California Press
Berkeley and Los Angeles, California

University of California Press, Ltd.
London, England

© 2011 by The Regents of the University of California

Library of Congress Cataloging-in-Publication Data

Bridges, Khiara M.
   Reproducing race : an ethnography of pregnancy as a site of racialization / Khiara M. Bridges.
    p. cm.
   Includes bibliographical references and index.
   ISBN 978-0-520-26894-4 (hardcover : alk. paper) — ISBN 978-0-520-26895-1 (paperback : alk. paper)
1. Alpha Hospital (New York, N.Y.)   2. Hospitals—Maternity services—New York (State)—
New York.   3. Discrimination in medical care—New York (State)—New York.   4. Minorities—
Medical care—New York (State)—New York.   I. Title.
   [DNLM: 1. Alpha Hospital (New York, N.Y.)
2. Maternal Health Services—standards—New York City.   3. Maternal Health Services—
standards—United States.   4. Anthropology, Cultural—New York City.   5. Anthropology,
Cultural—United States.   6. Healthcare Disparities—New York City.   7. Healthcare
Disparities—United States.   8. Hospitals, Municipal—standards—New York City.
9. Hospitals, Municipal—standards—United States.   10. Prenatal Care—New York City.
11. Prenatal Care—United States.   12. Socioeconomic Factors—New York City.
13. Socioeconomic Factors—United States. WA 310 AN7]
   RG501.U6B75 2011
   362.19'82009747—dc22

2010041690

20 19 18 17 16 15 14 13 12 11
10 9 8 7 6 5 4 3 2 1

To Clive R. Bridges and Deborah A. Bridges,
who have loved me flawlessly

CONTENTS

ACKNOWLEDGMENTS   IX

INTRODUCTION   I

PART ONE
CLASS

1 / Alpha Hospital: Unique, But Not Singular   21

2 / Pregnancy, Medicaid, State Regulation,
and Legal Subjection   41

3 / The Production of Unruly Bodies   74

PART TWO
RACE

4 / The "Primitive Pelvis," Racial Folklore, and Atavism in
Contemporary Forms of Medical Disenfranchisement   103

5 / The Curious Case of the "Alpha Patient Population"   144

6 / Wily Patients, Welfare Queens, and the
Reiteration of Race   201

EPILOGUE   251

NOTES   259

BIBLIOGRAPHY   273

INDEX   287

ACKNOWLEDGMENTS

I begin by thanking the wonderful mommies and mommies-to-be who sat down with me (and my mini tape recorder) and shared their fascinating stories. I hope this work reflects at least some of the complexity and beauty of their lives. I would also like to thank the physicians, midwives, nurse practitioners, registered nurses, and other hospital staff members who let me observe them, ask them questions, and generally get in their way. I thank the four special ladies who worked at the front desk of the "Alpha" Women's Health Clinic; they took me into their fold and made every single day I spent in the clinic fun and interesting. Thanks are also owed to the women who helped me get approval for my research from the "Omega University" Institutional Review Board. My appreciation for them is in no way dulled by this requisite cloak of anonymity. I owe a debt of gratitude to "Dr. Christine Johnson," the Director of Ambulatory Care at "Alpha Hospital." She answered my unsolicited phone call, listened to a hasty, inarticulate description of my project, and agreed to help me realize my fieldwork. A special thanks goes to Rayna Rapp—an exceedingly kind individual. But for Professor Rapp, this project probably would have remained a figment of my imagination.

I would like to acknowledge the Wenner-Gren Foundation for Anthropological Research for providing me with a generous grant that supported my fieldwork, as well as the Center for Reproductive Rights (in conjunction with Columbia Law School) for the fellowship that supported me through portions of the revision process. Moreover, the process of publishing this book has been mercifully easy. Thanks to Reed Malcolm, my editor at the University of California Press, for the experience. A special heartfelt thanks goes to Stan Holwitz, who set me up for success. Thanks are also owed to John Hoberman.

I am deeply indebted to the professors who have taught me over the years. Nicholas De Genova has guided this project from its inception. I thank him for his willingness to respond to my anxiety-filled e-mails, to engage with my work, and to scribble crushingly intelligent insights in the margins of my drafts. Neni Panourgia introduced me to Foucault and shared her magnificent brilliance with me. Brinkley Messick believed I could actually write this book—even when I was just a student in law school. Kendall Thomas sparked the desire in me to emulate him. Carol Sanger was a reliable source of advice and encouragement throughout my long journey into academia. David Leebron has had unending confidence in me. Finally, the late E. Allan Farnsworth was so much more to me than just a Contracts professor. I am grateful to them all.

I would like to thank my colleagues and friends in Columbia University's Department of Anthropology—specifically Adriana María Garriga-López, Ayça Cubuçku, and Danielle DiNovelli-Lang. I could always count on them for motivation and laughter.

Thanks as well to my ballet instructors—specifically my mentor and coach, Kat Wildish, for lovingly (yet relentlessly) torturing me over the years. I am also grateful to the scores of dancers with whom I have had the pleasure of training and working. I thank them for their inspiration and for always looking really shocked and disbelieving when I told them I was also an academic. Thanks are also owed to Joe Risico, for everything.

I am ceaselessly indebted to my family. I am indebted to my grandparents—Grandma, Church Grandma, and my two Granddaddies—whose strength and perseverance are the conditions of possibility for any success I may have in this life. Thanks as well to my extended family—specifically my "Uncle J," James Bridges, for insisting in his own special way that I be exceptional. Thanks to my sister, Algeria Bridges, who has supported me since the days when we shared a mural-painted bedroom and wore matching yellow Easter dresses. I have been awed by the intellect of my brother, Khari Bridges, since the time when he used to wear the yellow suit version of my Easter dress. Finally, my love for my parents, Clive R. Bridges and Deborah A. Bridges, defies articulation. Their love and encouragement lie behind every word that I write.

Introduction

Diana, Yessica, and Evelyn—all physician assistants, or Patient Care Associates (PCAs)—are chatting in one of the nurses' triage rooms during a lull in a typically chaotic day in the "Alpha" Women's Health Clinic. Diana, an outspoken, funny young woman of Haitian parentage who has been working for over six months in the clinic as a temporary employee, sits on an examination table and plays with the creases in her uniform. On the other side of the cramped space, touching up her carefully applied makeup, sits Yessica, thirty-five and Dominican Republic-born, who has been working at Alpha for close to five years. Evelyn, an older woman who had immigrated to the United States from Jamaica, and who has been a PCA at Alpha for over a decade, leans against a chest of drawers, arms angrily folded over her chest. Evelyn has just finished escorting a patient to the physician for her examination. The patient, in the final months of her pregnancy, had complained loudly and persistently about the long time she had waited for her appointment that day.

The incident with that disagreeable patient has sparked a conversation among Diana, Yessica, and Evelyn about the "problem" with patients generally. Diana brushes a piece of lint off of her shirt and remarks, "They don't even have good insurance. They come in here with their little lousy Medicaid and be the main ones raising up in the hallway."

Yessica and Evelyn laugh, commenting that Diana's statement is "so true." Encouraged, Diana continues, "They have more money than we do. They have two or three baby daddies that they get child support from. They have Section 8, so they pay $100 in rent. They have food stamps; they have WIC. And then they stroll in here with their Coach bags." More laughter, accompanied by a smattering of "I know" and "she's right." Diana continues, "That's why they have kids. For real. That's why they have them. And then us—we bust our behinds working everyday, and we have holes in our socks. Can't even afford to buy a bottle of water if we get thirsty." More laughter, but this time, Evelyn interjects, "But, we have a better quality of life than they do." Yessica disagrees, "No, we don't. That's why they *choose* to live their lives like that. Some people don't like to work." Diana, nodding her head, concurs, "My cousin could have collected welfare and just sat at home. She had two kids. But, she chose not to. She chose to get a job. And now, she's just like us."

⌁

In an article written almost two decades ago about Alpha's emergency room, the writer describes the care Alpha gives to its patients as "war-zone medicine":

> It also sees the worst wounds of the city: crack addicts, bullet holes from drug-related assault guns, AIDS patients, the homeless who have no place to go for care, teen-agers who need severed limbs reattached after being run over by subway cars, inmates from city prisons whose manacled ankles protrude from stretchers.
>
> At Alpha, battlefield images fit like bandages on a wound.
>
> Drugs are found in two out of three patients who are shot, stabbed or hit by a car, doctors say. One-fourth of the trauma cases involve people who have mixed two or more intoxicants, usually alcohol and cocaine.
>
> The homeless seek treatment for such ills as frostbite and rotted feet similar to soldiers who suffered trench foot, a disease caused by prolonged exposure to wet, cold and inactivity. (Dvorchak 1990)

⌁

Julie, a twenty-four-year-old, soft-spoken, self-professed Rastafarian who recently moved back to the United States from Trinidad, exits the secured door separating the waiting area from the examination rooms and empties the contents of her bag onto the front desk. "The midwife lost my clinic card!" she cries, referring to the card Alpha issues to every patient stamped with the patient's name, address, and a seven-digit number that identifies the patient throughout every clinic and department in the hospital. Patients must present this card at every appointment. If lost, the patient must get a new one issued in the Business Office located on the lobby floor of the ambulatory care building, a task that could take anywhere from fifteen minutes to two hours depending on hospital traffic that day. "She lost it! I know that she didn't give it back to me! Now she has me looking like I'm crazy!" Julie rustles through the pile of items she has poured onto the desk. "I don't have time to get another card! I have a lot of appointments to go to today! I have to go to Brooklyn. . . . I don't have time for this! The midwife—she's all smiles. But, when I tell her that she didn't give me my card back, all of a sudden, she's like, 'I have to go to lunch.'" Angry tears have begun to stream down Julie's face. "She should just say that she's sorry."

A middle-aged, African-American woman sits in the bustling waiting area in the Alpha Women's Health Clinic, waiting for a nurse to give her an injection of Lupron©—a medicine her physicians hope will help reduce the symptoms of her uterine fibroids. The physician who had attended to her on this day, Dr. Grenier, a very bubbly, young white resident, had prescribed an additional medicine to be taken orally. The patient attempted to fill the prescription at Alpha's pharmacy, which provides selected medications at no cost to the patient. However, Alpha's pharmacy did not stock the medicine Dr. Grenier had prescribed. And so Dr. Grenier consults with Dr. Ming, the attending physician, about what they can do for the patient. When the apparent answer is "nothing," Dr. Ming only half-mockingly says with a laugh, "We should close Alpha." Dr. Grenier, again only half-mockingly, responds, "Wait until I finish my residency! But, if they closed Alpha, where would they take all the prisoners who need medical attention? Or all the patients with tuberculosis? Or all the psychiatric patients? No hospital is going to see them. We always say that, after Alpha, if they put us in a *good* hospital, we wouldn't know what to do. But, if they put us in the jungle, we would be fine."

The doctors continue to debate how to treat the patient. Dr. Ming suggests, "We could give her the money to take the prescription to an outside pharmacy and have it filled." By this time, Trisha, a dour West Indian registered nurse not known for her tact has wandered over. She remarks, "Where is that money going to come from? The thing that kills me about these patients is that they don't have three dollars to pay for medication, but then they have Dooney & Burke bags and all this stuff that I can't afford—stuff that, if I bought it, I wouldn't be able to eat. But, they buy it because they think, 'Someone at Alpha will give me money.'" Dr. Ming simply smiles and says, "That's why I like working at Alpha—because it keeps you thinking." Trisha agrees: "You'll never get Alzheimer's here. Because your brain is always working."

In 1964, New York City began constructing a new building for Alpha Hospital. Important people understood the project to be a significant one; a director of the hospital had called the construction of a new building vital, as the hospital's "physical surroundings will match its staff's ambitions for patient service" (Opdycke 1999, 168). In response to the announced plans, a surgeon who had interned at the hospital offers a healthy dose of realism and skepticism by publishing a "tribute" to Alpha in a local paper, affirming his faith that the spirit of Alpha would not be "corrupted" by any expensive, elegant building the city might erect for it:

> She resists improvements as her bacteria resist antibiotics and in the end, virulent, she survives. So let the city fathers move in with their millions of dollars. Let them build new buildings, hire more help, buy more syringes, do their damnedest to destroy her personality and make her a replica of every other white, cold, sterile and efficient citadel of healing. She will resist that standardization. And I am willing to wager that when the last new building has been built, the last technician hired, the last dollar spent, there will still be no scissors on Ward M5. (Opdycke 1999, 168)

Dr. Veronica Rose—an intimidating, older white attending physician whose brashness, rudeness, and insensitivity make it difficult to appreciate that she is probably a very competent OB/GYN—exits her examination room, only to see a pile of patient charts in the box outside. She flips through them and asks Yessica, the PCA assisting her that day, "Who keeps putting all these walk-ins in my box?" Yessica, who was talking to a patient, stops that conversation to respond, "I'm not sure, Dr. Rose." Dr. Rose, dissatisfied, continues, "Is there anyone precepting today?" Yessica answers, "I think Dr. Silverstein is." Dr. Rose thrusts the charts into Yessica's hands and says, "Well then, let Dr. *fucking* Silverstein do them." She marches off, white coat swaying, the sound of her heels against the tile floor echoing. The patient to whom Yessica was speaking before her exchange with the doctor watches Dr. Rose, the physician she is scheduled to see that day, go around the corner and disappear.

❧

The above vignettes offer a pithy slice of life at Alpha Hospital, a place that is a "legend in American medicine—one of the country's busiest, wildest, most able hospitals, and one of the remaining few where ability to pay is not a prime consideration" (Zuger 2001). In these scenes, one can see the contours of major themes that frame the hospital and will recur throughout the ethnography: an ancillary staff, composed primarily of first-generation immigrants of color, whose distrust and dislike of the patients they serve cause them to echo the arguments made by conservative pundits in favor of dismantling the existing welfare state; well-trained, elite physicians struggling to provide the most technologically sophisticated health care to society's most destitute and most marginalized; patients, predominately poor persons of color, who are both the victims and the beneficiaries of Alpha's underfunded, overburdened nature, struggling to receive that most technologically sophisticated health care; the thinly controlled chaos that threatens to burst forth—and, occasionally, does indeed do so—despite the best efforts of the staff, physicians, and administrators to prevent it.

THE ROAD TO ALPHA

My path to the Women's Health Clinic (WHC) at Alpha Hospital had been quite circuitous. My first contact with Alpha was through an article in the "Sunday Styles" section of the *New York Times* about the author's struggle to be correctly diagnosed with (and ultimately treated for) Lyme disease (Cooper 2003). After having been seen by some of the most esteemed and status-rich physicians in Manhattan, none of whom could identify the origin of the "high fever, headache, generally altered consciousness, and . . . large necrotic wound" (Cooper 2003, 3) on the back of his leg, Cooper became desperate:

> In August, I started calling City Health Department numbers and ended up at the Poison Control Center, somehow persuading the operator to connect me with an actual doctor. I told him my story, and just when I thought the nice man on the other end of the phone was humoring me, he told me to meet him at Alpha's emergency room so he could take a look.
> Alpha? As in, leather restraints on the gurneys?
> Indeed. I endured a line 20 people deep just to see the triage nurse.
> Alas, it took a public city hospital like Alpha to cure me of the exotic ailment I had picked up outside of New York. (Ibid)

After being tested for Lyme disease at Alpha, and after the disease had been positively identified, Cooper continued his treatment there and was ultimately cured. He wrote of the irony that the most acclaimed of Manhattan's physicians could not do what a lowly staff doctor at the city's much maligned public hospital could. How peculiar, he wrote, that in a place evoking images of straitjackets and urban decay he found the cure that previously eluded him.

When I read this article that introduced me to Alpha, I had been living in New York City for several years, and had long thought of myself as a *New Yorker*. I remember feeling a bit ashamed after reading this piece, as it challenged that status: a "true" *New Yorker* would not have been oblivious to Alpha Hospital and the images it ought to conjure. While it was difficult to adjust to the idea of thinking of myself as merely *living in New York*, the article had appropriately introduced me to Alpha, which I now understood to be: 1) a psychiatric hospital, 2) a paradigmatic beleaguered public/poor person's hospital, and 3) a place where one received quality health care only after having endured bureaucracy and excessive wait times alongside the "tired, poor, huddled masses."

My second encounter with Alpha came a couple of years later. I was in midtown Manhattan on a Saturday evening, having just celebrated a college friend's birthday, when a young man who looked no older than sixteen approached me and asked, "Which way is Ninth Avenue?" Pleased that I could demonstrate my knowledge of all things Manhattan and help someone out in the process, I pointed a deft finger westward and said,

"Cross the street, walk another block. You'll see Ninth Ave." Smiling and thanking me, the kid took off across the street. Moments later, a livery cab running a red light struck him. In shock, I saw his body flying through the air, the sound of metal hitting flesh and bone seeming louder than anything I had thought possible. Some onlookers ran to his aid; others called 911 from their mobile phones. I could only stand motionlessly on the sidewalk. Eventually, I began to cry. I wept until the ambulance arrived minutes later, wept as I asked the paramedic where they were taking him, wept as he responded, "Alpha."

I did not know at the time that it was a foregone conclusion that he would be taken to Alpha, as the hospital received the bulk of trauma-related injuries that occurred in Manhattan. All I knew was that I could not free myself from the image of the airborne kid or the memory of the sound. In the cab on the way to Alpha, I tried to steel myself for the news he had died, that I was the last person who had heard him talk and seen him smile. I do not remember arriving in Alpha's emergency room, although I do have vague recollections of being told that because I was not a relative, the staff was prohibited from giving me any information regarding the boy's status. But I refused to leave without knowing if he had lived or died, and so I sat, defiantly, in a waiting room chair, hoping one of the workers would have pity on me. I would have sat there forever, but there was no need: an hour or so later, I saw the kid limping down the hall in a hospital gown, still smiling, but this time missing a front tooth.

On that first visit to Alpha, I bore witness to the hospital at its best—an institution that stood ready and able to put the pieces of an unlucky young man back together. I also bore witness to sights that might be anticipated (but for which one is never really prepared) in an emergency room of a public hospital on a weekend night: a man handcuffed to a stretcher, eagerly eating a mystery meat sandwiched between two pieces of white bread; another man sitting on a gurney with cuts all over his face, being interviewed by a policeman; an elderly man, completely and utterly alone, sitting in a wheelchair facing the wall. I do not remember witnessing the stepped-up security that has come to be a sign of the times since September 11, 2001 in New York City public institutions. One hospital administrator remarked that since that day, the hospital has hired more security officers and has restricted points of entry. She feared turning the building into "a fortress," saying "I still want to maintain this as a place you want to come to if you are sick. I still want that fuzzy, patient-centered feeling" (Becker 2002). On that first visit, I did not get the sense that the hospital had achieved that coveted "fuzzy, patient-centered feeling," but neither did I feel I had entered a fortress. (That only came after I began my research there and had to flash hospital identification every day when I came into the building.)

On that first visit to Alpha, I also do not remember bearing witness to the other aspect (besides legendary medical care) for which Alpha's emergency room is known. As one journalist put it, Alpha's "admirable characteristics, however, do not always translate into smooth or serene health care delivery, a fact well known to both Alpha's staff and its patients. The ground floor emergency area can be a sea of confusion and flaring tempers—doctors hollering at doctors, nurses at nurses, both of them at aides, at one another, at patients, and patients right back at everyone else" (Zuger 2001). Although I would witness countless verbal and near-physical confrontations during my fieldwork in the WHC, on my first visit to Alpha, the ER was fairly tranquil.

The next time I set foot in Alpha was in the early summer of 2005—this time with the purpose of studying race as a process. At some point during my studies in law school and graduate school, I had grown impatient with what had become a mantra within academia: "race is a social construction." I stood in complete agreement—of course race is a social construction. The truth of the definition of race offered by the American Anthropological Association (1998) seemed indisputable to me: surely race was a biologically arbitrary, socially constructed ideology about physical differences among humans, with a "race" being a socially salient, hierarchically ordered category. However, what bewildered and frustrated me was the absence of studies demonstrating *how* race was socially constructed. I wanted to know by what processes race had endured as an omnipresent social fact with powerful material repercussions despite its lack of moorings in biology (Crenshaw et al. 1995). And so, I dreamt up the present research project as an investigation of the construction of race during the event of pregnancy—an event that continues to engage racial discourses. In short, I wanted to write an ethnography of pregnancy as a site of racialization.

What I discovered when I finally began ethnographic research in the Alpha WHC exceeded my carefully crafted research questions. Indeed, when I began my fieldwork, I had to reformulate all of them. Initially, I had imagined that I would conduct my fieldwork for the project in Delta Hospital, a smaller public hospital located in central Harlem. Because I had envisioned the project as an ethnography of pregnancy as a site of the racialization of African American women specifically, Delta Hospital (which because of its location attends to large numbers of African and African-American people) was an ideal site. I spoke with the director of the Obstetrics and Gynecology clinic at Delta six months or so before I was to begin fieldwork, and he affirmed his commitment to providing Delta as my field. However, when the time arrived for my fieldwork to actually begin, he stopped returning my phone calls. I found myself field-less (and devastated). Six months later, after sending my research proposal to every director of obstetrics at every private and public hospital in Manhattan, Brooklyn, Queens, the Bronx, and eastern New Jersey, I still had not found another site. On a whim, I sent an e-mail to Rayna Rapp,[1] who I had never met, but whose acknowledgements in her book *Testing Women, Testing the Fetus* revealed her to be well-connected to those with the power to grant a humbled anthropologist access to that which lies behind hospital walls. To my utter surprise and delight, Professor Rapp responded and put me in touch with Dr. Christina Johnson, the Director of Ambulatory Care at Alpha Hospital. Dr. Johnson responded positively to my research proposal, and so began my extended love affair with Alpha.

And so also began the rearticulation of my research questions. The sheer racial and ethnic diversity of the patients seen within the Alpha WHC made insincere and artificial any insistence upon focusing on the racialization of African Americans alone; the heterogeneity of Alpha's patients forced me to broaden my project from one inquiring into the racialization of Black women to one inquiring into racialization processes more generally. Moreover, that which was common to the subjects of my study would no longer be race—as it would had I conducted fieldwork at Delta—but rather socioeconomic class, as all Alpha obstetrics patients came within Medicaid income limits. If the Alpha obstetrics clinic was to be my field, I had to directly confront the Medicaid apparatus. Additionally, it foregrounded my consideration of the relationship between race and class, as I found that to "get to" questions of race, I had to "go through" issues of class. This is not to say that class always precedes race, that race must come subsequent to class in every instance, or that race is an epiphenomenon of class; however, to pursue my investigation, the analytic of race had to be folded into an analysis that began with class. Thus, class is the point of entry for the first three chapters of the book, thereby enabling me to address questions of race in the last three chapters.

The book proceeds from the assumption that race is a discursive phenomenon; race is ideas about difference that become visible and tangible as they are made to be reflected in the material conditions within society

(Haney-López 1996). Material and societal conditions appear to affirm the veracity of ideas about race. And the unfortunate dialectic continues. I wanted to examine this dialectical process of race formation *as it occurs during women's pregnancies* because pregnancy engages racial discourses to such a dramatic extent that pregnancy can be described as a racially salient event. Roberts (1997) has made such an argument. Noting that scientific racism's primary supposition was the genetic basis of race and, consequently, superiority and inferiority, she argues "[b]ecause race was defined as an inheritable trait. . . . [r]eproductive politics in America inevitably involves racial politics" (9). Further, pregnancy has remained racially salient even though, prior to the recent reinvigoration of biological notions of race, there was a waning of ideas about racial biology; this is because Black mothers are thought to transfer to their children the "deviant lifestyle" that explains their persistent social inferiority. Expounds Roberts:

> As both biological and social reproducers, it is only natural that Black mothers would be a key focus of this racist ideology. White childbearing is generally thought to be a beneficial activity: it brings personal joy and allows the nation to flourish. Black reproduction, on the other hand, is treated as a form of *degeneracy*. Black mothers are seen to corrupt the reproduction process at every stage. . . . They damage their babies in the womb through their bad habits during pregnancy. Then they impart a deviant lifestyle to their children through their example. This damaging behavior on the part of Black mothers—not arrangements of power—explains the persistence of Black poverty and marginality. (1997: 9)

That white women are largely exempt from discourses that censure and condemn their reproduction *on the basis of their race* increases the racial salience of the event of pregnancy. Moreover, pregnancy is a focused occasion to interrogate racial processes because it directly implicates the material bodies of women. This is important because, historically and presently, the material body has been understood as the primary sign of racial difference (Schiebinger 1993; Wiegman 1995).

Although pregnancy is fairly described as a racially salient event, one of the greatest ironies I encountered during my fieldwork with pregnant women at Alpha was the absence of explicit discussions of race—even though it was obvious to me that race was essential to any explanation of *why* Alpha is the way it is and *how* it persists as such. That race is a powerful organizing principle at Alpha was suggested by the racial geography of the WHC: although several of the providers who worked in the clinic can be described as persons of color, most of them were white. Yet, the providers were assisted by a support, or ancillary, staff that was entirely composed of women of color. Moreover, during the period in which I conducted my fieldwork, most of the ancillary staff persons were first-generation immigrants to the United States. Thus, there was a fascinating, racially significant chain of command in the clinic: white persons, with the most power and prestige in the clinic, sat at the top of the clinic hierarchy with their non-white assistants populating the ranks below them. Furthermore, the racial dynamic within the clinic was made even more fascinating by the racial composition of the patients served there; although many white patients sought obstetrical and gynecological care at Alpha, the large majority of Alpha patients were racial minorities. This meant a predominately white group of providers practiced medicine upon a largely disempowered, disenfranchised, marginalized, and importantly, non-white group of patients. Although it was difficult to ignore or dismiss the racial geography of the clinic, very few of the persons with whom I spoke during my fieldwork actually commented upon it. Indeed, I was frustrated for many months by the refusal and/or inability of any of my interlocutors to offer race as a relevancy—despite the fact that race could not and should not be ignored as a salient category that has produced Alpha as the underfunded, discursively maligned, frequently polemical space that it is.

THE QUESTION OF PSEUDONYMS

In the final months of my research at Alpha, another anthropologist previously unknown to me also began fieldwork in the obstetrics clinic. Although I was initially apprehensive about the prospect of sharing "my" field with a "competing" anthropologist, she eventually became a valued colleague with whom I could compare notes. One afternoon, we began contemplating life after Alpha and the practicalities of writing up our research. I asked her if she would employ a pseudonym when she referred to Alpha in her scholarship. She replied that she probably would not, as she did not believe her argument to be hypercritical of the hospital such that a pseudonym was warranted. Then she smiled and said, "But, I think *you* should definitely use a pseudonym for Alpha in the stuff that you plan to write."

And so, my colleague interpellated me as the author of a work offering a relatively unforgiving critique of the Alpha WHC and the legislation and policies it is compelled to effect—the author of a critique so trenchant that, to protect the hospital (as well as my relationships with the people who enabled me to conduct my fieldwork there), I should employ a pseudonym when referring to it in my scholarship. However, I have also been identified previously on numerous occasions as a person whose politics lie far left of center. Thus, I recognized the contradiction: I am the author of a work that relentlessly critiques a generous, laudable moment in this country's "safety net": a moment of universal health care, no less. On other occasions, this is a moment I would vociferously defend. Therefore, I must recognize and concede the contradiction resulting from my reproving a place and policies whose nonexistence I would also reprove with the argument that the lack of commitment to state-subsidized or universal health care leaves the most vulnerable most exposed.

I insist the New York State Prenatal Care Assistance Program (PCAP), the Medicaid program upon which the overwhelming majority of pregnant Alpha patients rely, is an example of universal health care because its relatively high income limitations (a woman can earn up to 200 percent of the federal poverty line and still qualify for the program) and its availability to undocumented immigrant women enable health care to be provided to a significant number of persons who would not otherwise have access to it. Moreover, PCAP mimics universal health care insofar as the health services available under it are not limited to obstetrical care. Medicaid/PCAP-insured women can avail themselves of dental, optometric, dermatological, and general medical services (among others) should the need or even desire arise. However, the Medicaid/PCAP program should be considered a limited instantiation of universal health care, mainly because men and non-pregnant women are excluded from its ambit, but also because the generous insurance coverage given to the pregnant woman terminates just eight weeks after she gives birth. As I thankfully acknowledge the radical nature of the PCAP program—one midwife I interviewed insisted upon characterizing the program as "revolutionary"—I find myself in the awkward position of criticizing the revolution.

Now, one of the reasons the revolution has been launched in the obstetrics clinic of New York public hospitals is because the uninsured, pregnant poor have been conceptualized by decision makers as an "at risk population." That is, the "at risk population" served within the Alpha WHC would not have access to the health care I critique if those who are responsible for implementing Medicaid/PCAP had not imagined the "population" served by the program as having characteristics that demand a state response in the form of government-subsidized health care. Despite the failure of the United States to commit itself to providing medical services to the other millions of "medically indigent" individuals who are unable to afford private health insurance, there was something about this "at risk population" served by Medicaid/PCAP that produced results. Ironically, the racism, xenophobia, classism, and sexism that inform discourses about "risk" and "populations" in effect enable the realization of a universalized, though circumscribed, system of health care within a country that presently stands uncommitted to implementing a program of universal health care.

However, a problematic "state of exception" results from the engendering of this finite moment of universal health care, a moment that is designed for and only accessible to a bounded group. Which is to say: although one could make a persuasive argument that everyone should receive government-subsidized health care, the group of individuals that does, in fact, receive state-funded care becomes exceptional. When a radical moment of universal health care is realized within an otherwise privatized system, the group that benefits becomes understood as radically in need of the exception— they become particular, peculiar, unusual. They also become discursively constructed as even more likely vectors of disease and pathology. Significantly, the construction does not exist only at the level of discourse alone; it is made material through the manipulation of the physical bodies of Alpha patients. The production of the poor, PCAP-insured/uninsured pregnant women as exceptionally pathological would not necessarily occur if the United States actualized a system of unbounded, unlimited, and universal health care. Within a system of nationalized medicine, there would be no need to imagine a segment of society as somehow being more "at risk" for certain lamentable outcomes (and, therefore, uniquely deserving of the suspension of the system of privatized medicine) before health care is provided for them; the state's subsidization of their health care would be the expectation, not the deviation.

THE QUESTION OF METHODOLOGY

For the first couple of months of my fieldwork, I sat in the Alpha WHC waiting area and simply observed clinic traffic, attempting to make sense of what appeared to be barely controlled bedlam. I remember thinking this place that was to be my field for the next year-and-a-half was incredibly familiar, yet undeniably strange. It was familiar because, in many respects, it resembled the numerous doctors' offices I have frequented over the years—with the televisions broadcasting educational shows about nutrition and exercise, the nurses calling out names in the waiting area, the magazines sitting on tops of tables with the addressee information scribbled out with black marker, and the friendly, though intimidating, doctors with their white coats and stethoscopes. Yet, the WHC remained strange because hospital policy required identification upon entry. Thus, one got the distinct feeling after passing through security that one was entering into a potentially dangerous, but secured place—like a courthouse or airport. It remained strange because Alpha is *the* place in New York City where the indigent, homeless, or otherwise dispossessed go when they are injured or sick. Thus, on the way up to the WHC, one may hold the elevator for a bandaged homeless man. It remained strange because of the sheer diversity of the patients who seek prenatal care there. Thus, on any given day, one can overhear patients in the waiting area speaking English, Spanish, Mandarin, Cantonese, Polish, Arabic, Bengali, Urdu, Hindi, and French.

After I had familiarized myself with the space and the staff—and, importantly, after the staff had familiarized themselves with me—I eventually moved behind the front desk and began the "participant" portion of my participant-observation of the clinic. On those days, I worked behind the front desk and did intake—answering telephones and questions, greeting patients, making appointments, administering urine pregnancy tests, etc. About a year into my fieldwork, I moved to the nurses' triage rooms where I observed women's preparations for their medical examinations. After some time, I "participated" in these rooms by taking and recording women's weights and blood pressures and by testing the pregnant women's urine for the presence of glucose and protein, dipping a pH stick into the tube of collected urine they provided at the beginning of each visit.

Over time, as the required female presence in the room, I was able to observe patients' examinations by male providers. I also observed patients' consultations with social workers, nutritionists, Medicaid financial officers, health educators, geneticists, and nurses. I watched several ultrasound scans and several more labors and births in the labor and delivery room. Moreover, I conducted over 120 hours of in-depth interviews with eighty patients—something I was able to do while the women waited inordinately long periods of time to see their providers during their scheduled appointments—and fifty hours of in-depth interviews with thirty providers and staff persons. As a counterpoint to my fieldwork in Alpha Hospital, I also spent several weeks observing the obstetrics clinic in Sigma Hospital, a smaller public hospital located in the Lower East Side of Manhattan. Moreover, my research led me outside of institutional walls as I attended baby showers thrown in honor of the women I met at Alpha, audited birthing classes offered by non-hospital-affiliated organizations, interviewed women at their homes, and volunteered at a nonprofit organization dedicated to lowering the maternal and infant mortality rates in Northern Manhattan.

THE ARGUMENT TO COME

Chapter 1 provides a robust description of Alpha Hospital's location within the larger public health context. Alpha Hospital is a distinctive institution with a long and colorful history within New York City and the nation. This chapter provides that color. In truth, Alpha Hospital is arguably the best public hospital in the country; moreover, it is one of the few places in the nation where poor people have access to first-rate, outstanding health care. A vigorous acknowledgment of the uniqueness of Alpha Hospital—as an institution impressive in light of both the quality and breadth of the services it provides to the poor—raises the stakes of the critique that is to come. Given this institution is, perhaps, the best shot the poor have at getting quality health care, what does it mean that it (and the services it provides) can nevertheless be criticized as excessive in its technology, intrusive in its demands for knowledge, pathologizing as an equalizing move, demeaning to its patients, and perpetuating of racial and social inequalities? A vigorous acknowledgment that the program of universal prenatal care offered within Alpha Hospital may be the best version available makes more trenchant the critique of the U.S. political economy and racial politics that follows. But although Alpha Hospital is unique, it should not be understood as singular: to the extent that Alpha is a site wherein poor, pregnant women's bodies are excessively problematized and racial inequities are reiterated, this is a product not of some curious quality of Alpha, but rather that Alpha as an institution depends upon public dollars to deliver health care to uninsured, marginalized persons in the United States. Consequently, the critique is not of Alpha as such, but rather of the nationally circulating discourses, politics, policies, and practices that also affect Alpha and the people who populate it.

As mentioned earlier, the large majority of patients who receive their prenatal care from Alpha rely upon Medicaid/PCAP to cover their medical expenses. As a condition of receipt of this aid, women were required to meet with a battery of professionals—namely, social workers, health educators, nutritionists, and financial officers—who are legally obliged to inquire into areas of women's lives that frequently exceed the realm of the medical. This fact, coupled with interviews I conducted with women who described their experiences with this inquisitive apparatus, led me to conclude that Medicaid mandates an intrusion into women's private lives and produces pregnancy as an opportunity for state supervision, management, and regulation of poor, otherwise uninsured women. I explore this aspect of Medicaid in Chapter 2.

In Chapter 3, I direct my attention to the medical technology provided to indigent pregnant women as a matter of course within Alpha Hospital—a teaching hospital renowned for the highly sophisticated medical care that it can and does deliver to its patients. This chapter describes the prenatal health care that poor, pregnant women receive and notes that it is delivered within an abundantly technological, biomedical paradigm of pregnancy. I argue what Medicaid-insured, pregnant women's bodies receive is excessive in the sense that it goes beyond any necessary and appropriate medicalization, as well as that offered to privately insured women. This chapter concludes that the result of this excessive medicalization is that poor women are produced as possessors of "unruly bodies." Because the uninsured poor are universally produced as such, the consequence is a medicalization of poverty, with the poor being treated as biological dangers within the body politic. The excesses of Medicaid's medicalization, which can be understood as a suspicion of poor women's bodies as especially "at risk," provides an important basis for the argument that the "high risk" the patients receiving prenatal care from Alpha are thought to embody coalesces them into an apprehensible "population"—the interpretation offered in Chapter 5.

Prior to making that argument, however, Chapter 4 takes up the question of how the personally held racist beliefs of physicians may contribute to health disparities between racial groups. In essence, this chapter grounds the less-overt medical disenfranchisement of women of color discussed in the book with a robust discussion of its more-overt predecessor. It begins this task by discussing the largely unrecognized, yet still influential, racist oral tradition in medicine. This "racial folklore"—notably consisting of beliefs about the obstetrical and gynecological hardiness of Black and other purportedly "primitive" women—has long conditioned the reception of pregnant Black women in the United States. This chapter argues that notions of the obstetrical and gynecological hardiness of the marginalized have exhibited a remarkable hardiness of their own as they have managed to persist over the decades. This chapter demonstrates this persistence of racial folklore by offering observations and stories culled from ethnographic fieldwork alongside interviews conducted with obstetricians practicing in the Alpha clinic. The chapter then puts the ethnographic data in conversation with the literature documenting the persistence of racial disparities in health. It goes on to offer the personally held racist beliefs of physicians as an explanation. Physician racism has been shielded from critique, largely as a consequence of notions of the personal privacy of physicians. This chapter will attempt to continue to explode notions of doctors' personal privacy—notions that have functioned to hide the racism that may contribute to health disparities in the United States.

Chapter 5 investigates the use of the term "Alpha patient population" to refer to the individuals who received Medicaid-subsidized prenatal care from the clinic. This chapter considers how it is that the vastly heterogeneous group of women who seek prenatal health care from Alpha can be referred to as a single "population." The chapter argues that the shared poverty of the pregnant women who become patients at Alpha Hospital enables them to be seen as "high risk"; further, it is this imagined shared risk that enables the elision of individual differences and the apprehension of a unitary "population." The chapter then juxtaposes "Alpha patient population" with a figure that staff, providers, and administrators offered when speaking about the imagined "average" Alpha patient: that of the undocumented, uneducated immigrant. Several interviews with staff and physicians are reported in which the implicitly racialized, undocumented, uneducated immigrant is offered as a representative of all women who receive prenatal care from the hospital. These interviews support the conclusion that "Alpha patient population" operates as a deracialized racialist discourse that allows the providers, staff, and administrators who evoked it to speak race tacitly, yet avoid its explicit mention.

Chapter 6 begins with an examination of the acrimony characterizing the relationship between the clinic staff and their pregnant patients, suggesting that the acerbity of this relationship is rooted in employees' perception of the patients as uneducated. yet somehow incredibly shrewd, manipulators of the Alpha "system." It explores this construction of the health care-seeking subject—a figure I call the "wily patient." The chapter argues that the "wily patient" parallels the figure of the "welfare queen," similarly constructed as an uneducated, yet again somehow incredibly shrewd, manipulator of federal and state governments. It compares the figures of the wily patient and the welfare queen and notes a departure between the two: although the welfare queen is implicitly racialized as Black, the wily patient appears to be un-raced. A genealogy of the welfare queen is conducted to discover the origins of her Blackness. The chapter discusses the genesis of the stereotype of the "welfare queen" at the hands of Ronald Reagan in the 1980s and analyzes why he was able to get so much mileage out it. This history, which explores the racialization of categories of the deserving and undeserving poor, enables the argument that the wily patient also possesses an implicit racialization: one that is thoroughly non-white. The argument is that the operation of race successfully produced an entire population of women as racially Other-ed possessors of despised fertility. The chapter concludes with a discussion of how the discursive non-whiteness of the wily patient affects the experiences of those material wily patients who are racialized as white. This chapter is followed by a brief epilogue.

PART ONE

Class

ONE

Alpha Hospital: Unique, But Not Singular

George Washington was only a toddler when Alpha Hospital first opened its doors in the early eighteenth century (Opdycke 1999). Since then, Alpha has become arguably the best public hospital in the country. It is one of the few places in the nation where poor people have access to first-rate, outstanding health care. Indeed, the hospital is one of the most widely recognized medical institutions in the United States. The programs it provides top several lists: emergency medicine, neurology/neurosurgery, cardiovascular medicine, nursing, and, most notoriously, psychiatry. Alpha's reputation as a psychiatric hospital par excellence may be due to its counting many famous figures as former clients, including Edie Sedgwick, Norman Mailer, Charles Mingus, Allen Ginsburg, John Lennon's killer Mark David Chapman, and, more recently, Courtney Love, who was taken to Alpha after she was seen confusedly ambling around her Manhattan neighborhood. She was later photographed handcuffed to a gurney in the hospital—what may be standard procedure for those who resist treatment (*People* 2004). Yet one does not have to be a celebrity to be granted entry to Alpha's psychiatric ward. "If you're in Manhattan and you happen to be unfortunate enough to decompensate in a manner that involves an imminent threat to yourself or those around you," you are most likely going to Alpha—that "single word that, for more than a century, has told the rest of New York City that there is now one less person on the streets about whom it has to worry" (Harris 2008).

Alpha's status as a psychiatric hospital is so recognized that it has become embedded as such in the cultural imagination of the nation. This partially explains how Alpha has become a pop culture referent. Alpha was the site to which Barney Miller shipped everyone he considered mentally unstable when he encountered them during his travails in the Twelfth Precinct. In *Miracle on 34th Street*, Alpha Hospital was the temporary home for Kris Kringle as he awaited a court hearing to determine whether Santa Claus really existed. In one, not uncommon, heated exchange between Alice and Ralph in *The Honeymooners*, she tells him, "I'll go fix my lipstick. I won't be gone long, Killer. I call you Killer 'cause you slay me." Ralph, a jibe always on the tip of his tongue, replies, "And I'm calling Alpha 'cause you're nuts!" However, "spokesmen for the hospital will remind you, with the dogged patience of those who have had to say it again and again, that Alpha is much more than a psychiatric center" (Harris 2008). By most accounts, it is an excellent hospital that provides superb, wide-ranging care.

Alpha is unique for two distinct reasons: first, the quality of the medical care it offers in many respects is the world's best. Alpha's program for the reattachment of limbs has global renown (New York City Health and Hospitals Corporation 2009). Should the president of the United States or any manner of foreign dignitary require medical care while visiting New York City, he or she most assuredly will be whisked to Alpha Hospital (New York City Health and Hospitals Corporation 2009). When police officers or firefighters are injured in the line of duty, Alpha's record of offering the best in trauma care assures that they will be rushed to Alpha's emergency room (Dvorchak 1990); indeed, Alpha's record of excellence in providing trauma medicine explains why its ER was inundated with patients after the explosion in the basement of the World Trade Center in 1993 (Zuger 2001) and why its ER would have been similarly inundated in 2001 had there been more survivors following the collapse of the Twin Towers. Moreover, Alpha's history has included pioneering innovations and Nobel-Prize–winning research (Opdycke 1999, 12). The history continues to the present, as Alpha is the site of a number of studies that may very well shape the future landscape of medicine and technology. Accordingly, Alpha is frequently cited in medical journals as the hospital at which research was conducted and important (read: publishable) results were found.

Furthermore, it is a referral center for "high-risk" pregnancies, providing cutting edge maternal-fetal medicine to those who require it (NYC.gov 2010). It also offers women enjoying "low-risk" pregnancies the option of a midwife-assisted, natural childbirth in a picturesque, Jacuzzi-fitted birthing center. Wrote one journalist, "The lavish birthing room hardly squares with the image of Alpha. . . . Luxury and Alpha might never have appeared in the same sentence, but the new birthing center is gleaming, beautiful, and luxurious" (Fein 1998). Between the birthing center and the traditional labor and delivery ward, close to two thousand babies were born at Alpha in 2007 (NYC.gov 2010).

The second reason for Alpha's uniqueness is that because of the generosity with which New York City's public hospitals have been funded, it is able to offer the world-class medical care described above to more people who otherwise would have no access to health care at all, let alone state-of-the-art health care. "[N]owhere else in the United Stated does there exist a public hospital of such scope and generosity" (Opdycke 1999, 12). Indeed, when the federal government began subsidizing health care for the poor via the Medicare and Medicaid programs, millions of persons across the United States gained access to health care that they had been unable to afford in the past. However, this increased access to health care enabled by Medicare/Medicaid was not as dramatic in New York City, in which universal access to health care was already close to being realized—due in part to the city's expansive network of public hospitals and clinics. (Opdycke 1999, 139). "New York City has provided hospital care in its public hospitals as a mandatory service, not a discretionary service" (*U.S. News & World Report* 1975). Alpha Hospital is a significant part of this story, as it has always been the oldest and largest of all the public hospitals and clinics in New York City, the flagship institution providing care to more of those in need than any other public hospital in the area.

However, Alpha's status as a (if not "the") premier institution of public health in the nation and perhaps the "best shot" the poor have for obtaining quality health care raises the stakes of the critique that is to come. In the following chapters, I will argue that the institution (and the services it provides) demeans its patients and perpetuates racial and social inequalities. In the process of supposedly equalizing the poor and their non-poor counterparts, Alpha nonetheless pathologizes and stigmatizes the former. Indeed, because the program of universal prenatal care offered within Alpha Hospital may be the best version available, and Alpha may be the closest the nation has come to universal health care, the critique of U.S. political economy and racial politics I offer becomes all the more critical.

. . . BUT NOT A SINGULAR ONE

Though the uniqueness and extraordinariness of Alpha Hospital should be recognized, the hospital ought not to be understood as singular. Which is to say, to the extent that Alpha is a site where poor, pregnant women's bodies are excessively problematized and racial inequities are reiterated, this is a product not of some peculiar quality of Alpha, but rather a product of an institution that depends upon public dollars to deliver health care to uninsured, marginalized persons in the United States. Consequently, the critique is not of Alpha as such, but rather of the nationally circulating discourses, politics, policies, and practices that also affect Alpha and the people who populate it.

Alpha is a site of racialization—a racialized and racializing institution—because it is a hospital that is firmly located on the second tier of the U.S. two-tier health care system, a second tier disproportionately populated by poor people and people of color. "For years, New York City's public hospitals have been known as health care outposts of last resort. If the Health and Hospitals Corporation, which runs them, had advertised their medical services, it would have been considered akin to Albania hawking its tourist attractions: they may exist, but who would want to go there?" (Steinhauer 2000). While we may see within Alpha "the contrast between public care and private at its purest" (Opdycke 1999, 12), this is a contrast that is present throughout the nation. Alpha is unique in that it does an exceptional job of providing medical services to a large group of persons who must rely upon public health care, but the hospital is far from singular: numerous institutions throughout the United States replicate the job that Alpha endeavors to do for the poor. In every major city in the United States, one will find a relative of Alpha, a distant cousin perhaps—a public hospital existing alongside its private counterpart, providing the care the latter either cannot or will not provide. And so, the ethnography I offer might have been written about any of these other laudable institutions of public health.

Further, although Alpha is world renowned for its research and innovations, such achievements do not exempt it from its status as a public hospital; Alpha must still depend on government dollars, which seem to always be in short supply. The result is that Alpha is plagued by problems affecting many public institutions: it is underfunded and understaffed.

Moreover, the equipment that the staff and physicians use may be in short supply, or may have been superseded by newer, better versions—versions that remain out of the hospital's fiscal reach due to budget constraints. A chief resident, Gloria Vance—a soft-spoken, pleasant white woman who was looking forward to finishing her residency and beginning a new position as a general OB/GYN at a large private hospital in Boston—explained it to me in the following way:

> Anywhere from the actual machine for a CAT scan to the X-ray machine is better at Omega [the private hospital with which Alpha is affiliated] than it is here. It has a higher resolution. So, for example, if we're ruling out a pulmonary embolism—which we do a lot, because in pregnancy, people are at an increased risk for getting blood clots—they will often call it a poor study here, whereas, at Omega, they never do. One time, I asked the radiologist why that was so, and he just said that the actual scanner [at Omega] is a better quality machine. So, there is just the equipment level. And then there's the number of scanners and the number of staff—so that makes it easier to scan, or MRI, or whatever, over at Omega than to do it here. And it's not always true that one is going to be better than the other. It's just that, in terms of the overall, it's easier to get a scan there. And it's better quality. . . .
>
> [Alpha] is a teaching hospital. And for somebody who has no insurance, it's a tough world. And they feel like this is a place where they can come. But, if you compare what is here versus what is at Omega, there are just more restraints here—because it's all based on budgets.
>
> Another procedure, for example, that we could do at Omega is a procedure called endometrial oblation. There are all different types of techniques to do it. And we don't have all that technology [at Alpha] to do that.

These challenges, which may affect the quality of health care that Alpha can deliver to a patient on any given day, are mirrored in the experiences of other public hospitals throughout the nation.

Moreover, if I had not had the good fortune of stumbling upon Alpha in New York but instead ended up patrolling the halls of the obstetric clinics at Chicago's Cook County Hospital, Los Angeles' County General, or Atlanta's Grady Memorial Hospital, I would have still been able to write some version of the ethnography of pregnancy as a site of the racialization contained within. That is, because public hospitals serve those marginalized elements of society private hospitals can refuse, public hospitals have in turn become marginalized (Opdycke 1999, 194). It is the Alpha Hospitals of the nation that have served those groups that the vicissitudes of history have marked with stigma: individuals dying from tuberculosis, babies born with crack cocaine metabolites in their bodies, gay men and intravenous drug users suffering from AIDS, and so on. During the mid-1980s, when ignorance of HIV and AIDS caused "the fear of contagion" to grip the United States, Alpha treated more people suffering from AIDS than any other hospital in the country; this was not because the providers and staff at Alpha were exceptionally heroic or courageous, but that "the city's municipal hospitals, and Alpha in particular because of its location in Manhattan, must accept any AIDS patient, many of who are referred by private hospitals" (Sullivan 1985). At the time, many were aware of the stigma that AIDS patients brought to the institution that cared for them. "Faculty members expressed concern that treating a disproportionately large number of AIDS patients could stigmatize Alpha and upset an overall patient mix that traditionally has offered Omega-Alpha residents a classic postgraduate training in medicine in a major big city hospital." (Sullivan 1985). Yet, there was nothing Alpha could do to avoid its patients and the stigma they brought; as the hospital of "last resort," it admitted them and cared for them in the best way it could. That public hospitals serve the stigmatized in part explains their continued existence; Alpha and like institutions survive because they meet "social needs that private providers have been unable or unwilling to address" (Opdycke 1999, 10).

THE ROLE OF MEDICAID

Medicaid and Medicare threatened to undermine the segmentation, and simultaneous racialization, of the U.S. health care system by allowing for the integration of the two tiers. When Medicaid and Medicare were first introduced in 1965, many commentators believed public hospitals would find themselves invigorated as they would no longer have to absorb the health care cost of the previously uninsured who now had Medicaid/Medicare. Other commentators believed public hospitals would find themselves deserted in the advent of Medicaid/Medicare, as the formerly uninsured who depended on them would take their Medicaid/Medicare insurance to more prestigious private hospitals. (Opdycke 1999, 140). Many of them did. However, public hospitals—and Alpha Hospital specifically—did not find themselves deserted wastelands as every indigent former patient flocked to the more privileged private hospital down the block. This was because there still remained a large number of persons who did not qualify for Medicaid or Medicare and, uninsured, would continue to depend on public hospitals for their health care. One can still find stories of uninsured patients who were turned away from private hospitals only to end up at Alpha Hospital and have their lives saved there. The *New York Times* reported the story of a French woman who had sought care for abdominal pain from one of the more prestigious private hospitals in Manhattan.

> Pelvic cancer was suspected, and she was admitted to the obstetrics and gynecology floor, where the diagnosis was confirmed. A private doctor, along with the house staff, attended to her. The doctor concluded that she needed surgery within several weeks followed by chemotherapy. The woman had no insurance. The senior physician discharged her, and left a note on the woman's chart saying that she had instructed her to obtain health insurance or go to a public hospital.
>
> Investigators determined that when the woman left the hospital, on Manhattan's West Side, she had barely been able to walk. That same day, she went to Alpha Hospital, a city facility, where surgeons operated immediately. (Kleinfield 1999)

Moreover, private hospitals are still able to choose which services they will provide and which they will deny. Accordingly, "the exodus to the private sector did not represent a cross-section of the municipal caseload— more white patients than black found a welcome in the private system, more Medicare than Medicaid, more acutely ill than chronic, more ex- pectant mothers than drug addicts, more sober employed than homeless derelicts." (Opdycke 1999, 146). Instead of undermining the segmentation that characterizes the U.S. two-tiered health care system, Medicare/Med- icaid actually functioned to exacerbate the polarization. "[T]he arrival of Medicare and Medicaid had further narrowed the circle of New Yorkers who had to depend on public care, leaving behind, once again, the people with the least choices and least resources." (Opdycke 1999, 146). These people are, for the most part, Alpha's patients.

Further, private hospitals not only could select which services to pro- vide, but also choose whether they would accept Medicaid/Medicare in- surance at all. When reimbursements offered by private insurance compa- nies, especially managed care plans, were cut and became comparable to those paid by Medicaid/Medicare, many private hospitals were happy to open their doors to the publicly insured (Steinhauer 2000). The president of the Health and Hospitals Corporation, which manages the public hospitals in New York City, described the situation: "Right now, Medicaid and Medicare are like gold cards in every hospital in the city. They all are trying to attract those patients" (Steinhauer 2000). Indeed, part of the motivation for the construction of the birthing center at Alpha was to stem the exodus of Medicaid patients from the public hospital to their private counterparts. The former director of obstetrics and gynecology at Alpha said upon the opening of the center, "We've got to dispel that *Midnight Cowboy* image of Alpha. People are going to see this center, they're going to stop and say, 'This is Alpha?' And they're going to look at the whole hospital in a new way." (Fein 1998). [Dustin Hoffman's character in *Midnight Cowboy*, Ratso, was a poor, likely uninsured street hustler who refused to seek medical care for what was probably tuberculosis. He tells his friend, "Just get me on a bus. You ain't sending me to Alpha." He ultimately dies on the bus, having avoided at all costs the stigma attached to being an "Alpha patient."]

However, this is where Alpha's story diverges from the stories of other public hospitals with affiliations with private hospitals: the private hospital with which Alpha is affiliated, Omega Hospital, refuses to accept Medicaid insurance. As a consequence, there is no blending of patient populations between Alpha and Omega as there might be between public and private hospitals that both accept Medicaid. The segregation of populations accomplished by Omega's refusal to accept Medicaid insurance increases the likelihood that the Alpha patient will be poor and, consequently, a racial or ethnic minority.

THE EXOTICIZED PUBLIC SIBLING

That Alpha has an affiliation with a private hospital attached to a private medical school is not unique. Alpha's affiliation with the elite Omega University School of Medicine (OUSOM) is an example of the relationships between private medical schools and public hospitals that can be observed throughout the nation. In literature made available to the public, Alpha boasts that its half a century-long academic affiliation with Omega enables Alpha patients to receive cutting-edge care from the most select of medical experts (NYC.gov 2010). This was a relationship the city brass actively sought, believing that an official relationship between Alpha and OUSOM would be desirable because the "private affiliates would help attract top-level physicians; at the same time, the private institutions would bring to the public sector the same disinterested commitment to excellence that they were thought to pursue in their own facilities" (Opdycke 1999, 111). From OUSOM's perspective, a relationship with the public hospital was beneficial because the latter offered greater opportunities to its faculty for teaching and research and its students for observing pathology they might not see within private hospitals. Many physicians I interviewed commented positively on the fact that due to the lack of regular medical care brought on by the absence of health insurance, patients seen at Alpha tend to present themselves to the hospital with disorders and diseases that are in more advanced stages than their privately insured counterparts. Comments made by Dr. Renee Escueta, a young but senior attending physician who began her medical career as a resident at Alpha, exemplify this. When I asked her why she chose to work in Alpha as opposed to a more prestigious private hospital, she responded, "The patients are very interesting. They are much more interesting than private practice. Because of the level of pathology in them. You don't see. . . . A lot of it is unfortunate because they haven't taken care of themselves. So, things that can be caught early, or things that can be treated go many steps further. So, by the time they get here, it's a big deal. But, you can learn from it."

The result is that public hospitals in symbiotic relationships with private medical schools offer themselves as the "very interesting," exoticized complements to private teaching hospitals. Moreover, within the racial logic of the United States, exoticization is simply a degree or two removed from racialization. The relationship between exoticization and racialization is made explicit in a *Los Angeles Times* article written about Alpha almost two decades ago. The journalist quotes an ER physician, "We're kind of a field hospital. This is war-zone medicine." He continues, "We see everything here. We are the window to the world. You will never go anywhere else in the world and see something we haven't already seen at Alpha. . . . It's like a Third World situation." (Dvorchak 1990). Alpha's status as a site for the observation of the exotic, the rare, and the unusual is evident in the doctor's first comments; the seamless addition of the descriptor "Third World" in his final comment expertly exemplifies that exoticization is not far removed from racialization. To the extent that Alpha's status as the exoticized antipode to Omega Hospital's norm set in motion the processes by which Alpha and the patients it serves are racialized, variations on these processes are likely evident in the scores of other public hospitals across the nation with academic affiliations with private medical schools.

Before I dive into an analysis of these processes, however, I must provide a bit more background to the place and the people who are the substance of the ethnography.

The Alpha WHC is housed in an aesthetically pleasing, recently constructed ambulatory care building that was annexed to the primary hospital building—an older, visibly more decrepit structure that can be fairly described as having passed through "obsolescence into decrepitude" (Shonick and Price 1977, 236). The ambulatory care building boasts an eight-story skylight and glass walls, which allow each of the five floors to be flooded with natural sunlight. The WHC, located on the top floor, shares its waiting area with the dermatology clinic, ultrasound clinic, and financial services desk—at which every patient must check in before seeing a doctor in any of the clinics located on the floor. There is a lot of open space in the connected waiting areas; at times, that open space is put to good use as it accommodates long lines of patients. Because the building is open and airy, sound travels easily; a person on the top floor can hear everything occurring in the spacious lobby on the ground floor, from a symphony playing classical music to commemorate the events of September 11th to an argument between a security guard and a distressed woman attempting to visit a loved one who has been rushed to the emergency room.

The large majority of the patients seen within the WHC are poor women of color receiving Medicaid/PCAP insurance to cover the cost of their prenatal care. I met only one woman during my tenure at Alpha who was not receiving Medicaid or any other government-subsidized health insurance. This woman was ineligible for Medicaid because her income exceeded the limits set by Medicaid guidelines. Since becoming pregnant, she had become a full-time employee at her place of employment (as opposed to a "contractor" to the business that she had been in the years preceding her pregnancy), and had signed up for the health insurance offered by her employer. However, the employer-based health insurance—and the other private insurance plans she had subsequently researched—refused to pay for her prenatal care expenses, claiming her pregnancy was a "preexisting condition." Thus, she paid for her prenatal care (and labor and delivery) expenses entirely out of her own pocket. Save for this relatively unlucky woman, all other patients I encountered at Alpha relied upon Medicaid for their health insurance during their pregnancies.

Moreover, the majority of patients attended to within the WHC are Latina—many U.S.-born, many others documented and undocumented immigrants. The WHC also sees many women hailing from other parts of the globe such as South Asia, Africa, Asia, and Europe. Finally, although they are a minority, there are still quite a number of U.S.-born Black and White patients. Accordingly, the Alpha "patient population" is comprised of a diverse group of women in terms of ethnicity, racial ascription and identification, level of educational achievement, health status, history of substance abuse, prior relationship to the state and its regulatory apparatuses, familiarity with the biomedical establishment and biomedical discourse, ideas held about pregnancy and childbirth, desire for medical intervention, etc. And while all were poor (with the exception of the unlucky outlier mentioned above), it is also imperative to note that some were poorer than others.

The WHC offers three categories of medical providers of gynecologic and obstetric care: 1) medical doctors, 2) midwives (certified nurse practitioners who have completed midwifery training and certified nurse midwives), and 3) nurse practitioners (nurses whose extensive training qualifies them to perform a host of medical procedures—including Pap smears, vaginal examinations, biopsies, and insertion of laminaria as part of a pregnancy termination procedure). Medical doctors working in the Alpha obstetrics clinic can be divided into two categories: attending physicians and residents. Between the attending physicians and the residents, the approximately twenty-one residents who rotate through the Alpha WHC throughout the course of their four-year residency provide the bulk of services to obstetric and gynecologic patients. The residents are also present in Alpha's labor and delivery ward and thus care for women during labor. Residents split their highly coveted residency between the public Alpha Hospital and the private Omega Hospital—a split that, along with the perceived camaraderie among residents, is cited by the residents as the Alpha-Omega residency program's primary draw. Indeed, the Omega University School of Medicine advertises: "Alpha is a large municipal hospital with a diverse patient population; Omega is a large private university referral center drawing patients from a wide geographic area for all of the divisions in our department and the medical center. The combination provides an enviable mix of medical, surgical, sociological, obstetrical, and gynecological problems that cannot be found under the roof of any single institution."

Because the attending physicians at Omega deliver prenatal care to their patients in private offices outside of Omega Hospital, the residents do not attend to Omega's patients during their prenatal care. The first time a resident usually meets a pregnant Omega patient is when the patient arrives at the hospital to deliver her baby. However, at Alpha, the residents provide prenatal care to the patients as there are no "private offices" to which Alpha patients can go. Alpha attending physicians, who are Omega faculty or fellows undergoing postgraduate training in gynecologic oncology, maternal-fetal medicine, or reproductive endocrinology and infertility, also attend to patients; however, because there are fewer attending physicians than residents, patients assigned to a medical doctor as their provider (as opposed to a midwife or nurse practitioner) are more likely to see a resident than an attending physician. Attending physicians also perform an oversight function to the extent that they are consulted by residents about patient cases, and they authorize the courses of treatment the residents recommend.

While many of the residents and several attending physicians are racial and ethnic minorities, it is not incorrect to state that most of the providers working in the Alpha WHC are White. Indeed, all of the midwives and nurse practitioners during my fieldwork were White.

Assisting the providers is the "ancillary staff," a term used in the hospital to describe those categories of employees whose purpose is to support the providers by performing auxiliary but essential tasks. Included within the ambit of ancillary staff are: 1) Patient Care Associates (PCAs) who take the patients' vital signs, draw blood and collect urine samples, make follow-up appointments upon the request of the provider, and shuttle the patients in and out of examination rooms; 2) frontline staff, who from their post behind the front desk greet patients, take all relevant paperwork and distribute it to the relevant providers/PCAs, and make appointments; and 3) registered nurses, whose training allows them to provide some health care services to the patients—namely administering injections, dispensing prescriptions and other medications, taking medical histories, and performing colposcopies and other noninvasive procedures. Ancillary staff also includes nutritionists, social workers, HIV counselors, and financial aid officers—staff whose purpose and function I will discuss in greater detail in the following chapter.

The WHC is an extremely frenzied, oftentimes chaotic, not infrequently confused space. And it is the ancillary staff who are compelled to manage the bulk of this confusion. Accordingly, the job of the ancillary staff worker is a stressful, frequently thankless one. One journalist wrote that "[o]n a hectic Saturday night at Alpha, the staff can often be heard to wonder out loud just what it was that drove them into the so-called caring professions, dooming them to wade through the endless insoluble miseries of their fellow citizens, all the while entangled in an urban health care system seemingly tattered beyond repair" (Zuger 2001). In my experience, the ancillary staff in the WHC does not wait until a hectic Saturday night to engage in such musings; they tend to wonder about their lot daily—and for good reason.

During the course of my fieldwork, I was able to work behind the front desk and perform the tasks the frontline staff generally performed—answering incoming telephone calls, making gynecology and obstetrics appointments for patients who presented themselves at the desk or called the clinic's main telephone number, providing pregnancy tests to women who sought them, taking the relevant paperwork from women with appointments and making sure the providers with whom their appointments were scheduled received such paperwork, and doing whatever running around the clinic was required to ensure that patients' expectations were managed and the clinic continued to function. On the days I worked as a frontline staff person, I would leave for home at 6 p.m. completely exhausted, sweat staining my shirt—the smile and pleasant demeanor with which I tried to greet patients having disappeared hours beforehand. My feet would be sore from the incalculable number of occasions that called for me to run from the front desk to the back examination rooms. I would swab my hands with hand sanitizer, hoping that the ritual would somehow undo the countless times a patient had greeted me with an uncovered sneeze or cough instead of "hello." Yet, the women who perform this job—the job I volunteered to do for research purposes, a job from which I could throw up my hands and vow never to do again because it is "too much"—resided at the bottom of the clinic's hierarchy.

There was one occasion on which I did, indeed, vow never again to work as a frontline staff person. It occurred during my first month of conducting patient intake. By that time, I had observed innumerable belligerent interactions between staff and patients and had placed the blame for any and all hostility in the hospital squarely on the shoulders of the ancillary staff workers. I felt that if the staff were more patient and explained more things more carefully to the patients, tempers would not flare. So, on this day, I sat behind the front desk, indirectly offering myself as a model of how staff *should* treat the patients they serve.

All went well during the morning. During the afternoon, however, I was approached by a relatively nondescript, racially and ethnically ambiguous young woman who said that she needed prenatal care. Beginning prenatal care at Alpha was a complex procedure: A woman had to first take a hospital-administered pregnancy test. The following day, she would call for her test results; if positive, she would then schedule a Prenatal Care Assistance Program (PCAP) appointment, during which she met with a nurse, health educator, nutritionist, social worker, and financial aid officer. It was only after meeting with those professionals on that day that she was given an appointment to *return* to see a physician, midwife, or nurse practitioner. As a result, on the whole it usually took two to three weeks after a woman first presented herself at the hospital before she really "began" prenatal care by getting a physical examination. I started to explain the procedure to the patient—confident that if she were informed about the hospital requirements, she would not become angry at some point down the line when her expectations were not met. However, I did not have a chance to go through more than half of the procedure when the patient interrupted me: "I'm not stupid. Just give me the pregnancy test." Taken aback, I recovered quickly and handed the woman a test tube, rubber stopper, paper cup, and plastic bag. I began explaining that she should urinate into the cup, pour the urine into the tube, firmly plug the tube with the stopper, place the tube into the bag, and bring the bag back to me. She interrupted me again: "Are you an idiot? I know that already." She stalked off toward the restroom. Five minutes later—during which I had replayed the scene over and over in my head, trying to figure out where I had gone wrong—she returned with the plastic bag, shoved it across the front desk, and asked, "Am I going to get my prenatal care today?" I said no and told her that she had to call back the following day to confirm her test results. Displeased, she called me a bitch, told me, "Your fucking system is stupid," and sauntered away.

A former chief psychologist at Alpha once said of the staff who worked beside him in an "emblem of urban government's catastrophic inattention to its own public institutions" that "I don't know if it was a kind of masochism or a kind of macho—and that applies to the women as well—a sense of pride in being able to do the most difficult jobs in the most difficult place and do them well" (Harris 2008). The ancillary staff who worked in the WHC did possess a sense of pride born from having endured the daily disorder and occasional abuse that can be expected in the clinic and from having acquired a certain competence regarding how to manage a far-from-ideal situation. It is the ancillary staff women who are simultaneously pushed and pulled in varying directions, who are called upon to assuage the tempers of both the patients and the providers to whom they must answer, and who are regularly faulted for the clinic's shortcomings. Comments made by second-year resident Dr. Francie Howard are representative of many:

> There are many days when the ancillary staff is not doing their job. And you're like, "You're not doing your whole job. I'm doing my job and your job." And it causes some tension.
>
> When I think about the labor floor [at Omega], you have young—not just young—but, young, motivated, committed, energetic people who are really good at their job and take pride in their work. And here at Alpha, a lot of times, you have people who don't take pride in their jobs, don't want to be there, don't feel committed to it. And it ends up that they are. . . . I hate to use the word "lazy," but I'm going to have to say "lazy."

A chief resident articulated a similar sentiment during another interview. An intern present in the room during the interview felt so strongly about ancillary staff incompetence that she interjected herself into the conversation.

> CHIEF: For them [the ancillary staff], it's just a job. And they don't have any repercussions. I mean, how often do nurses get sued? They don't. If anything happens to the patient, they don't have any accountability. And they don't care. For them it's a paycheck, and there's a union. And it's like: "I have my job. I have to work 9 to 5. I have to take my break! I have to take my break! Wait! Lunch! I can't go without lunch!" Yet, all these patients are supposed to get seen and we [the doctors] are still working. But, you know, it's lunchtime! [laughs] Like, I said, it's just—you know, they don't care about the patients like we do.
>
> INTERN: The problem is that we don't pay them that well, so we don't hire good people to begin with.
>
> CHIEF: Well, you'd be surprised at the benefits that I think they have. So, I don't know how much they get paid or not. . . . When I talk to [other physicians], our job is not just a job. For me—and I think it's the same for most of us—we don't say, "I want to make this money." I mean, we're here for a different reason; because we actually care about the patients. Because we can put—we make a lot of sacrifices. We put aside this, put aside that. . . . But, the ancillary staff—they don't care at all! They don't. Of course not. They don't care. It's just like I said: It's because it's just their job.

Not only is the ancillary staff faulted for most things that go awry in the clinic, but it is also on their heads that the curses and threats hurled by frustrated patients first land. And it is the ancillary staff who has only an hour-long lunch break during which they may step away from the bedlam and disorder and re-center themselves, finding comfort in a lunch brought from home and a salary that just barely separates them from the maligned, problematized, and marginalized women they serve.

The ancillary staff's proximity (in terms of racial ascriptions, immigration histories, and socioeconomic status) to the stigmatized and scorned patients they assist—patients whose receipt of government assistance during their pregnancies causes them to be apprehended within political and popular discourse as "lazy" welfare recipients growing fat off of government largesse—goes a long way toward explaining the ancillary staff largely figuring in the ensuing ethnography as overwhelmingly negative forces with which patients must contend. However, it is important to argue at an early stage that the ancillary staff ought not to be unfairly condemned. Yes, many of these staff workers were rude and tactless; several of them uttered lamentable racial and ethnic stereotypes of the diverse group of patients they served. At many times, they expressed a plain contempt toward their indigent charges. These bare facts should not be ignored. But, the staff's bad behavior should not be conceptualized as unfortunate peculiarities of the individuals—as bad people behaving badly. In truth, much of their bad behavior ought to be understood as structural: a response to their duty to perform jobs that are highly stressful, yet for which they receive very little compensation. Furthermore, that behavior should be understood as a rational mechanism that distances the actors from the discursively maligned patients they serve.

Consider a story Yolanda told me approximately a year into my fieldwork. Yolanda was a heavyset woman in her fifties when I first met her, someone who had immigrated from Jamaica decades before. She was an Alpha veteran; not only had she been employed by the hospital for over thirty years, but she had given birth to her two now-grown children there. During my time at the hospital, she conducted patient intake at the front desk—taking paperwork from patients who were scheduled to see a provider that day, creating new patient charts, making appointments, dispensing urine tests, answering phones, etc. Although she laughed and joked with her colleagues, she rarely smiled at anyone else. Her reputation for being impolite, brusque, and downright mean to patients was known throughout the obstetrics clinic. Whenever a staff person leaned over and whispered to a colleague, "Guess who got into a fight with a patient this morning?," more often than not, the colleague would guess in response, "Yolanda?" And more often than not, that person would be right.

Even though it frequently infuriated me to observe Yolanda's hostility to patients, and although I remain convinced that she should never have been given a job that required her to interact with them, I grew quite fond of her over time. And, eventually, after more time the feeling became mutual. So, one afternoon when the clinic had slowed considerably, Yolanda turned to me as I sat next to her behind the front desk and said, "I tried to get food stamps yesterday." I laughed: I thought she was kidding. This was the same woman who would look with disgust at a pregnant woman approaching the desk and say contemptuously (and not entirely out of the woman's earshot), "These women here are too busy. Too too busy. And me and you both gotta pay for their babies." So, when Yolanda told me that she had tried to get food stamps, I thought that she was joking—that she would never accept the government assistance I believed to be the fuel behind her antipathy toward Alpha's patients. When I realized she was serious, I tried to save myself by asking, "What did you say? You went where yesterday?" She continued, "I went to the old building [the primary Alpha Hospital building] and asked for food stamps—because, you know, Alpha doesn't pay me nothing. And you know how they say that you can have a house and a car and a train and you can still qualify for food stamps? Well, they wouldn't give it to me. They said I earned too much."

In this two-minute aside, Yolanda revealed just how close she was to being one of the patients she assisted everyday. She was needy enough to at least *believe* that she might qualify for government assistance; further, her circumstances were such that she actually *acted on* that need by inquiring into the program. Moreover, had Yolanda been thirty years younger and pregnant, there is no doubt that she would have qualified for all the government assistance that most Alpha patients receive, because, as mentioned earlier, the income limitations in New York State for Medicaid insurance during pregnancy are quite high. So, while Yolanda might have "earned too much" as a single woman to qualify for the food stamp program, she likely would not have earned too much as a pregnant woman to qualify for Medicaid (and the Women, Infants, and Children (WIC) vouchers that provide pregnant women and mothers with children under the age of five with milk, cheese, cereal, fruit juice, and the like). Accordingly, Yolanda's poor treatment of Alpha patients must be accounted for with a measure of interest in her specific subjectivity and subject position. She was called upon to serve—under impressively stressful conditions and with a professedly unimpressive compensation packet—a group of patients whose races, ethnicities, nationalities, and socioeconomic statuses closely mirrored her own. As such, I suspect that Yolanda's animosity (and the staff's animosity more generally) is intensified by a recognition of her own similarity to the patients' profile and her desire to disavow the discursively disparaged patient as an abject version of herself.

In such a light, consider a story told to me by Minnie, a middle-aged woman born in Puerto Rico, who had been working at Alpha Hospital for twenty-seven years at the time of my fieldwork there. Minnie was trained as a PCA and therefore could work more closely with providers "in the back" as she prepared patients for their examinations; however, she tended to be at the front desk, conducting patient intake alongside Yolanda. Minnie was a pleasant, jovial woman whose ability to speak Spanish was greatly appreciated by both the Spanish-speaking patients and her non-Spanish-speaking colleagues. I was quite fond of Minnie, who took to calling me *nena*, a term of endearment in Spanish that literally translates as "doll." Although Minnie was exceptionally nice to me and, for the most part, kind to the patients who sought her assistance, she could also be very nasty to patients when she was frustrated, tired, or annoyed.

A couple of months after I began fieldwork, Minnie became ill and was unable to come to work for several days. When she returned, I asked her if she was feeling better. She said yes and continued,

> I have been taking medicine for my high blood pleasure for four years, *nena*. I take the same medicine—it hasn't changed. Now, when I went to get my prescription filled the last time at the pharmacy, I noticed that the medicine they gave me dissolved really quickly when I put it in my mouth. And it left a bitter aftertaste. And then, *nen*a, I started getting these terrible headaches. Really terrible. So, you know, I figured that the pharmacy had made a mistake and gave me the wrong medicine. So, I went back there and I told the pharmacist that, you know, they had made a mistake. And do you know what he says to me, *nena*? He says, 'It's probably all in your head. How often do you go see the doctor? Maybe you don't go often enough." I was shocked. He didn't know I was a nurse—that I've been working in the hospital since before he was born.

I asked him why he was getting an attitude with me. And he says, "Well, it seems that you are just repeating yourself." And I said, "Well, that's because you don't seem to be understanding me." So, I left. I wasn't going to stand there and argue with him all day. I went to another pharmacy and I had the prescription refilled there. The pills they gave me there were like the ones I've been getting for years now. And the headaches went away. So, I'm feeling much better now.

The incredible irony of Minnie's story was that the rude pharmacist treated her in a manner similar to the way she has treated more than a few patients at Alpha. I have observed her become aggravated on innumerable occasions by patients who seem to be repeating themselves pointlessly, but who are actually trying to reiterate a complaint that appears to be falling on unhearing ears. *She* has been the rude pharmacist who is unable or unwilling to understand the difficult patient who will not just go away. I have no doubt the pharmacist Minnie encountered had dismissed her as an irritable old lady with a Spanish accent who stalked into his pharmacy with an attitude, erroneously believing that her Medicare card entitled her to make unlimited demands on his time. Differently stated, the pharmacist saw in Minnie a version of what Minnie sees in Alpha patients. Like Yolanda, at least some portion of the hostility Minnie demonstrated toward her patients can be explained as an attempt to create distance between herself and them such that they could not, or no longer, be considered abject forms of herself.

Having provided what I hope is sufficient background information about the place and the major players who populate it—and having hopefully exonerated, to some extent, the ancillary staff from being unfairly blamed for the unfortunate role they play in the analysis that is to come—I now turn to the critique. In the next chapter, I begin by exploring the deluge of requirements that follow a woman's receipt of government subsidization of her prenatal health care costs. That is, as a condition of receipt of Medicaid coverage of prenatal care expenses, poor, uninsured pregnant women are compelled to meet with a battery of professionals—namely nurses, nutritionists, social workers, health educators, and financial officers—who inquire into areas of women's lives that frequently exceed the purview of their medical care. This chapter argues that, as a result, Medicaid mandates an intrusion into women's private lives and produces pregnancy as an opportunity for state supervision, management, and regulation of poor, uninsured women. In essence, the receipt of Medicaid inaugurates poor women into the state regulatory apparatus.

TWO

Pregnancy, Medicaid, State Regulation, and Legal Subjection

INTRODUCTION

For my first weeks in the Alpha obstetrics clinic, my "field" appeared to me as a swirl of bodies barely contained by a space that struggled (and frequently failed) to maintain an air of sterility and restraint. However, over time, patterns began to emerge. I learned the bodies could be dichotomized into categories of "patient" and "employee." Of the "patient" bodies, some were "obstetric patients" and some were "gynecology patients"; some sought abortions and others infertility services; some were "medically high risk" and would be seen by doctors specializing in maternal-fetal medicine, and others were "low risk" and would be seen by midwives. . . . It would be a long time before I learned all of the myriad ways in which patient bodies could be classified.

Similarly, it would take months before I understood the different employee bodies. I came to realize that in addition to the nurses and doctors, a host of professionals worked in the obstetrics clinic: abortion counselors, patient advocates, geneticists, HIV counselors, nurse/health educators, nutritionists, social workers, and financial officers. I eventually learned that many people were located in the clinic because all pregnant patients at Alpha are required to meet with them upon beginning prenatal care.

The requirement that pregnant patients consult with at least four different kinds of professionals in order to receive prenatal health care from

Alpha is not hospital policy—it is a Medicaid policy that the hospital enforces. For the indigent patient, Medicaid coverage means that she can receive health care during her pregnancy at no cost to her. For the hospital, Medicaid coverage held by its pregnant patients means that the hospital will not have to assume the costs of patients who cannot pay for services rendered to them. As a public hospital and member of the New York City Health and Hospital Commission,[1] Alpha Hospital is required by legislative mandate to provide services to any patient, with or without health insurance, who presents herself at the hospital—a fact about which Alpha professes pride. In numerous advertisements for the hospital, statements that "more than 80 percent of Alpha's patients come from the city's medically underserved populations" are followed with the declaration, "No one in need is ever turned away from Alpha."

Moreover, that Alpha Hospital cannot and will not refuse service to any patient who presents herself at the hospital is known by many patients. A woman once approached the Women's Health Clinic (WHC) front desk and said, "I'm pregnant. . . . I don't have insurance. . . . I need prenatal care. . . . Did I mention that I don't have insurance?" I ran into this prospective patient that evening on my walk to the subway station. She recognized me from the hospital, and we made polite conversation as we walked. Eventually, we began talking about her pregnancy, and I asked her, "So, what made you come to Alpha for your prenatal care?" She responded, "I was laid off from my job last month and I lost my health insurance. My friend told me that I should go to Alpha because they have to see you. Even if you don't have any health insurance, they have to see you. They can't turn you away." Her friend was absolutely correct: Alpha Hospital does not refuse to provide health care to anyone, regardless of the patient's ability to pay. Therefore, Medicaid coverage held by Alpha patients means that the state and federal governments will reimburse Alpha for the cost of services it must provide anyway. Accordingly, it is in the hospital's financial interest to ensure that all the patients it serves have Medicaid.

Moreover, before the hospital can be reimbursed by the state for the services it renders to pregnant patients with Medicaid, the hospital itself must be qualified as a Prenatal Care Assistance Program (PCAP) provider—meaning the state has approved it to provide prenatal care services to Medicaid recipients.[2] And it is the New York Medicaid statute that mandates that a patient meet with a nurse/health educator,[3] HIV counselor,[4] nutritionist,[5] social worker,[6] and a financial officer.[7] In order for Alpha to be reimbursed through Medicaid for the prenatal services it provides, it must guarantee that the patient meets with the above professionals. Hence, the bureaucratic apparatus in place in the obstetrics clinic is mandated by the state.

Because all pregnant patients at Alpha are expected to be or to become Medicaid recipients, all Alpha prenatal care patients are expected to meet with the PCAP professionals. Even if a woman has no interest in applying for Medicaid (instead opting to use her own private insurance[8] or pay out-of-pocket for her prenatal care) she must still meet with all the people before being scheduled to see a provider for a medical examination. This policy is in effect because the hospital apparently chooses to err on the side of fiscal caution, presuming that every patient receiving health care within the obstetrics clinic will eventually become a Medicaid recipient. In the event that a patient ultimately receives Medicaid coverage, the hospital can be reimbursed for its services as it has satisfied all the PCAP requirements for Medicaid reimbursement for that patient. Alternatively, in the event that the patient ultimately does not receive Medicaid coverage but instead pays for her prenatal services through private insurance or out-of-pocket, the hospital is not disadvantaged in any way, the only consequence being that the consultations with the PCAP professionals would have been made unnecessary. As a result, all pregnant patients at Alpha are compelled to meet with the PCAP professionals and to provide private information that far exceeds the purview of their medical care—information that, importantly, opens their lives to regulation and the possibility of intervention by the state. I elaborate more extensively on the forms the state intervention can take in the "Some Concluding Thoughts" section at the end of the chapter.

The requirement that, as a condition of their receipt of public assistance in the form of state-subsidized health care, poor women make themselves vulnerable to the state by divulging both intimate and banal details of their lives with a battery of professionals is profoundly different from the experience privately insured pregnant women can expect upon beginning prenatal care. This chapter explores how, in demanding patients to meet with a constellation of officials who inquire into women's personal lives, Medicaid renders pregnancy an opportunity for state supervision, management, and regulation of poor women. In essence, this chapter analyzes how the receipt of Medicaid might be understood as an occasion for the initiation of poor women into the state regulatory apparatus and a circumstance for making poor women into disempowered legal subjects.

Although this chapter discusses the specifics of the New York State version of Medicaid, the critique offered within is, with a caveat, applicable to all states participating in the Medicaid program. As a bit of background, in 1965 Congress created Medicaid, a federal–state cost-sharing program through which states are reimbursed for expenditures for medical services provided to qualified persons. Individuals qualify for the program when they are uninsured and their combined incomes and resources are deemed by law to be insufficient to meet the cost of necessary medical care. In 1986, Congress established PCAP at the federal level to reimburse states that opted to offer prenatal care to pregnant women whose incomes exceeded Medicaid eligibility standards (Swift 1995). The following year, in the Omnibus Reconciliation Act of 1987, Congress amended the Medicaid statute to require states to offer Medicaid coverage of pregnancy-related services (United States Congress 1987). Although the amendment required each state to extend eligibility to women whose incomes are up to 133 percent of the federal poverty line, states can opt to extend benefits to women whose incomes are up to 200 percent of the poverty line.

In 1989, New York State enacted its own version of PCAP, which extended prenatal care services to women with incomes between 100 and 200 percent of the federal poverty line. For women who meet the income limitations, PCAP coverage in New York commences at the beginning of the pregnancy and terminates sixty days after the woman gives birth. Moreover, New York has opted to make undocumented immigrant women eligible for PCAP (New York City Human Resources Administration 2009). As the children of these undocumented women have been born within U.S. borders, they are citizens and therefore eligible for continued Medicaid coverage. However, if the mother was not a citizen or permanent resident before the birth of the baby, her status is not changed by giving birth; consequently, sixty days after delivering, she is no longer eligible for government assistance and finds herself, once again, without Medicaid or any other health insurance.

Because New York State has elected to fund and administer its PCAP program through the state Medicaid program, I use "Medicaid" as a proxy for "PCAP"—although other states electing to participate in the Medicaid program may not similarly administer and fund their prenatal care programs. Nonetheless, to the extent states such as New York mandate the inclusion of the "extra-medical" within their prenatal care programs—that is, to the extent other states also require pregnant women seeking prenatal care to meet with nutritionists, HIV counselors, social workers, nurse/health educators, financial officers and the like—the critique offered here is relevant.

Before describing the consultations as experienced by the women they affect, I first situate the apparatus within the theoretical frame of Foucauldian biopolitics.

ALPHA OBSTETRICS AND THE FOUCAULDIAN BIOPOLITICAL PROJECT

Much has been written about the government's interest in the production and management of health, both of the individual and of the population.[9] Perhaps the most famous excursus is that of Foucault, who elaborated upon this state interest via his notion of "biopolitics": whereas in the classical age, state power was demonstrated in the exercise of producing death—that is, in *killing* its subjects—in the modern age, "this formidable power of death . . . now presents itself as the counterpart of a power that exerts a positive influence on life, that endeavors to administer, optimize, and multiply it, subjecting it to precise controls and comprehensive regulations." (1978, 137). Foucault describes a "power over life" that

> focus[es] on the species body, the body imbued with the mechanics of life and serving as the basis of the biological processes: propagation, births and mortality, the level of health, life expectancy, and longevity, with all the conditions that can cause these to vary. Their supervision was effected through an entire series of interventions and *regulatory controls: a biopolitics of the population.* (139)

Following Foucault, prenatal care presents itself as an occasion par excellence for the state to "administer, optimize, and multiply" life, to subject the body to "precise controls and comprehensive regulations," and to ultimately gain a modicum of control over "the level of health" of the population.

Yet, pregnancy alone does not put the pregnant woman within the jurisdiction of the biopolitical state. Although the state may desire to exercise its "power over life" by submitting the expectant mother and her fetus to "an entire series of interventions and regulatory controls," the pregnant woman is not compelled to surrender herself to such a state project. Again, this is because at present pregnancy—absent other circumstances (such as the woman's incarceration, her enrollment in a state-sponsored drug rehabilitation program, etc.)—does not enable the state to reach the woman and her pregnant body with its biopolitical power.

The biopolitical state could achieve the regulation of every pregnant woman and every pregnancy by creating a law mandating that women receive prenatal care. However, at present such a law does not exist. Indeed, there is no law in the United States that makes criminal or otherwise penalizes a woman's failure to submit herself to any kind of prenatal care during her pregnancy. Should a woman endure the forty weeks of pregnancy without ever having sought and/or received medical care from a physician, nurse practitioner, midwife, or other professional whose services are intended to ensure the birth of a healthy baby and the continued health of the mother, no law punishes this behavior (or lack thereof). In some states, a woman who exposes her fetus to controlled substances may be found to have neglected her child and, consequently, lose custody of the infant.[10] And, of course, once a baby is born, many laws can be used to punish a woman for directly harming or failing to protect her infant. But there is no law penalizing a woman for "failing to protect" her not-yet-born child by neglecting or otherwise refusing to undergo a medically managed pregnancy.

However, the power of moral sanctions imposed upon pregnant women who fail to receive prenatal care should not be underestimated. Many of the pregnant women I encountered at Alpha Hospital were very much aware of the "immorality" of a pregnant body unsupervised by a member of the medical establishment. On the unlikely occasion that a woman is not aware that a pregnancy unmanaged by medicine opens her up to moral condemnation, the WHC employees often provide this education.

To explain: although the majority of patients at the WHC begin their prenatal care shortly after discovering their pregnancies and deciding that they want to carry them to term (usually within their first twelve weeks), many others come to Alpha after becoming dissatisfied with the care they have been receiving at another hospital. These patients, usually quite far along in their pregnancies, are expected to bring along with them documentation of their previous prenatal care. This holds true even though Alpha repeats all laboratory tests, ultrasounds, vaginal examinations, and the like that may have been conducted elsewhere. Hence, asking a woman for her records from another hospital frequently functions only to "educate" women about the immorality of an unsupervised pregnant body, shame those women who cannot produce such documentation, and provoke the latter into defending their documentation-less status.

Moreover, there are many patients who, for various reasons, have not received any prenatal care, yet seek such care from Alpha during the later stages of their pregnancies. I have observed on numerous occasions the women who work behind the front desk at the clinic—Minnie, Yolanda, and two women who answer the clinic's incoming telephone calls—exchange looks of disapproval when a visibly pregnant woman seeks to begin her prenatal care at the hospital while being unable to produce proof that she has been receiving care elsewhere. On one occasion, a prospective patient (who, I eventually learned, had recently arrived in New York City from the Dominican Republic) saw the disapproving glances and overheard someone ask rhetorically, "She doesn't have any papers?" The patient, Jessenia, answered back defensively and insolently, "I was going to the doctor in my country, so don't even worry about that!" Whether Minnie, Yolanda, and Alpha employees in general actually believe the accounts women give to explain their lack of documentation is another story altogether. Minnie once said to me, "These patients tell you this and they tell you that. Who knows what they did in their country? Who knows how they got here [to the United States]? That's not my business. My business is to help them."[11]

Moreover, the phenomenon whereby Alpha staff routinely request documents from patients to verify their receipt of prenatal care at another location can be analogized to another issue that impacts the lives of many patients seeking prenatal care at Alpha: immigrant "illegality." A person with a work or student visa, "green card," or other paperwork affirming her authorized position within the borders of the United States—that is, a person with proper documentation—is said to be a "documented," and therefore "legal," immigrant to the United States. Conversely, a person without such papers becomes identified as "undocumented," or an "illegal alien." Thus, the presence or absence of documents determines the "legality" of a person. One might say that a similar operation is at work in the prenatal care context: Those persons who can produce proper documentation of their prenatal care have "documented," or "legal," pregnancies." Those without such paperwork have "undocumented," or "illegal," pregnancies. In light of this, Jessenia's encounter with the rhetorically posed question, "She doesn't have any papers?" deserves some reconsideration. Without contextualization, the inquiry "She doesn't have any papers?" might be understood as an inquiry concerning not simply Jessenia's pregnancy but her immigration status—to which Jessenia's defensive response might also invite ambiguity. That is, her response might be understood as a defense against an imputation of "illegality" onto her pregnancy and more generally her immigrant body.

To return to the question of morality, law, and the interest of the biopolitical state in optimizing "life," although moral sanctions are a powerful and effective force—which, at the very least, inform women that failing to receive prenatal care is commonly viewed as irresponsible behavior, but also likely induce pregnant women who are not so inclined to actually submit themselves to prenatal care—these moral sanctions are not "law." Undoubtedly, because a woman's feelings of guilt due to moral condemnation of her unsupervised pregnant body may cause her to seek prenatal care, such moral sanctions might and should be understood as assisting the state's biopolitical project of administering, optimizing, and multiplying (i.e., regulating) life. This is especially true if the only medical care a woman can afford is subsidized by the state; in such circumstances, the state finds itself a newly visible subject upon the poor, pregnant woman's acceptance of state-subsidized care, brought forth by acts of extralegal morality. Nevertheless, morality is not law. That is, although moral sanctions may be analogized to the law insofar as both may compel people to act (or refrain from acting), the state is not invested in moral sanctions and cannot directly use them to comprehensively regulate the pregnant body and the pregnant woman.

Although moral sanctions do not create legal subjects located within the state's biopolitical enterprise, Medicaid might. At Alpha Hospital and other facilities that accept Medicaid insurance coverage for prenatal care, state subsidization of a pregnant woman's medical expenses via Medicaid functions as a carrot that entices women to submit themselves to biopolitical supervision, management, regulation, and discipline. Women are offered a contract where, in exchange for the state's payment of medical bills, they are obliged to open their lives to the possibility of state intervention. A description of the process of initiating prenatal care at Alpha Hospital illustrates the point.

However, before turning to this description, one last note on the question of whether the pregnant woman, when poor, is always already located within the reach of the biopolitical state: during an interview, a patient told me that a WHC social worker, Carmen, informed her that a woman will "get into trouble" if she gives birth to a baby at Alpha and lacks a record demonstrating that she has attended more than four prenatal care appointments. When I asked Carmen if this was true, she laughed a bit and said:

> If somebody comes . . . to deliver and it seems like they haven't been getting prenatal care here or elsewhere, what happens is that they will hold the baby until they can get a nurse to go to the home and see if everything is taken care of there. And once they get clearance, then the

lady can take the baby home. It's not like they get in trouble. It's just that we have to clear the air because if she wasn't prepared enough to come to prenatal care, who says that she's prepared enough to take care of a baby? That's neglect. Why haven't you been getting your prenatal care? That's neglect. It can cause birth defects and all sorts of things like that. It's not that they lose they baby. It's just that we hold the baby long enough so that the nurse can check to see if there is a crib and things like that. . . . We want to clear the air. After that, we let them go. But, we don't want Alpha to be on the front page of the paper—saying that some lady took her baby home and bad things happened to it.

As noted above, many visibly pregnant women such as Jessenia present themselves for the first time to the WHC without medical records of earlier prenatal care. If these women cannot manage to be seen by a provider four times before delivering their babies, those babies will be held at the hospital until "the air is cleared" at their homes. Although the hospital's intent in refusing to release these newborns to their mothers may not be punitive, it is difficult to conceptualize the inability to take one's newborn home as anything other than "getting into trouble." In this way, poor, simply pregnant women do have a relationship with the state: in light of the hospital's prerogative to retain custody of the baby until a social worker has observed the home, a kind of *legal* enforcement is in place— even absent a specific law explicitly addressing prenatal care. That the pregnancies of the poor may be, from their inceptions, within the jurisdiction of a biopolitical state that can punish or otherwise discipline the pregnant woman for having failed to receive prenatal care (while the pregnancies of non-poor women are not so jurisdictionally located) might suggest that, in a society uncommitted to universal health insurance, the uninsured poor who rely upon the government for health care are located in a peculiar state of exception.

PRENATAL CARE ASSISTANCE PROGRAM: INITIATION INTO THE STATE REGULATORY APPARATUS AND THE PROCESS OF LEGAL SUBJECTION

At Alpha, a woman must first take an Alpha Hospital-administered urine test to confirm her pregnancy (without regard to whether she has already confirmed her pregnancy with an at-home test) before she is given her initial PCAP appointment—the appointment during which she meets with the battery of PCAP professionals. Interestingly, the Public Advocate for the City of New York released a report in May 2007 describing the requirement that a woman reconfirm her pregnancy with a hospital-administered pregnancy test as a "barrier" to prenatal care (Gotbaum 2007). The Public Advocate conceptualized the requirement as such because a woman must be physically present in the hospital to reconfirm her pregnancy in this way; consequently, the requirement prevents women from making prenatal care appointments over the phone.[12] Yet, the problem is even more severe than the Public Advocate's report reveals insofar as women cannot simply make the desired appointment on the day they physically present themselves to the hospital. Rather, they must also wait another twenty-four hours (or one business day) after submitting their urine for pregnancy testing—when the results are inputted into the computer system. A woman can bypass the additional waiting for the results of the hospital-administered pregnancy test only if she has documentation from another hospital or clinic confirming her pregnancy; then, upon her initial presentation at the clinic, she is immediately given a date to return for her PCAP appointment.

There was some controversy in the clinic as to whether visibly pregnant women were required to take an Alpha Hospital-administered urine test to confirm their pregnancies. One contingent of the staff believed that hospital policy required all women, regardless of physical condition, to be tested for pregnancy. Another contingent believed no confirmation was required when a woman was "showing." Thus, whether a visibly pregnant woman had to take a hospital-administered pregnancy test depended on who sat behind the front desk when the prospective patient made the inquiry.

On the day of her PCAP appointment, a woman meets with a registered nurse/health educator, HIV counselor, nutritionist, social worker, and financial officer, each of which is described in the following sections. Notably, the Public Advocate also described as a "barrier" to prenatal care the necessity that women meet with this coterie of professionals prior to having a medical examination. She says:

> Requiring multiple visits prior to the first prenatal care appointment not only delays entry into prenatal care for pregnant women but also may discourage women already struggling to juggle the demands of work and/ or childcare or overcome other barriers to appropriate health care, such as immigration, language, or transportation issues, or stigmatized behavioral issues. While social workers, HIV counselors, and nutritionists

provide valuable services, meeting with them should not be a precondition for prenatal care. . . . (Gotbaum 2007, 13)

It should also be noted at the outset that the PCAP appointment day tends to be an extremely long one, principally because the woman must meet for long periods with several people. Frequently "PCAP patients," which is their moniker on the day of their PCAP appointment, have to wait long periods before even beginning the individual meetings with each professional. If the patient does not speak English or Spanish (most of the Alpha PCAP professionals know enough Spanish to conduct their portion of the PCAP visit with patients who speak Spanish only), this language barrier tends to lengthen the visit as the employee must then use the "language line"—a telephone with two receivers connecting the employee and patient to a translator over the phone. The necessity of waiting for a translation of every question and response almost doubles the length of the visit and potentially delays the ability of the employee to begin her session with the next scheduled PCAP patient. Thus, women who have arrived on time for their PCAP appointments may end up waiting another hour or two before they begin their sessions. And once begun, their sessions may last two or three hours.

I stress the length of the PCAP day because it might be understood as training women to accept a common characteristic of "public" institutions: hideously long waiting periods. Accordingly, the PCAP day teaches women that public institutions (which Alpha exemplifies) are frequently too under-staffed to effectively and efficiently meet the needs of those who depend on them. Insofar as the poor are compelled to rely upon public institutions more than their non-poor counterparts, the length of the PCAP appointment day might be understood as educating PCAP patients about how the poor are commonly treated and the expectations the poor should have when negotiating these institutions. More forcibly, it communicates to women that their time is not highly valued; the exorbitant length of the PCAP day, and the excessive waiting periods that can be expected more generally within the Alpha WHC, abundantly demonstrates the state's conception of their time as being something utterly negligible.[13]

Registered Nurse / Health Educator

During the PCAP patient's meeting with the nurse, the latter takes the woman's medical history, asking if she has ever had any of a number of medical problems (e.g., diabetes, hypertension, heart disease, gynecologic surgery, anesthetic complications, and uterine anomalies). The nurse also records information about any past pregnancies a woman has had—whether any were ectopic or multiple, whether she carried the pregnancy to term or had a spontaneous or induced abortion, and whether she suffered any complications during the pregnancy, labor, or delivery. The nurse documents whether the woman has had any history of mental illness; whether she has experienced trauma or violence in the past; and whether she consumes tobacco, alcohol, or any other "illicit/recreational drugs" (and, if so, in what amounts). All of this information is recorded on a standardized form produced by the American Congress of Obstetricians and Gynecologists (ACOG)[14]—the ACOG Antepartum Record. The form solicits sociological data such as birth date, age, marital status, and, interestingly, race. Additionally, the nurse draws blood and takes a urine sample from the patient in order to conduct a battery of tests, including blood type, Rh type, and hemoglobin electrophoresis.

The nurse also refers the patient to the Women, Infants, and Children Program for Pregnant, Breastfeeding, and Postpartum Women (WIC) by completing a medical referral form. WIC is a federal program, administered by the New York State Department of Health (NYSDOH), whose mission is "to safeguard the health of low-income women, infants, and children up to age 5 who are at nutritional risk by providing nutritious foods to supplement diets, information on healthy eating, and referrals to health care" (United States Department of Agriculture 2008). WIC participants receive food vouchers for "foods [that] are high in one or more of the following nutrients: protein, calcium, iron, and vitamins A and C. These are the nutrients frequently lacking in the diets of the program's target population. Different food packages are provided for different categories of participants." (United States Department of Agriculture 2006). The patient must take the forms the nurse gives her to the WIC office (conveniently located in another part of Alpha Hospital) to receive food vouchers, which can be redeemed at grocery stores and farmers' markets that have been approved by the NYSDOH.

The nurse's final task is to provide the patient with what is called "education" involving a number of matters that could conceivably affect the patient's pregnancy (e.g., sexual activity, exercise, travel, domestic violence, seat belt usage, and the use of any medications, "including supplements, vitamins, herbs, or O[ver] T[he] C[ounter] drugs"). At a prenatal care visit that takes place later in the pregnancy, patients are "educated" about the "signs and symptoms of preterm labor, anesthesia/analgesia plans, fetal movement monitoring, circumcision, breast or bottle feeding, postpartum depression, and newborn car seat." Patients are also educated about "postpartum family planning/tubal sterilization." The language used by Alpha employees and on Alpha forms is "education." For example, a list of the employees with whom the patients meet on the day of their PCAP appointment appears on the "Patient Education Flow Sheet"; the matters they discuss are broken down into "1st Trimester Education Topics," "2nd Trimester Education Topics," and "3rd Trimester Education Topics"; further, the Alpha employee must document that each topic was discussed by checking a box marked "health education/literature given." Alpha Hospital's use of the term *education* in reference to the vast quantities of information given to women during their PCAP appointments and over the course of their pregnancies mirrors the language of the ACOG Antepartum Record forms, which label the topics that should be discussed with the patients as "Plans/Education." Then again, ACOG articulates the objective of the organization on its Web site as the promotion of "patient education." Nevertheless, the use of this term may be problematic insofar as Alpha employees inform their patients about only one—albeit the dominant and most powerful—model of pregnancy and childbirth: the biomedical model. Thus, it might be more appropriate to regard the program of knowledge given to the patients by Alpha employees as *training*. Indeed, historian Barbara Duden has made this argument elsewhere: "Each prenatal visit to the clinic serves as a training session for the forthcoming game" (1991, 25).

HIV Counselor

As per NYSDOH guidelines, all PCAP patients must receive counseling as to the "benefits of HIV testing as early in pregnancy as possible to reduce perinatal transmission" and the "meaning of the test results for both mother and newborn."[15] Further, all patients receive an "explanation that all cases of HIV infection and names of all partners known to the provider will be reported to the NYSDOH for epidemiological and partner/spousal notification purposes only." Hence, all PCAP patients meet with a counselor who discharges this duty. If the patient assents to the test, the blood drawn by the nurse is tested for the presence of HIV-antibodies. If the woman does not assent, the counselor must document the reasons the woman gives for declining testing.

One patient with whom I developed a rapport over the course of her pregnancy declined testing at Alpha because, since becoming aware of her pregnancy, she had been twice tested for HIV at other health care facilities. From notations made in her chart, it appears that employees at Alpha asked her for her consent to HIV testing at every prenatal care visit—that is, until she produced documentation of the negative test results from one of the other facilities. This patient's experience suggests that HIV testing is highly encouraged at Alpha. It is not unreasonable to interpret this policy as premised on a presumption of infection/contagion until proven "innocent"—that is, "safe" and unthreatening to the body politic (and the physicians who must care for her).

Nutritionist

Each patient meets with a nutritionist who records any known food or non-food allergies, notes whether the patient has had any difficulty eating due to nausea or vomiting, and provides information to the patient about the nutritional needs of pregnant women. Furthermore, during the meeting with the nutritionist, patients are asked to record (in exacting detail) what they ate for breakfast, lunch, and dinner the day before. Afterwards, they are given a chart with an itemization of foods (e.g., milk, cheese, meat, eggs, fruit, cereal) and asked to circle the number of times per day (or alternatively, per week) these foods are consumed. After the assessment, they are given information about the prenatal diet's relationship to a "healthy baby," dietary recommendations for pregnancy, and "tips" on how to increase or control weight gain, as needed. Should the nutritionist find the patient's diet unsatisfactory, she checks a box labeled "inadequate/unusual dietary habits" and asks the patient to make a verbal commitment to meet the nutritional needs of herself and her fetus.

The nutritionist's assessment of the patient's diet has a direct relationship to a woman's eligibility for WIC. Because, by statutory caveat, WIC food vouchers are only available to those pregnant women who are at "nutritional risk," it is in the interest of a patient who wants to receive WIC vouchers that the nutritionist find fault with her diet and, concurrently, enable her eligibility for WIC.[16] Bracketing the stigma that may be associated with the receipt of WIC—as one patient who had been approved for WIC but who refused to pick up her vouchers told me, "I'm okay [financially] for now. When the baby comes, I'll use it, but, not really for that [the milk and cereal that WIC provides women]. Just for, like, formula, because that's expensive"—the process of becoming eligible for WIC through a requisite consultation is not without its demeaning elements. Consider the following nutritional evaluation, recorded in a patient's chart: "Diet needs improvement—limited intake [of calcium] food, protein food, fruits and juice." However, the patient appeared (to the lay observer) to have an adequate diet and a healthy appetite; the previous day, the patient drank tea for breakfast; ate a sandwich with turkey, cheese, lettuce, tomatoes and mayonnaise for lunch; ate rice with broccoli in garlic sauce for dinner; and snacked on a banana post-dinner. Moreover, although the nutritionist noted that the patient had only a "limited intake" of calcium, protein, fruits, and juice, the patient indicated that she consumed milk, cheese, eggs, and beans more than four times per week, drank juice as often, and ate fruits and vegetables at least twice a day. Nevertheless, per a notation in her chart, the patient's diet was deemed insufficient, and she was referred for and enrolled in WIC. This, together with a score of similar evaluations in patient charts, suggests that as a practice, the nutritionist summarily deems a patient's diet insufficient in order to qualify her for WIC.

Irina, the one patient I met who was ineligible for Medicaid and was paying for her prenatal care out-of-pocket, is a revealing outlier. Because of her relatively high income, Irina was not entitled to enroll in WIC, and in her chart, the WIC medical referral form was blank, save for the nurse's scribbling of "PT REFUSED." Nevertheless, the nutritionist had indicated that Irina's "diet needs improvement . . . . Limited in protein food, fruits, juice and vegetable. Eats sugar cereals." The nutritionist had also checked a box indicating that Irina was at "moderate risk" due to her "inadequate/unusual dietary habits." Yet, like the case cited above, Irina had consumed an ostensibly healthy amount of healthy foods over the course of the previous day: Cheerios with soy milk, orange juice, a roll, an egg, two servings of cheese, several glasses of water, beet soup, bread, avocados, bean sprouts, lettuce, a glass of soy milk, vegetable soup, yogurt, peach cobbler, decaffeinated tea, and Corn Pops. During our interview, Irina provided more color to her session with the nutritionist: "The nutritionist told me that I wasn't eating enough dairy or something and I was like . . . . Cottage cheese has been my craving and that's my—really, my first trimester craving was cottage cheese with Thousand Island dressing on it. Now I'd probably vomit if I ate that. But it was delicious at the time." Irina's case would seem to indicate either that the nutritionist deemed her diet insufficient only because the nutritionist did not know that Irina was not entitled to enroll in WIC (and if she did know, would not have found fault with her diet), or that the nutritionist summarily disapproves of every patient's diet. Either way, the presumptive condemnation of women's diets can be understood as a moralistic gesture—even when done with the design of enabling WIC eligibility. One could imagine an alternate scenario where, for instance, WIC eligibility is not endangered by a nutritionist's honest and reasonable finding that a woman's diet is indeed healthy as it is.

Although many women welcome their meetings with the nutritionist and appreciate the information given to them, just as many found the coerced consultation offensive. When I asked a patient, Willa, about hers, she said, "I get really uncomfortable talking to nutritionists." When I asked her why, she said:

> WILLA: I don't like to do it. It makes me really uncomfortable.
>
> KHIARA: Really? Why is that—do you think? Has it always been that way?
>
> WILLA: Yeah. Because it's always been such an issue of tension. And my family has always been so much about healthy eating—but, we're all fat. So, it really stresses me out. Like, we're all overweight. Yet, we're always so educated. So, it makes me angry. . . . And I always feel like I'm not really eating the way I should. . . . No—it's true. I don't like talking about it. It's weird. Can we change the subject, please? [Laughs.]

Although I was happy to oblige Willa by immediately asking her a question about a different topic, it seems self-evident that she could not so easily "change the subject" during her required meeting with the nutritionist.

On another day, I made polite conversation with a woman, Gladys, whom I had interviewed earlier in her pregnancy. She told me about recent developments in her life and her excitement about her baby's upcoming birth. She also told me that she had been informed at her last prenatal care visit two weeks prior that she would have to meet with the nutritionist again that day, which she did. She said:

> She [the nutritionist] was trying to tell me that I had gained too much weight. Just a couple of weeks ago, they were trying to tell me that I wasn't gaining enough weight. Now, she's trying to tell me that I'm overweight. I'm not overweight; I'm normal. Hello?! I'm Black. I have hips. I have a butt. [Laughs.] I'm supposed to go back to see her today, but I'm not going to.

Gladys' comments are remarkable because she invokes a problematic notion of race—a possibly biological one in which body type is determined by racial type—in order to critique the normative assumptions of the hospital personnel. Her statement can be understood as denying the universalist claims made by a biomedical and biopolitical discourse concerning "proper weight gain"—asserting that such claims must be qualified, as they only apply to non-Black persons. Moreover, Gladys' and Willa's experiences should serve to emphasize that obliging a woman to confess her dietary habits to a nutritionist is not always a benign affair. As Gladys and Willa are aware, a "nutritional assessment" that tends to end with a condemnation of their diet entails a compelled and, at times, unwelcome scrutiny of women and their bodies, as well as a presumptively pejorative judgment about them.

Social Worker

Although oddly paired, the screening the nutritionist performs is identified as a "Nursing Nutrition/Psychosocial Assessment." Thus, after the nutritionist asks the patient questions about food allergens, diet, and eating problems, she determines whether the patient has any of the "risk factors" identified on the "Alpha Hospital Psychosocial Screening" form. These factors are: "unwanted pregnancy; teen pregnancy; foster care/surrender for adoption planned; HIV positive; [history of] or current substance abuse; high risk medical problems/poor [obstetric history]; anxiety; lack of familial/environmental support system; marital/family problems; domestic violence; depression; concern [regarding] capacity to care for a newborn; retardation; [history] of psychiatric treatment/or current emotional disturbance; lack of entitlement/benefits; homeless/shelter resident." There is also a box to check if "no referral [is] necessary at this time." If the nutritionist deems a social work referral appropriate for a patient, she escorts the patient to the social worker's office. The social worker then acquires more information from the patient about the "risk factor," and if necessary, puts her in contact with additional professionals who can assist her.

In practice, the list of risk factors on the Psychosocial Screening form is not exhaustive, and the expectation is that the social worker will see *all* of the PCAP patients who come through the obstetrics clinic. As explained to me by one of the social workers, Tina, Medicaid eligibility is sufficient to establish the woman as "at social risk," thereby making a social work referral appropriate. Thus, the seemingly incongruent coupling of the nutritional and psychosocial assessments is exposed to be still more perfunctory, serving to merely establish that there was some cause to compel the woman's evaluation by a social worker.

Accordingly, all PCAP patients meet with a social worker and are encouraged to divulge personal information. Tina gave me an exhaustive list of the questions she asks patients during their social work screening:

> Was this pregnancy wanted and do you want to have this baby? Do you have any experience? . . . If you're a first-time mom, do you have anybody who can teach you how to take care of a baby? Is the father involved? Do you have a place to live? Money to buy things for the baby? A social support system? Do you have anything in your history that might make the parenting difficult? There might be things that surface for you at a time when you need to be at your best for your baby. Is there any child abuse, sexual abuse, domestic violence? . . . Is there any substance abuse? Does she consider it a problem? Is she in a program? Has she been arrested? Has she ever had any children taken away from her—which means that she has a history of poor parenting? Are you breastfeeding, bottle-feeding? Did you apply for WIC? . . . After you deliver this child and are taking care of a newborn, do you plan on having another baby right away? If you're not, it's easier to not [become pregnant again] if you [choose a contraceptive that you could leave in place for long periods of time]. Do you know what options are out there? Are you going to breastfeed? If you are, there are [contraceptives] that are better while you're breastfeeding. Do you have everything that you're going to need to know? Do you want parenting classes? Yes—you can go here for them. Do you have everything that you're going to need for the baby? No—try going to this place. Maybe they can help you. You have to be in the best condition that you can be in for your baby. So, maybe you should get counseling. Here are some places that you can go.

To a pregnant woman expecting solely routine prenatal care during her visit to the hospital, it may seem relatively counterintuitive that, prior to having a standard medical examination by someone qualified to do so, she must meet with a social worker and detail intensely personal and intimate facts about her life.

Although all Alpha patients are required and expected to meet with a social worker, the social workers are not always successful in meeting with all of the patients. Tina explained to me (with a great degree of frustration) that this is primarily because Alpha PCAP patients must meet with a number of staff members on the day of their PCAP appointments. The meetings with the social workers are commonly viewed as less important than the numerous blood and urine draws, the nutritional assessment/WIC referral, and the Medicaid subscription process with the financial officer. Hence, the social worker is not infrequently bypassed. Tina explained, "Yes, we miss a lot of people, which is a problem, because we're supposed to see one hundred percent. It's a really bad situation because everyday there are PCAPs. Everyday, there are new patients. So, it's difficult as it is to catch all of the new ones each day. So, if you miss one, well—you may catch her at her next visit. But, on her next visit, there's a whole set of new patients, which you have to see all of. So, missing a patient—yeah, it's a bad situation." She added that she and the other social worker were not penalized—"other than the embarrassment"—for failing to see all of the PCAP patients. However, all women who deliver at Alpha Hospital are required to meet with a social worker prior to being discharged from the hospital and taking their babies home with them. Tina noted, "If there isn't already a database on them, then they'll create one then." Accordingly, it appears difficult for a patient to avoid the confession that is simultaneous with a social work consultation.

The invasive nature of a coerced meeting with a social worker may be mitigated by two things. First, many patients seek and appreciate the services of the social worker. On subsequent visits to the clinic, some patients request to speak with the social worker with whom they met during the initial PCAP visit. For example, one patient, who had become homeless and was placed in temporary/emergency housing by the New York City Department of Human Services (DHS), had been transferred to another shelter that she believed was unsanitary and located dangerously far from Alpha. She sought out the social worker, who documented that conditions at the shelter were unsatisfactory, with "bedbugs and poor kitchen amenities in which to refrigerate the milk she receives from WIC and to cook and adequately feed herself/baby." Time was of the essence; if the patient stayed in the shelter for more than forty-eight hours, it was to be deemed a "permanent placement," thereby making it difficult for her to be reassigned to another shelter. To assist the patient, the social worker obtained a letter of "Medical Necessity" from the patient's provider requesting the patient "be transferred for medical necessity and the health of her child to a facility suitable for a pregnant women [sic] and closer to our facility." Due to the assistance of the social worker, the letter was obtained on the day the patient requested it, and the patient was moved to a more hygienic shelter that was, indeed, closer to Alpha.

Second, the invasive nature of a requisite meeting with a social worker may be mitigated by many of these meetings being uneventful. The following record of one such meeting is similar to many of the notations the social workers make in patients' charts, and is, therefore, characteristic of the exceedingly mundane quality of a large portion of the social workers' interactions with patients:

Pt [patient] is a 29 y/o, Polish, married, female who is pregnant [. . .]; EDD [expected date of delivery] 7-3-07. Pt was referred from HRC [High-Risk Clinic] to be seen for a routine psychosocial assessment. Pt is seen in High Risk clinic diagnosed with Thyroid since two years ago. Pt uses Thyroxin 125mg. Pt states her mother has High Blood Pressure. Pt has Medicaid and Metro Plus number [. . .]. Pt states that she and husband [. . .] 28 y/o are happy about this unplanned pregnant [sic]. Pt cell phone number is [. . .] and home phone number is [. . .]. Pt reports a stable marriage for five years. Pt lives with husband and he is only support system. Pt is alert and participated. Parents are in Poland with one sister. Pt is the youngest child in the family, born and raised in Poland. Pt completed 5 years of college education in Poland, can read and write in English and Polish. Pt is employed part time as a Bookeeper [sic] and earns $128.00 [per week]. Husband work [sic] as an electrician his salary is $400.00 a week. Pt. denies any history of substance and sexual abuse, arrest, psychological problems or domestic violence.

Pt was referred to social work from PNC [Prenatal Clinic] to be seen for a routine psychosocial assessment. Pt is domiciled and undocumented. Pt was alert and oriented. Pt has an [sic] limited support system. Pt was receptive to social work intervention and answered all questions asked. Pt will breast and bottle feed the baby. Pt will think about contraceptives and CNS for well care baby. Pt was counseled on the importance to comply with appointments and preparations for the birth of baby such as crib, car seat and clothing. This interview was conducted in English. Pt will continue [prenatal care] at Alpha Hospital.

When a woman has "no issues," as is true of many women such as the one above, such social work referrals may be perceived as just another bureaucratic hurdle a woman must overcome before having a medical examination. Tina explained that a patient with "no issues" simply will be given a packet of information on physiological changes she can expect during pregnancy and social services available to pregnant and parenting women.

Even so, Tina acknowledged that the intervention she is required to make by Medicaid may be perceived as odd:

TINA: A lot of times, the patients don't know why they have to see a social worker. It's really strange. But, it's required by PCAP—their insurance.

KHIARA: Most of the time, do patients volunteer—well, let's say that [the nurse] brings [a patient] over. Would she be receptive to social work? Most of the time, do you find that?

TINA: Very rarely—usually when they decline, there's something to hide. But generally, even if they're not thrilled—if they didn't come to the hospital and say, "OK, I want to see a social worker!" . . . Even if that's not how they're coming, once they are here, they participate. And then once you give them the packet of information, they're appreciative. Even the experienced mom is appreciative of the information packet.

Alternatively, social work referrals may be perceived as a gross, unwelcome imposition into matters seemingly irrelevant to the desired prenatal medical examination—which, it deserves underscoring, is the principal reason pregnant women present themselves to the WHC. One patient's file revealed such a polemical encounter, per the social worker's notation recorded in the medical record:

Pt [patient] is a 32 y/o Hispanic, single, female who is pregnant . . . ; EDD [expected date of delivery] 6-10-07. Pt was seen for a follow up on ACS [Administration for Children's Services—the municipal bureau that investigates child abuse and neglect] cases. This worker tried to get information from patient regarding the new case that ACS worker Mr. Jones mention [sic] to this worker but patient just stated that there is nothing new to report. Mr. Jones did not allow Ms. Jane Doe the new worker on the case [to] talk to this worker. Ms. Doe's tel. Number is [. . .] Mr. Jones telephone number is [. . .]. This worker discuss [sic] the case with Supervisor, Hannah Williams who is going to follow it.

In this instance, the patient, Rhonda, was discovered to be the subject of an investigation by ACS. Rhonda appears to have viewed the social worker's inquiries into the ACS investigation as an annoyance about a tangential issue and, consequently, refused to cooperate. The social worker, in turn, contacted the ACS caseworkers directly, and, when they failed to cooperate, referred the matter to her immediate supervisor, who "is going to follow it." This is a remarkable sequence of events when considered in its context—a woman's presentation at a hospital for routine prenatal care.

I had the pleasure of speaking with Rhonda at length during an in-depth interview. She explained to me that she had become the subject of an ACS investigation as the culmination of a succession of unfortunate events: Her youngest son was born at twenty-four-weeks gestation, and as a result, is severely physically and mentally disabled. He is under the care of a specialist in Alpha Hospital, who is committed to seeing her son walk one day. (At present, he is confined to a wheelchair.) When Rhonda became ill due to her immediate pregnancy and was unable to take her son to one of his regularly scheduled doctor's appointments, the physician reported her to ACS, with the rationale being that she was "neglecting" her son by failing to bring him to his therapy. Rhonda was not angry at her son's physician for reporting her to ACS (although one must wonder about the frequency with which the privately insured get reported to ACS for missing doctors' appointments). She says that her son's physician jokingly told her, "You know I called the peoples on you. But, it's because I want to see my boy walk." She also says that the visit to her home by ACS investigators was without incident; they "looked around and left." But, she was fearful that the social worker from the WHC would reactivate ACS's interest in her by making unnecessary inquiries into a matter that had already been resolved.

Obligatory social work consultations are potentially less problematic when they are designed to empower the woman by providing her with information and services of which she may avail herself. Yet, on many occasions, it becomes obvious that the social worker is instead situated antagonistically to the woman; that is, the social worker reveals herself to be acting as the agent of a potentially punitive state. This is not to argue that the social workers are *always* acting as agents of a potentially punitive state; instead, social workers always have the potential to *become* agents of that state. Accordingly, it is rather invidious to compel a woman to divulge information about herself to an individual who has the option of using that information against her. Below, I quote at length a portion of an interview I conducted with a patient, Ashley, and her boyfriend, Paul:

KHIARA: And you spoke to the social worker. How was that meeting with the social worker?

ASHLEY: Yeah. I didn't like her. . . .

KHIARA: What didn't you like about her?

ASHLEY: I thought she was very forceful. And I didn't like her attitude. They were like—I have some mental health issues . . . . And I told her about them—just being honest and everything. And she was like, "You know, you're going to have to go see the psychologist. And if the psychologist thinks—recommends drugs, you're going to have to take them or else your baby's going to be taken away." I was like, "Don't scare me like that!"

PAUL: Total scare tactics.

ASHLEY: Total scare tactics. And I didn't appreciate it. And she was, like, pushing, like . . . . If I don't want to take Prozac, I don't have to. I can do without it during my pregnancy. But, she was so, like, forceful. And then, Paul was sitting outside. [Initially], she didn't want him to be there. And then she was like, "Do you want me to bring him in? Do you want me to tell him?" What? [Laughs.]

PAUL: "You have to take your medicine!" [Laughs.] . . .

KHIARA: The interesting thing is that, had you not mentioned. . . . You volunteered the information and the mental history that you have. And because you volunteered it, she sort of ran with it.

ASHLEY: Yeah, it was very strange because I volunteered it because—because I wanted help and I wanted to do this properly. But, I don't want to be pushed drugs and pushed someone else—encourage someone else to push drugs on me. That's one of the reasons why I came here: because I didn't want the epidural! [Laughs.] I don't want it pushed on me.

KHIARA: Ironically.

ASHLEY: I didn't appreciate her. It left me feeling very sour that day.

KHIARA: . . . Did she actually force you to go see the psychologist?

ASHLEY: I wanted to. That's one of the things I wanted to do. Yeah, she did set that up for me.

KHIARA: And have you met with that person?

ASHLEY: Yeah, I see her every week.

KHIARA: Does she push drugs?

ASHLEY: No! Not at all. No.

KHIARA: I wonder why it is that [the social worker] felt compelled to be heavy-handed. . . .

ASHLEY: She was quite heavy-handed. I just don't—I didn't understand. But, like, at first I was fighting with her. I was like, "No!" You know? Like, I was coming up with all these arguments about why it's not right. And then I was like, "Oh, just shut up! She's not going to get it."

One may find the social workers' interventions with Rhonda and Ashley unproblematic, even laudable as an indication of Alpha Hospital's commitment to all aspects of the health of their pregnant and unborn patients. The theory might be that prenatal care involves more than ensuring that the pregnant woman's amniotic fluid level remains stable and the fetus grows at an appropriate rate; it also means ensuring that the social environment into which a woman brings her newborn is healthful and life-affirming. However, one must bear in mind that this "holistic" approach to prenatal care—which, in practice, may be more punitive than affirming—is made compulsory for patients who do not have private insurance but merely optional for their private insurance-holding counterparts. That is, while private insurance-holding expectant mothers can forego a social work assessment by electing to receive prenatal care from a private hospital or physician that eschews such a requirement, the poor-qua-public-insurance-holders have absolutely no choice in the matter.

Medicaid Financial Officer

Patients are required to meet with the financial officer only if they do not have Medicaid when they present themselves to the hospital for prenatal care. Because some Alpha prenatal patients have Medicaid insurance coverage prior to the pregnancy that brings them to the Alpha obstetrics clinic, not all PCAP patients meet with the officer.

As noted above, the PCAP appointment day can be extremely lengthy; accordingly, some patients who ought to meet with the officer sometimes do not have the opportunity to have their consultation before the end of the business day. These patients are instructed to stop by the Medicaid office whenever they are in the hospital during regular business hours (e.g., at subsequent prenatal care appointments). As mentioned earlier, the expectation is that all of the prenatal care patients seen at Alpha will have Medicaid during their pregnancies. To meet this expectation—that is, to identify all those patients who have somehow slipped through the cracks—several times throughout the day, a Medicaid financial officer makes the rounds through the Alpha WHC waiting room, asking patients, "Do you have insurance? Are you pregnant?"

During the consultation, the financial officer explains to the patient that she needs to submit documents establishing proof of pregnancy, identity, address, and income in order to qualify for Medicaid and have her medical expenses covered by the state. Proof of pregnancy is established by the submission of an Expected Date of Confinement (EDC) letter—a document stating the woman's projected delivery date, calculated based on the date of the woman's last menstrual period. This letter is usually given to the patient after she meets with the nurse/health educator. Proof of identity may be established by a state driver's license or ID card, school or other photo identification, birth certificate, U.S. or foreign passport, or a permanent resident alien card ("green card"). Proof of address may be established via a postmarked envelope, utility bill, or rent receipt (complete with the patient's home address and signature from the landlord). Lastly, proof of income may be established via two pay stubs, a signed and dated letter from the employer on company letterhead, or a 1040 form with wage statement. If the patient has no income, she must submit a "Letter of Support" with proof of address from the supporter.

It may be stating the obvious to describe the process of applying for Medicaid as stressful and anxiety-producing, especially for those patients who are in the country "illegally" (i.e., without proper documentation). One patient, a Polish woman residing in the United States without documentation, tearfully approached me one day after meeting with the Medicaid financial officer and showed me the list of the documents she would have to submit to receive Medicaid coverage for her prenatal care medical expenses. She said, "I don't have these papers! It's too complicated! Too much!" I could only assure her that every patient with whom I had spoken had managed to get Medicaid coverage and that she would not be the exception. But although I encouraged this patient to be optimistic about her application, there are numerous reasons for her to be pessimistic. Establishing proof of income may be nearly impossible for those women who either work "off the books" at businesses or who receive cash as payment for work performed informally, such as babysitting or housecleaning. A woman in such a situation must then acquire a letter from a person who she can claim financially supports her—although she very well may support herself. Moreover, a requirement as simple as establishing proof of address may be difficult for those patients and families that have recently moved or expect to move within the upcoming weeks or months. One patient explained to me that she had all the paperwork she needed in order—except for the proof of address; she had been staying with her sister but knew that would have to end soon.

It bears repetition that women with private insurance or those who can afford to pay for health care out-of-pocket—that is, wealthier women—can escape the necessity of having to reveal information about the sources of their income before receiving prenatal care. The question of how they make their money (and how they arrived in the country) is made irrelevant every time the private insurer is billed for services rendered or the check with which she pays for directly billed services clears.

—

What the above description should demonstrate is that much is extracted from the poor woman when she finds herself pregnant and in need of government assistance with her medical bills. The state essentially says to her, "We will pay your bills in exchange for state surveillance of your pregnant body and the private arena in which it exists together with the possibility of a sustained, regulatory relationship." It is quite an exchange to make—considering that women with private insurance are not similarly compelled to assent to a relationship with the state. Indeed, government subsidization of medical services becomes a kind of recruitment device that enlists poor women into the welfare bureaucracy.[17]

Again, some may find state intervention into women's private lives completely unproblematic and potentially desirable—understanding it as a laudable effort to provide pregnant women with a wealth of information they can use to make their pregnancies healthy events on multiple levels. Indeed, this is the rationale given by some of the Alpha Hospital employees who actually provide the services mandated by the state. Social worker Tina enthusiastically describes her job as that of providing valuable services to women who need them. She argues that pregnancy might be an ideal time to make interventions in women's lives. She says, "There may be child abuse, sexual abuse, domestic violence. For a woman in an abusive relationship, she could be raped by her spouse and wind up pregnant. The pregnancy is a good reason to leave the house and come to the hospital. For a woman in that situation, this [the meeting with the social worker] could be an opportunity to get help." Even for women who have not experienced traumatic events in the present or past, Tina thought that her role remained important and useful nevertheless, as she could ensure that those women are connected to all the social services they might want to use.

However, subsequent to all meetings with patients, Alpha Hospital employees must make a written notation inside the patient's medical record of the topics discussed. Upon review of these notations, it is difficult to squelch skepticism toward hopeful articulations that Medicaid-mandated services are provided for the benefit of the woman alone. A common notation reads as follows:

> Information delivered: 1st Trimester: orientation to facility, rights/responsibilities of pregnant patient, pregnancy danger signs, common discomforts, drugs/ETOH/smoking OTC drugs, enrolled in WIC, occupational concerns, contacts after clinic hours (emergency), domestic violence, toxoplasmosis[;] 2nd trimester: pregnancy danger signs, common discomforts, sexuality, fetal movement, physical activity/exercise, signs/symptoms pre-term labor.
>   Patient Response: PT VERBALIZED UNDERSTANDING.

Consider another patient's encounter with the "Breastfeeding Teaching Protocol": within this protocol, the nurse is required to articulate to the patient the benefits of breastfeeding—among them, "economic, convenience, safety, health . . . , nutrition[al], immunity, [and] development[al]" benefits. The "outcome" of the meeting: "The patient will verbalize commitment and desire to meet her infant's nutritional and nurturing needs via breastfeeding." Indeed, all documentation of employee meetings with patients is punctuated with a statement attesting to the patient having verbalized an understanding of the information or a commitment to follow the instructions delivered.

A skeptical observer could reasonably understand these notations as doing nothing more than offering written proof that the hospital provided the meeting pursuant to the requirements of Medicaid. Indeed, if the services were for the benefit of the woman alone, there might be no reason to document they were delivered; as long as the pregnant woman received the information, the hospital's mission would be accomplished. Alternatively, documenting that the patient verbalized understanding or a commitment to act in accordance with the "education" might be read as protecting the hospital from future litigation initiated by the woman. For example, a woman who smokes cigarettes during her pregnancy and subsequently gives birth to a low birth-weight baby would have a difficult time suing the hospital for failing to inform her about the causal relationship between smoking and birth weight if she had "verbalized understanding" about the matter early on in her pregnancy. The same might be said about a range of other issues that endanger the health of the fetus.

Remarkably, this skepticism about the hospital's program is shared by some Alpha employees. On one occasion, I saw a patient's medical record sitting on a chair in one of the triage rooms. I picked it up and, noticing its volume, remarked to one of the nurses in the room, "It's so thick! That's a lot of paperwork." She said, "You know why, right? Litigation. Patients can't sue us." This nurse's somewhat flippant statement is descriptive of a troubling predicament in which the pregnant Alpha patient is left: at the end of her PCAP visit, and after having traversed the terrain of bureaucratic requirements, she is left with no legal recourse against the hospital.

Moreover, it is not all women whose lives are intervened into and regulated in the way mandated by the Medicaid/PCAP apparatus, and it is not all women who are left without legal recourse against the institution providing their care. Rather, it is only poor, uninsured women's lives that are rendered accessible to state intervention, regulation, and management. As a consequence, Medicaid coverage of prenatal care could be construed as a carrot that attracts poor women into the state regulatory apparatus and an occasion to make woefully disempowered legal subjects of women.

SOME CONCLUDING THOUGHTS

To distill the central theme of the above exposition: for the uninsured poor, state regulation occurs simultaneously with prenatal care. Foucault's theorization of the carceral is helpful in understanding the significance of this fact. In *Discipline and Punish*, Foucault (1975) argued that the classical-era scaffold, which could demonstrate the immense power of the sovereign only by destroying the body of the prisoner, was replaced by the instrument of the modern-era prison—the consummate vehicle for acting on the heart, thoughts, will, and inclinations of the prisoner. It produced docile bodies through a technique combining constant surveillance with the precise management of the prisoner's body in space (both physical and temporal). The Panoptican, the prison par excellence, dramatized and epitomized the operation of power in the modern age: the prisoner, whose body is always capable of being seen, bears this knowledge and, in turn, becomes the agent of his own discipline and oppression.

In the final chapter of this seminal tome, Foucault explained that the work accomplished by the prison has been disseminated to a range of institutions:

[M]oving still farther from penality in the strict sense, the carceral circles widen and the form of the prison slowly diminished and finally disappears altogether: the institutions for abandoned or indigent children, the orphanages . . . , the establishments for apprentices. . . . And then, still farther, there was a whole series of mechanisms that did not adopt the "compact" prison-model, but used some of the carceral methods: charitable societies, moral improvement associations, organizations that handed out assistance and also practiced surveillance, workers' estates and lodging houses. . . . (1975, 298)

The result of this dissemination was the creation of a "carceral archipelago" that "transported [the technique of the prison] from the penal institution to the entire social body." (Foucault 1975, 298). Indeed, "this great carceral network reaches all the disciplinary mechanisms that function throughout society" (298). Thus, bodies incarcerated in penal institutions are not the only ones subjected to constant surveillance and management, performed with the intent to "correct" the desires of the subject; rather, all bodies caught within the "carceral net"—frequently indigent, disenfranchised, and importantly for the purposes of this study, female—are thus subjected.

The observation that the bodies that tend to be caught within "carceral nets" have specific racial, class, and gender ascriptions may require an amendment to Foucauldian theory, which arguably speaks at a broad societal and historical level without concerning itself too much with social distinctions. Anna Marie Smith's work (2007) paves the way for this amendment. In an insightful and scathing critique of the U.S. attempt at "welfare reform" in the form of Temporary Assistance for Needy Families (TANF), Smith argues that modifications need to be made to Foucault's schema of biopolitics, which posits that modernity in the West witnessed the advent and subsequent dominance of the confessional mode of discipline. Writes Foucault:

We have become a singularly confessing society. It plays a part in justice, medicine, education, family relationships, and love relations, in the most ordinary affairs of everyday life, and in the most solemn rites; one confesses one's crimes, one's sins, one's thoughts and desires, one's illnesses and troubles, one goes about telling, with the greatest precision, whatever is most difficult to tell. . . . One confesses—or is forced to confess. When it is not spontaneous or dictated by some internal imperative, the confession is wrung from a person by violence or threat;

it is driven from its hiding place in the soul, or extracted from the body (1978, 59).

Foucault argues that the purpose of the confession was not to punish the confessor, but to reveal the "truth" of the confessing subject and, consequently, to transform him. The confession was "a ritual in which the expression alone, independently of external consequences, produces intrinsic modifications in the person who articulates it: it exonerates, redeems, and purifies him; it unburdens him of his wrongs, liberates him, and promises him salvation" (62).

Smith sees something entirely different at work in the TANF regulatory apparatus. Although welfare beneficiaries are required to assume confessional postures with state agents and to expose the details of their sexual lives to the state, Smith argues that these are not Foucauldian "confessions." They exist not to "produce intrinsic modifications in the person," but to *punish* the woman who asks the state for welfare assistance. TANF's requirement that a woman seeking benefits divulge the details of her intimate life to a caseworker is not a corrective dialogue; instead, the statute requires that caseworkers take " 'case histories' not to prepare the ground for therapeutic counseling, but to punish applicants who commit fraud or violate time-limit rules" (Smith 2007, 55). TANF applies " 'continuous monitoring' to the recipient population and the paternafare payers, but it does so to advance social control" (55). Moreover, TANF's requirement that a beneficiary of the program find employment outside of the home, without regard to whether the job provides her with financial stability or the opportunity to mother her child, is a demand of a state interested not in "moral-disciplinary transformation" but punishment. Smith concludes, with regard to TANF, "The soul craft that Foucault teaches us to search for in disciplinary technologies is largely absent; we are left instead with crude, superficial, and impersonal modes of correction" (55).

Smith's observation about TANF is also true for the Medicaid/PCAP health insurance program upon which the overwhelming majority of Alpha patients rely. The program asks a woman to confess the details of her economic situation to a financial officer not because it expects any "intrinsic modifications" will be produced in the woman, but because it wants to know whether she qualifies for assistance by meeting the baseline level of indigence. The program asks a woman to confess the content of her diet not because it wants to educate her about the foods that are good and bad for her, but because it wants to shuttle her off to another federal program that will feed her. The program asks a woman to confess the details of her social history to a social worker not because it expects the dialogue will be therapeutic to the woman, but because the state wants to know if, when the baby is born, it is justified in removing him or her from the woman's home. PCAP/Medicaid appears to be as much about social control and as little about the creation of a disciplined subject as is TANF.

And so, it would appear that Foucauldian notions of "discipline," and even "power," need to be productively revised. That is, power and the promise/possibility of discipline might not be as ubiquitous and random as Foucault suggests. There might be an intentionality to power and discipline that would allow them to be directed toward certain subjects thought *worthy* of discipline. Power, discipline, and all of the conceptual tools that Foucault presciently described take place within a world shot through with stratifications in the name of nation, citizenship, class, race, gender, disability, etc. It may be simply naïve to expect the abandoned Uighurs in Guantanamo Bay would be affected by power in the same way as are monied policy makers in D.C. Similarly, it may be wrong to expect the marginalized expectant mothers at Alpha are "disciplined" in the same way as their privately insured counterparts at Omega. Likewise, it may be mistaken to insist that those with race, class, and gender privilege will be caught up within "carceral nets"—within the regulatory reach of the biopolitical state—to the same extent as those who lack such privilege.

Accordingly, one can understand Medicaid coverage of prenatal care as an apparatus that attracts poor, pregnant subjects onto the carceral archipelago. That the state pays the medical bills accrued by pregnant women for their prenatal care is benign, in and of itself; however, the endeavor appears more disciplinary, surveillance-intensive, regulatory, and punitive when one considers what the state requires the woman to give in exchange: access to her private life.

All of this is to say: the pregnant women who decide to attempt prenatal care with state assistance find themselves, along with their male partners, most decidedly within the reach of the disciplinary, regulatory, and biopolitical state. (Information about boyfriends and husbands is gathered by the nurse, social worker, and possibly, financial officer. Accordingly, after a woman has completed her PCAP appointment, the hospital—and state—will know her male partner's name, his telephone number and address, his race and citizenship status, his place of employment and salary, whether he is supportive of the pregnancy, if he has ever abused her physically or otherwise, and sundry other details the woman happens to share. Hence, women's extraordinary visibility before state authorities effects the extraordinary visibility of the males with whom they have relationships.)

In sum, the fact of pregnancy alone may not bring a woman within the jurisdiction of the state. Yet, pregnancy combined with the woman's attempted receipt of state aid not only does so, but becomes an opportunity for the state to create a legal subject whose private life is exposed to supervision, surveillance, and regulation. In this way, Medicaid and the PCAP program bring pregnant women within the grasp of the biopolitical state, making them and the previously invisible, private elements of their lives visible, exposing them to state oversight, and ultimately baring them to the potentiality of state-sanctioned violence.

"State-sanctioned violence" refers to violent acts committed by the state—violent acts that are only understood as legitimate because they are perpetrated by the government through legal means. So defined, I view the ability of the state via ACS to demand entrance into a woman's home and survey its contents—as was the experience of Rhonda (discussed above)—as an act of state-sanctioned violence. Moreover, I view the state's ability to take custody of a woman's children as a gross act of state-sanctioned violence. That the hospital will refuse to release a newborn into her parents' custody when the mother is discovered to have harbored an "undocumented pregnancy" ought to be understood as a demonstration of this type of state-sanctioned violence. Yet more extreme demonstrations occur. I spoke with a postpartum patient, Victoria, who recounted her experience: When she went into labor in the early hours of the morning, she brought her two children, ages seven and twelve, with her to the hospital, opting not to leave them unsupervised in the home. However, because no other adults were present with Victoria upon her arrival at Alpha's labor and delivery ward, and because minors are not allowed into the delivery rooms, her children were placed in foster care while she delivered her infant son. It was only after she was discharged from the hospital that she was able to regain physical custody of her older children.

Victoria's experience might be understood as an exceptional, almost spectacular, demonstration of poor women's vulnerability—a vulnerability that is produced by the state as a result of poor women's negotiation of this arguably revolutionary moment in universal health care. However, in the next chapter, I will take up a more prosaic demonstration of poor women's vulnerability—that is, the production of their pregnant bodies as "unruly."

THREE

The Production of Unruly Bodies

INTRODUCTION

In Chapter 2, I demonstrated that attempting prenatal care with the assistance of state aid coerces poor women into an expansive state regulatory apparatus that far exceeds the purview of that care. In this chapter, I suggest that this attempt produces the bodies of poor women, as a class, as problematic entities in a distinctly medicalized sense. That is, the state, through the vigorous, intensely scientific, and excessive program of prenatal care it requires physicians, nurse practitioners, and midwives to give to Medicaid recipients, produces poor, pregnant women as possessors of unruly bodies.

A brief note: there might be a tension in my suggestion that the program of prenatal care provided under Medicaid is excessive—the tension resulting from the fact that many of the poor, pregnant women whose bodies are the objects of the excess of technology desire the manipulation of their bodies in the manner effected by Medicaid; some of the women with whom I spoke would not have it any other way. Indeed, Medicaid/PCAP-insured pregnant women who receive their prenatal care at Alpha Hospital can and do avail themselves of the most current and sophisticated health care available on the market. (The availability of the technology that is used for Alpha patients despite its exorbitant cost is due, in large part, to Alpha's status as a teaching hospital and its relationship to the Omega University School of Medicine.) Within the logic of capitalism, this most expensive technology offered within Alpha would be least available to the women who receive their care there—those who represent the most marginalized element of society. Once again, then, I risk the contradiction of critiquing a hopeful moment that both defies the logic of capitalism and capitalist distribution and is very much desired by some of the women. I accept this tension without trying to resolve it.

Moreover, although I criticize the excessiveness of the medical technology brought to bear as a matter of course on the bodies of the pregnant women within the Alpha WHC, I am careful to distance myself from those who see only the tyrannical and oppressive aspects of medicalization. Scholars who focus on medicalization as a repressive mechanism (as opposed to a productive mechanism in the most Foucauldian of senses) generate scholarship that ignores the more beneficial effects of medicine and medicalization and the desire many individuals have for it. Consider Lupton's comments on the matter: "In their efforts to denounce medicine and to represent doctors as oppressive forces, critics tend to display little recognition of the ways that it may contribute to good health, the relief of pain and the recovery from illness, or the value that many people understandably place on these outcomes. They also fail to acknowledge the ambivalent nature of feelings and opinions that many people have in relation to medicine, of the ways that people willingly participate in medical dominance and may indeed seek 'medicalisation'" (1997, 98). Accordingly, I acknowledge the favorable effects of the program of prenatal care practiced at Alpha and the willingness with which many of the women I encountered participated in the medicalization of their bodies and pregnancies. That is, my critique of PCAP/Medicaid does not prevent me from seeing the many salutary and therapeutic effects of the apparatus I criticize. Here, I acknowledge, wholly, that the medical gaze directed at Alpha patients did not prevent the realization of healthy outcomes for women and their infants; in fact, in many instances, I am confident that it aided such outcomes.

One last note: when I argue that poor women are "produced" as possessors of unruly bodies, I use the word "produce" in a conscious effort to evoke imagery of manufacture and industrial processes. It is an effort to analogize the treatment of women's bodies at Alpha—and wherever bodies are managed according to a general program of medicine without regard to their individual specificities—with the methodical creation of a product. In the case of pregnant women's bodies subjected to the course of medical treatment mandated by New York's Medicaid program (as they are at Alpha and at other New York hospitals accepting Medicaid insurance), what is ultimately produced is an unruly object that is most competently managed by trained professionals. Moreover, to say pregnant women's bodies are produced as unruly, in lieu of describing their bodies as "treated" or "seen as" unruly, underscores that there is more at stake in the Alpha WHC than the mere representation of poor women's bodies. Women's bodies *behave* as unruly when they are constantly measured, quantified, weighed, gauged, or otherwise assessed within a technology that speaks in terms of normal and abnormal. Variations from the norm become anxiety-marked occasions for further surveillance and the possibility of disciplining the body back to normality. In sum, the bodies produced by the Alpha obstetrics clinic through the nine-month gestation of the fetus are not merely conceptualized or regarded as unruly; they act accordingly.

THE INTEMPERANCE OF THE MEDICAID PRENATAL CARE PROGRAM

The course of medical treatment required by the New York State Medicaid program produces the pregnant body in a very specific, highly medicalized way. Per the protocol PCAP providers must follow, the pregnant body whose prenatal expenses are paid by the state via Medicaid is one that:

1. Should be monitored every three weeks during the first two trimesters, every two weeks during the first two months of the last trimester, and every week during the final month of pregnancy; should be weighed at every visit to the clinic, and the body's blood pressure ratio should be measured and recorded;

2. Can benefit from prescribed prenatal vitamins;

3. Requires the visualization of its interiority via ultrasound between twelve and twenty-four weeks, a procedure during which all parts of fetal anatomy are identified, amniotic fluid levels are checked, and other physical abnormalities that can be seen (i.e., placenta previa, vasa previa, etc.) are detected;

4. Demands urine testing for glucose and albumin at each visit;

5. Should be given a Group B streptococcus culture at 35–37 weeks;

6. Should be hailed back to the clinic within eight weeks after giving birth to be given a final medical exam, to be assessed for any

additional "medical, psychosocial, nutritional, alcohol treatment and drug treatment needs of the mother or infant that are not being met," and to be given information on family planning and/or actual contraception if the preferred method has been identified (Office of Medicaid Management 2007, 14);

7. Should be given a referral enabling the woman's enrollment in WIC;

8. Requires the "glucose challenge test" at the woman's initial visit and again at twenty-eight weeks, which necessitates the woman having her blood drawn, then consuming a sugary beverage ("Glu-cola"), and having her blood drawn once each hour for three more hours to test how well the woman's body metabolizes glucose, and as a consequence, whether the body is diabetic;

9. Should be given a "repeat gonorrhea, chlamydia, syphilis and HIV screen during the third trimester, as clinically indicated," and once again at the post-partum visit; and

10. Should be vaccinated for Hepatitis B and screened for tuberculosis.

Items one through five of the above list are not particular to state-subsidized prenatal care; the privately insured undergoing medicalized prenatal care should expect similar treatment. However, the balance of the list differs from the care given to privately insured patients in the following ways:

1. Although privately insured women commonly receive a medical examination six to eight weeks after giving birth, their doctors do not assess their "psychosocial, nutritional, alcohol and drug treatment needs" unless given a reason to do so; neither do I expect providers attending to privately insured patients provide information on contraceptives to women at their postpartum visits—that is, unless a woman specifically requests it;

2. Women with private insurance most likely will not receive a referral for WIC as part of a general policy;

3. Administration of the "glucose challenge test" at the woman's initial prenatal care visit and again at twenty-eight weeks is reserved for

Medicaid recipients. The privately insured receive the test only once, when they are twenty-eight weeks pregnant;

4. Although all pregnant women—with or without private insurance—should expect a test for gonorrhea, chlamydia, and syphilis during the Pap smear they receive during their initial prenatal care visit, only Medicaid-recipients are tested for these sexually transmitted diseases again during their third trimester—and yet again during their postpartum visit;

5. The privately insured are not commonly vaccinated for Hepatitis B or screened for tuberculosis.

The general structure of prenatal care selected by privately insured women who desire a medicalized pregnancy and childbirth does not greatly diverge from the program of care mandated by Medicaid; frequent doctor's visits during which the body and its functions are measured, examined, and manipulated within sterile, white-walled spaces are as common for wealthier pregnant women with private insurance as for women with Medicaid. However, although the course of general treatment mandated by Medicaid is not unique to government-subsidized insurance or otherwise reserved for poor, uninsured women, where it does diverge from that given to the privately insured demonstrates the unique excesses of the program and clearly reveals the heaviness of the government's hand when it comes to managing the health of the poor. Thus, the reason one might find resemblances between the care given to the privately insured and that to the publicly insured is because the latter is a *caricature* of the former—with some parts of the former's program being grossly exaggerated and distorted while other parts are diminished and eliminated altogether.

At least part of the reason the health care provided to poor women at Alpha Hospital is excessive is because Alpha is a teaching hospital—a site where young residents can practice (in the most literal sense of the term) obstetric and gynecologic techniques. Accordingly, the residency program is most educative, thorough, and attractive to prospective students when it offers a wealth of opportunities to practice medical science. The effect of Alpha's status as a teaching hospital on the care it provides—and that this status often translates into Alpha providing a glut of intensely technologic and scientific care to its indigent patients—was noted by a journalist decades ago during the height of the AIDS crisis. Remarking on the happenstance that many people hit hardest by the AIDS epidemic at the time were poor, uninsured individuals whose only hope for and source of medical care were public teaching hospitals like Alpha, this journalist wrote:

> Because one of its primary missions is the training of doctors, Alpha's interns and residents have a strong incentive to employ a vast array of diagnostic tests and high technology, just to gain experience. According to some physicians at Alpha, the reality that all the tests and all the technology have failed to prevent a single death is now beginning to raise questions about whether most AIDS patients should be treated in teaching hospitals. (Sullivan 1985)

Although similar questions have not been raised about whether poor, pregnant patients should be treated at Alpha and other teaching hospitals, there still exists a strong incentive for residents (as well as for the attending physicians who train them) to employ a surfeit of diagnostic tests and high technology on the pregnant bodies of their indigent charges. This incentive must partially explain the excesses of the prenatal care program dispensed at Alpha. However, the incentive cannot entirely explain all the excesses, as all providers accepting PCAP/Medicaid insurance—without regard to whether the provider is associated or affiliated with a teaching hospital—must provide health care in line with the dictates of the New York Medicaid law. Which is to say: many of the immoderations of the program are dictated from above. Accordingly, an important explanation for the excesses is the vision of the poor, uninsured pregnant woman and her copious medical needs possessed by the legislators, physicians, epidemiologists, and other policy makers who imagined the program and encased it in law. (I discuss this phenomenon more expansively in Chapter 5.)

Many of the individual doctors, nurse practitioners, and midwives who enact the state's course of treatment on the bodies of their indigent patients recognize the excessiveness of the state's program. As one attending physician, Dr. Trisha Valencia, rather matter-of-factly said to me, "We test more than the average place." Dr. Valencia went on to explain that the aggressive testing conducted at Alpha was due, in part, to the Medicaid law's adherence to recommendations made by the American Congress of Obstetricians and Gynecologists (ACOG), which suggest that "epidemic institutions" offer the abundance of screenings and diagnostic tests actually offered to Medicaid patients at Alpha.

However, although Dr. Valencia seemed to be an enthusiastic supporter of the excesses of the Medicaid prenatal care program, believing it to be adept at uncovering diseases and conditions in the "high risk population" Alpha patients purportedly represent, her faith in the effectiveness of the vigorous program of screening for sexually transmitted diseases and infections appeared to waver. I asked her if the hospital found that patients were, indeed, becoming infected with gonorrhea and chlamydia during their second and third trimesters after having tested negative at the beginning of their pregnancies and prenatal care. She responded:

> Yes. Yes, we catch it. [long pause] It's hard to say because if you don't test for it, you won't catch it. But, because we test for it here, the odd one will come up. I will say for the most part, no: we don't find new cases [of gonorrhea and chlamydia]. But, the odd one will come up. And you don't want to expose the baby to it. If you are already there doing Group B strep[tococcus culture]—which everyone is getting done around the same time [during the thirty-sixth week of pregnancy]—then, it takes very little effort to do an additional test.

Other providers, similarly pointing to the fact that all pregnant women can expect a vaginal examination during the thirty-sixth week of pregnancy and the ease with which a screening for sexually transmitted pathogens can also be done during that time, diminished the fact that repetitive testing for STDs and STIs constructs poor women as uniquely vulnerable to sexually transmitted bacteria and viruses and, in so doing, suggests poor women are sexual gluttons—an interpretation I expand upon in Chapter 5.

Yet, the Medicaid law goes beyond the recommendations ACOG makes for "epidemic institutions" with regard to the third, postpartum screening of patients for STDs and STIs. I had asked Dr. Valencia to explain the policy of testing the patients, once again, for sexually transmitted pathogens six weeks after they had given birth.

VALENCIA: Yeah, that's more of a legal type issue. There are regulations that say that for the postpartum visit to be paid [reimbursed], these tests must be done. And it includes [screening for STDs and STIs].

KHIARA: And is that a Medicaid thing?

VALENCIA: Yeah.

KHIARA: Yeah, because when I think about it in my non-medical brain, I thought that it was a bit excessive.

VALENCIA: I know. Because you are not supposed to have been sexually active [during the first month and a half after giving birth]. So, if you were negative back when you were thirty-six weeks, you should be negative [during the postpartum visit]. But, it's a Medicaid requirement and they want that documented. I don't know if it will change. And I don't know how to change it—because that's how it's been for a while. And that's one of the requirements. Some of the things make sense. The Pap smear, I would do it again [during the postpartum visit] because a lot of times we have inadequate samples when they are pregnant. Just because of the way the pregnant cervix is. And sometimes these women lose their coverage, and they will not be back to see a doctor when the coverage for the obstetric care finishes. So, sometimes it's good to just do the Pap Smear again. But, the repeat [gonorrhea/chlamydia] screening—that doesn't really make sense.

Although Dr. Valencia found the treble testing for STDs and STIs illogical, she was like the other providers I interviewed inasmuch as she was not otherwise disquieted by this aspect of the program and its discursive construction of poor women.

GRADATIONS OF EXCESS

The prenatal care program required by Medicaid can be contrasted with two models. Only one model of prenatal care to which the Medicaid program might be compared is the one available to the privately insured when they elect to receive care premised on the constant surveillance and measurement of the pregnant body. The Medicaid program is excessive regarding this care in the important respects discussed in the previous section. But, even if one holds the two programs are more alike than different, one should bear in mind that when the privately insured receive care that resembles versions given to the publicly insured, it is because the privately insured woman has *chosen* such a program for herself. Women with Medicaid do not elect highly medicalized and technology-dependent care: it is elected by the state on their behalf.

The second model of prenatal care to which the Medicaid program might be compared is what the privately insured receive when they opt out of a paradigm of pregnancy as always and necessarily being a medical event. This model of prenatal health care, accessible to scores of privately insured women, is largely outside of the reach of the publicly insured. When compared to this program, the health care given as a matter of course to the poor is dramatically excessive. Consider the experience of Kamilah, an African-American woman with private insurance who I interviewed two weeks after she had given birth at her home to her third child:

KHIARA: So, did you have to go to, like, a clinic for your prenatal care appointments?

KAMILAH: For my appointments? No, I just went to [my midwife's] home.

KHIARA: So, you never had to go into a medicalized environment?

KAMILAH: Well, I went to a clinic the first couple of times. And when she referred me for sonograms, I did that. But, other than that, it was either in her home office or in my house. It's great because in your last month, [you have to go] more often. Thirty weeks—once you pass that, it's twice a month. And once you're thirty-six weeks, weekly. And those weekly visits, she comes to you. Partly to familiarize herself with your home. I mean, she knows my stuff because this is her third [child that she has delivered in my home]. But, you know, [she comes to your home in order] to familiarize herself with your home. And also, so that you don't stress getting to her. So, we had our visits here.

Kamilah did not recall being weighed at every visit with her midwife—especially the weekly visits she had during the last month of her pregnancy. Neither did she recall having her blood pressure taken repeatedly. Although her urine was tested for glucose and albumin at every prenatal care appointment, Kamilah herself would do the testing by dipping a pH stick into urine she had collected; she reported to the midwife whether the pH stick revealed anything abnormal. Kamilah was never prescribed prenatal vitamins; rather, her midwife recommended a vegan prenatal vitamin she could take if she felt she was not consuming healthy amounts of the recommended foods. Kamilah reports her midwife did conduct a vaginal examination during the thirty-sixth week of the pregnancy, but she was not tested again for sexually transmitted infections during that examination. She ultimately gave birth to her third child in her bedroom while her two young children slept.

Kamilah—and probably more than a few public insurance-holding women, if given the option—preferred to receive a course of treatment that refuses to view pregnancy as an ailment and that simultaneously empowers the pregnant woman to care for her own body. Yet, women receiving Medicaid cannot enjoy prenatal care delivered outside of a paradigm of pregnancy as a medical event requiring medical intervention. The prenatal health care provided to practically all Medicaid-insured women is premised on a constant, third-party surveillance of the pregnant body—a body whose health appears to be capable of failing at any given moment.

THE TECHNOCRATIC MODEL OF PREGNANCY

The Medicaid-insured woman receives prenatal care that is in line with what medical anthropologist Robbie Davis-Floyd (1994, 1127) termed the "technocratic model of childbirth"—within which "the female body is viewed as an abnormal, unpredictable, and inherently defective machine." I would expand Davis-Floyd's argument to encompass the nine months that precede labor and childbirth; hence, I propose that the regime of prenatal care described above is a function of a "technocratic model of pregnancy"; accordingly, Davis-Floyd's "technocratic model of childbirth" would represent the final stage of a larger ideology of the pregnant body. It is a body whose ability to process sugar may suddenly disappoint, whose blood pressure may dangerously climb, and whose weight gain (or lack thereof) may indicate some unspecified complication. It is a body deficient in nutrients, for both itself and the fetus it carries within; hence, prenatal vitamins are prescribed to it and it is enrolled in WIC to enable its acquisition of "iron-fortified adult cereal, vitamin C-rich fruit or vegetable juice, eggs, milk, cheese, peanut butter, dried beans/peas, tuna fish and carrots" (United States Department of Agriculture 2006). It is one that is always already susceptible to pathogens in the form of bacteria and viruses; hence, it must be tenaciously screened for their presence. Indeed, the pregnant body produced by Medicaid is so greatly susceptible to sexually transmitted pathogens (i.e., those that produce gonorrhea, chlamydia, syphilis, and HIV) that it must be doubly screened for their presence during pregnancy and once again six weeks after giving birth.

Moreover, the body produced by Medicaid, in line with the technocratic model of pregnancy, is one whose interior should be made visible to the naked eye via technological interventions; subsequent thereto, women are rewarded with fuzzy, black-and-white images of their insides. Interestingly, many of the interiors of Alpha patients are made visible via ultrasound several times over the course of their pregnancies. This is because, invariably, on the day of the woman's ultrasound appointment, the fetus is not in a position within the uterus that enables the technician to acquire images of all relevant parts of the anatomy. If the technician cannot acquire a satisfactory image of, say, the fetus' femur, the woman must return to have a rescan. Additionally, if there is a discrepancy between the woman's asserted date of last menstrual period (LMP) and the size of the fetus as indicated by the ultrasound, the woman must return to have a "growth scan," during which the technician determines how much the fetus has grown since the previous scan. If the sonogram indicates the fetus is smaller or larger than it should be based on its LMP, the physicians and technicians have to determine whether the LMP is incorrect or if there is a problem with the fetus. For example, instead of being abnormally small for the sixteen weeks it would be based on the date of the woman's LMP, the fetus could really be only twelve weeks gestational age. Most of the time, the woman has simply miscalculated or misremembered the date of her LMP and there is nothing wrong with the fetus. Nevertheless, one can imagine the anxiety a woman feels when she is told preliminarily, "Your fetus is too small." The result of suboptimal fetal positioning and LMP discrepancies is that patients find themselves with several ultrasound scans over the course of their pregnancies. This may serve to reiterate woman's dependency on medical technology or their belief in the "unruliness" of their bodies.

Although I endeavor to problematize the staggering and ostentatious technology (including ultrasound imaging) that is used to manage women's pregnancies inside of Alpha Hospital, many of the patients with whom I spoke absolutely adore the fuzzy black-and-white images of their fetuses with which they are rewarded after their ultrasound scan. Petchesky (1987, 72) has observed a similar phenomenon: "Women frequently enjoy seeing pictures of their fetuses, citing that it creates a feeling of intimacy, as well as a sense of predictability and control." At Alpha, the ultrasound technicians usually give the women at least two images of the profiles of their fetuses' faces. Although I found indecipherable many of the other ultrasound images (such as those of the feet or hands), I could usually relate the fuzzy images of fetuses' profiles with that of a baby—although Petchetsy notes "the photographic image . . . obscures the fact that that image is heavily constructed" (62). I have been present on numerous occasions where women create a scene of sorts when they are told by the technician that they would not be receiving ultrasound pictures, usually because the fetus was not in a suitable position for its profile to be "photographed." Additionally, I know many women who have created photo albums from their sonogram pictures, and several who have put the ultrasound images of their fetuses on their cell phones as screensavers. Nevertheless, patients' joy in the acquisition and possession of ultrasound images should not serve to diminish the critique of fetal imaging, nor should it serve to mitigate the critique of the excessive technology used to manage all women's pregnancies at Alpha.[1] As Petchesky observed, women's ways of seeing their ultrasound images may be affected by public images of fetuses. Similarly, patients' excitement over their ultrasound images, and enthusiasm about the medical management of their pregnancies, is far from a "natural" response; rather, it is one that is a product of a culture (perhaps coinciding with what can be identified as a "U.S. culture") that, for the most part, fetishizes the fetus and venerates medical science.[2]

Lastly, the look of the place should not be disregarded, as it helps to complete the description of the Medicaid-produced pregnant body. This body is one that should be led down white-walled, white-tiled corridors by gloved and uniform-wearing medical assistants. The body should be exposed, unavoidably, to the smell of disinfectants, cleaning solutions, sanitizers, and sterilizers. It is one that is appropriately treated in antiseptic examination rooms by physicians, nurse practitioners, and midwives who wear white coats. Indeed, one of the first observations I made upon beginning fieldwork at Alpha was how simple it was to identify a staff member with his/her occupation in the clinic. The staff is structured according to the following hierarchy: The medical assistants, or PCAs, are all women of color who wear beige nursing uniforms. The registered nurses are all women of color who wear white lab coats. The residents are the relatively young persons, usually white, who wear white coats. The nurse practitioners and midwives are more easily confused as they are all young, white, well-dressed women who do not wear coats. Finally, attending physicians are the older persons who wear white coats. The exception to this schema is the lone male midwife, Mark—an older, stately gentleman who opts to wear a white coat. Had I not had met Mark on my first day at the clinic and had a long, enjoyable conversation during which he described his occupation and background,

I would have wrongly assumed due to his age, gender, and white coat that he was an attending physician.

An Inauthentic Exit from the Technocratic Model of Pregnancy

Although women at Alpha Hospital may receive their prenatal care from midwives, this opportunity does not usually offer them an exit from the technocratic model of pregnancy. On the day of the PCAP appointment, after meeting with the host of staff members described in Chapter 2, and after completing all the urine and blood tests requested of them, women are given an appointment to return to the clinic and have a medical examination. This appointment—ironically called a "doctor's appointment" by Alpha staff—is the woman's first meeting with her physician, nurse practitioner, or midwife. Which one the woman is assigned to is a matter of chance, however, as the woman merely receives the next available appointment. If that is with the midwife, the patient will continue to be seen by the midwife for the duration of her pregnancy (unless a medical problem is later detected and she is transferred to the High Risk Clinic to be attended by a physician).

Few patients know three categories of providers exist in the Alpha WHC. In fact, when I asked women if they were being seen by a doctor, nurse practitioner, or midwife, I was usually met with bewildered expressions and/or attestations of "I have no idea." To clarify, I am not suggesting that these Alpha patients are somehow irresponsible for not having discovered the training and qualifications of the providers of their prenatal care; instead, I am emphasizing that many Alpha patients have not been given enough information to know that their providers' training and qualifications is a relevant inquiry. Further, even if patients are aware of the three varieties of care, few know they can request one of the three. It would appear that even the Alpha employees are surprised when they are approached by a patient who requests a certain type of provider. Wendy, a former eleventh-grade English teacher who when I met her was pregnant with her second child, told me that during her initial PCAP visit, she requested a midwife as her prenatal care provider. She says, "I remember [the nurse] telling me, 'Well, you're lucky that you ended up here, because we have a midwife program and you're interested in that.' And I'm like, 'I'm not lucky. I picked it.' [laughs] . . . . 'This is why I came here. 'Cause that's what I wanted.'" And further still, of the small group of patients who know they can choose among a physician, nurse practitioner, and midwife, very few realize the differences in the manner of care offered by midwives versus physicians or nurse practitioners insofar as midwives tend to ascribe to a paradigm within which pregnancy is not necessarily a medical event.

Undeniably, many patients who have had experiences with both the midwives and physicians appreciate that midwives take a different approach to the woman's health care. The patients frequently describe their midwives as "nice"; they say the midwives "take their time" during their meetings with the patients. Many patients report the midwives ask more questions and try to get them to talk more about their pregnancies. One patient's midwifery encounter exemplifies many of the stories women have shared about their experiences with the Alpha Hospital midwives: Before this patient had her first official meeting with (and examination by) the midwife, she had been informed the midwife would be Mark, the lone male. She was wary of being examined by a male and told me she would probably switch to a female physician for her subsequent visits. However, at her next appointment when I saw her in the waiting room and asked about her visit with Mark, she said, "He is so amazing! I love him. I went in there [the exam room] and told him that I was worried about the baby because I'm not showing that much. And I wanted to know if he thought that I was too small. And he says, 'You're just falling in love. And you're going to be doing this over the next thirty years. And you're just going to have to let go and stop worrying and enjoy the experience.' It was so unexpected! I totally didn't expect him to say that—to respond to my question in that way! I loved it." This patient's experience is to be contrasted with patient encounters with physicians, who are described as "rushed" and "fast," or alternatively, unremarkable. The adjective most frequently proffered by patients describing their physicians is "fine," as in: "How do you like your doctor?" "She's fine." Or, "How was your visit with the doctor?" "It was fine."

Another important difference between the midwifery practice and that of the physicians and nurse practitioners is that only the midwives' patients can deliver in the birthing center at Alpha Hospital; the patients of the physicians and nurse practitioners must deliver in the standard labor and delivery rooms. In the latter, patients must remain in a hospital bed, connected to an IV and external fetal monitor. Only two persons (eighteen or older) are allowed to join the laboring woman in the delivery room. Once the woman delivers, she and her newborn are transferred to a different postpartum room where they remain until they are discharged from the hospital. In contrast, patients who deliver in the birthing center are not confined to the bed. Because the patient has neither an IV nor fetal monitor, she may move freely within the room, which is equipped with a kitchen, Jacuzzi, large-screen television, and private bathroom, and offers expansive views of the East River. Moreover, there are no limitations on the number of persons (or their ages) who may join her in the birthing room while she is in labor. Finally, the woman may remain in the same room until she is discharged from the hospital.

I should also note that when there is actually a choice between proceeding within the biomedical paradigm of pregnancy, labor, and delivery, and an alternative one, midwives choose the latter. Wendy gave me an account of the birth of her son, who she had previously delivered at Alpha. She says the umbilical cord was wrapped around her son's neck for much of the last trimester of pregnancy. Instead of undergoing a C-section, however, her midwife heeded her wishes and attempted a vaginal delivery. Once her son's head was delivered, the midwife removed the umbilical cord from his neck. The rest of the delivery proceeded without incident. The patient said, "The only reason why I was able to avoid a C-section was because of the midwife; if I had had a doctor, they would have done the C-section. No questions asked." I wholly agree with this assessment. (In fact, I believe even most midwives would have advised her to undergo a C-section.) This patient's experience demonstrates that the Alpha midwives may perform fewer medical interventions than the physicians and nurse practitioners. But, and crucially, this situation only arises when the midwives have a choice.

And therein lies the fundamental reason the midwifery program at Alpha Hospital cannot and does not offer women a real exit from the technocratic model of pregnancy: the choices of the midwives are constrained by their status as PCAP providers. Midwives, like the other categories of providers at Alpha, must comply with the Medicaid protocol for PCAP providers; moreover, they have the institutional oversight that ensures they follow that protocol. Accordingly, patients who are seen by midwives must submit urine to be tested at every visit. They must endure the "glucose challenge test"; the triple screening for gonorrhea, chlamydia, syphilis, and HIV; and all required vaccinations. Their fetuses are screened for genetic abnormalities. Their bodies are constantly weighed, their blood pressure systematically checked, and their interiors regularly made visible via ultrasound or vaginal examinations. So, essentially, the unorthodoxy, or "alternative-ness," of Alpha's midwifery practice is severely constrained by the necessity of delivering care in accordance with the dictates of being a PCAP provider. This reading was affirmed by a midwife:

> We have to work within the system here. It's very limiting. We do a million tests that probably don't need to be done on these nice, healthy women. And we see them sometimes more often than I would like. It's a weird system. . . . It's a burden on them, I feel like.

A Real Exit from the Technocratic Model of Pregnancy

Although the midwifery program at Alpha does not offer a real escape from a technocratic model of pregnancy, there is an exit for the Medicaid-insured women—albeit a narrow one—from a regime of prenatal care that understands her pregnant body as appropriately managed by only the most vigilant of medical science. To explain: the lack of institutional oversight of midwives, physicians, and nurse practitioners who accept Medicaid insurance, yet who are not affiliated with a hospital, allows these caregivers relative freedom to provide prenatal care that is not premised on the unremitting surveillance and quantification of the pregnant body. Although as PCAP providers, such institutionally unencumbered providers are statutorily obligated to assess their patients as regularly and vigorously as does the providers at Alpha, the absence of institutional oversight enables these unaffiliated caregivers the discretion to ignore or avoid their legal obligations.

However, this exit from the regime of hypervigilance in practice is reserved for only the most savvy and resourceful of Medicaid-recipients. Because the caregivers who provide this health care do not have professional affiliations with institutions such as public hospitals or community clinics—places where Medicaid-insured women would easily find them—women desiring less technology-intense prenatal care must act as careful consumers and locate these providers through other channels (i.e., Internet searches, word-of-mouth, etc.). This is especially true because an institution such as Alpha views such alternative providers as competition for the patient-consumer who can very well take her "business" elsewhere. As one of the administrators at Alpha responded after I relayed a patient's request for names of other physicians from whom she could seek prenatal care, "She has to find that information on her own. We're not here to give away our business." Therefore, Alpha (and, likely, any similarly situated institution competing for insurance dollars) does not as a matter of practice inform women of other options; to do otherwise is simply bad business. The result is that only the most astute Medicaid-recipient—the woman who has the wherewithal to learn about the entire breadth of her options—can choose whether she will submit to the intensively medically managed pregnancy she will receive within institutional walls. All other women receiving Medicaid coverage of their prenatal care expenses virtually have no effective choice at all.

⌒

In sum, the body produced by Medicaid is one that is insistently and tenaciously medically managed. Although I suggest the course of treatment mandated by Medicaid exceeds "normal" medicalization insofar as Medicaid recipients are doubly and trebly tested for conditions for which the privately insured are screened only once, one need not accept this to appreciate that the prenatal care given to poor women who rely upon Medicaid can have especially disempowering effects. That is, even if one assumes for argument's sake that Medicaid recipients' prenatal care is not medicalized beyond the extent to which privately insured women's care is when the latter elects into the technocratic model of pregnancy, the intersection of this "normal" medicalization with a population entirely composed of poor women is uniquely problematic. In the following section, I discuss Barbara Duden's scholarship on the fetus and her critique of the medicalization of pregnancy generally. I then explore her critique in the context of the poor women this affects at Alpha Hospital.

THE DUDENIAN FETUS

The possibilities and problems associated with the biomedical paradigm of pregnancy are invariably at work in the Alpha WHC. The understanding of the pregnant body within biomedical discourse has been convincingly described as disempowering to the woman upon whom it is enacted. Historian Barbara Duden's work (1993) in this area is instructive. She argues that women's experiences of pregnancy in the modern era are held hostage by the fetus—a biological fact that is taken to be best dealt with within the biomedical paradigm. A woman's fetus, however, is only accessible to her via technological processes on which medical professionals hold a monopoly. Thus, the fetus "disembodies" a woman's perceptions and "forces her into a nine-month clientage in which her 'scientifically' defined needs for help and counsel are addressed by professionals" (4). Duden compares this experience of pregnancy with those of women who have been protected from the fetus by historical happenstance or for whom the fetus has been inaccessible due to their subordinated socioeconomic positioning within global capitalism. She describes the pregnancy of the mother of a poor recent immigrant living in Harlem as much more "sensual, warm, touchable, familiar" (27). Pregnancy—before the advent of photogenically produced fetuses and tests that can detect the presence of Human Chorionic Gonadotropic (HCG) hormone—was a more embodied, personal event. Knowledge of it resided with the woman who *sensed* it; further, a woman's pregnancy was only made known to others through her announcement of it. Duden argues that "the fetus" has altered this. Pregnancy is now a condition professionals first confirm, then manage for a woman.

On the issue of tests that can detect the presence of the HCG hormone in urine and, in so doing, determine the fact of a woman's pregnancy, Duden writes: "Today when I do not get my menstrual period, I wait a week, perhaps a few days more. Then I face a decision. I can cross a historically unprecedented threshold and enter the world of scientific 'facts' by obtaining a kit for a urine test. Seeing the result, I conjure up a fetus, and with it the abstraction 'life' " (53). She then goes on to say that once the fetus is thus conjured, submission to the biomedical establishment closely follows.

Duden's narrative about the closure of the universe of possibilities a woman can imagine about her pregnancy and pregnant body upon the acquisition of a "kit for a urine test" is particularly relevant at Alpha Hospital. Indeed, an exaggerated version of Duden's scenario is performed numerous times a day at the obstetrics clinic: prospective prenatal patients must submit urine to be tested for HCG in order to begin prenatal care at Alpha— this despite the large majority of prospective patients having already confirmed their pregnancies with at-home tests prior to setting foot inside of the hospital. Accordingly, if Duden is correct that the performance of a urine pregnancy test inscribes women within a specific model of pregnancy and the "fetus," Alpha's requirement that it be repeated serves to reinscribe and reiterate this model and its power. It educates women about the nature of the enterprise (i.e., one that is scientific and medicalized) into which they are entering by receiving their prenatal care from Alpha. Moreover, it effectively proclaims, "You're not really pregnant until we say so."

In sum, Duden's argument is that a woman now must depend on technically trained professionals to care for her during an event that is discursively constructed as something she is told she is intellectually and technically unprepared to manage for herself. Thus, pregnant women are disempowered and made dependent.[3]

THE DUDENIAN FETUS AT ALPHA

Duden's argument is applicable to all women living in the era of the fetus. Accordingly, all pregnant women, without regard to class, would be equally disempowered and equally made dependent by the fetus. However, the critique is exaggerated when it is extended to the women it affects in Alpha Hospital: poor, pregnant women. That is, a poor, pregnant woman may experience the disempowering and dependency-producing effects of a medically managed pregnancy as yet another demonstration of her powerlessness within society. Indeed, prenatal care so delivered may be understood as a disciplinary mechanism that educates poor, pregnant women about their status within society and the behavior expected of those who occupy that station. Specifically, being poor is about being dependent on others, about submitting oneself to surveillance, about being problematized. Being poor is about putting oneself within the charge of someone who can meet the needs one cannot satisfy for oneself.

Indeed, for non-poor women, the element of choice may temper the effects of the disempowering aspects of the Dudenian fetus and the concomitant medical management of pregnancy. Duden speaks of electing to put oneself within the charge of medical professionals by accepting discursive constructions of the fetus. She argues that women must "decide" whether to understand their pregnancies as the production of a fetus with needs only medical science may satisfy. Alternatively, women may reject this view and choose "aliveness"—a presumably more sensuous, corporeal embodiment outside of the biomedical construction of pregnancy. If the woman chooses the former, "she becomes the subject of a series of needs—for counseling, prenatal testing, diagnosis, prognosis, and management" (Duden 1993, 54).

> If a woman does not eschew the series of powerful suggestions that stamp her as the reproducer of a life, she cannot avoid patienthood under the gynecologist, sharing with him the social responsibility for the future of the life within her, including the decision about whether to remain its uterine environment or not. Once she consents to cooperate in prenatal

testing and the biotechnological care and management of her insides, she is caught in a series of unavoidable "decisions" that lead from amniocentesis to the interiorization of eugenics to the scientifically guided care of a modern infant.

But a woman can refuse to accept this state and put herself outside the framework that imposes such needs. Inevitably, she then exposes herself to a series of criticisms. Some will see her as a "primitive" who deprives herself and her infant of the benefits of modern medicine. Others will see in her the romantic who places good will, emotions, and irresponsible trust above the certainties of a modern institutionalized reality. And others will dismiss her as utopian. (54)

Yet, the poor, Medicaid-insured patient at Alpha Hospital—frequently ill-informed of those noninstitutional sites where she may enjoy demedicalized prenatal care—does not have the option of rejecting a scientific, technological model of pregnancy and putting herself "outside the framework that imposes such needs." She does not have the luxury of being viewed as a romantic or being dismissed as a utopian. She cannot even elect the title of "primitive." Insofar as no options outside of an intensely medically managed pregnancy exist for the large majority of poor, pregnant women accepting Medicaid, they are forcibly conscripted into the regime of biomedically produced and satisfied needs. I do not read Duden as arguing in favor of women foregoing medical treatment entirely—and neither would I suggest it. Rather, I understand Duden as acknowledging that a continuum of prenatal care exists, with the woman who refuses all prenatal care on one end. On the other end sits the woman who is the imperfect incubator for a fetus whose needs are satisfied only by the most relentless medical science. Medicaid recipients, for the most part, are forced to be with the latter or forego prenatal care altogether. Such a circumscribed choice may hardly be a choice at all.

Admittedly, even if given the choice, many poor women may elect to have a medically managed pregnancy. I have talked to many Alpha Hospital patients who enthusiastically express their happiness with the care they receive from the WHC. Indeed, many women choose to receive their care from Alpha (as opposed to a hospital closer to their residences) because they have heard it offers the "best" (read: most technologically intense and scientifically advanced) prenatal care.

This is in line with Fraser's (1995) study of obstetric and midwifery practices in the South, and can be read as a response to Davis-Floyd's work—which may be accused of promoting natural childbirth as the "good" or "right" childbirth experience. Fraser cautions that race complicates the narrative told by those scholars who conceptualize midwifery and natural childbirth as uniformly desired and desirable and medically managed pregnancy and childbirth as uniformly undesired and undesirable. Fraser shows that in the impoverished, predominately African-American community in which she did her fieldwork, medically managed pregnancies and childbirths were highly coveted. This was a community that, due to classism and racism, had largely been ignored by the medical establishment. That the women in this community now had the choice of receiving their prenatal care from obstetricians and delivering their babies in hospitals with the aid of anesthesia "signaled a symbolic if not fully realized inclusion in the field of vision of a health-care bureaucracy that had until then largely ignored the health needs of African Americans" (57). Fraser notes present-day critiques of medicalized pregnancies and childbirths, and the simultaneous lauding of midwifery and natural childbirths, have "emerged with the growth of a consumerist, choice-oriented social movement influenced in large part by middle-class (white) feminist theory and praxis" (55). Poor women of color—who previously have been excluded from both obstetrical practice and the generation of the feminist critique of that practice—might disagree with the problematization of the biomedical paradigm of pregnancy and childbirth and, indeed, want pregnancies administered in line with it.

Although Fraser's intervention is an important one, it is imperative that what women "want" is not naturalized. That is, we should not conclude that it is "natural" for poor women of color to want medicalized pregnancies and births without seeing those wants as being born out of a particular sociopolitical context. Indeed, if the poor women of color who were the subjects of Fraser's research desired medicalized pregnancies and births, their desires were in some part a product of the previous unavailability of those services—an unavailability dictated by racism and classism. We must bear in mind that what is hegemonic becomes desirable and desired; yet, hegemonic desires are hardly an essential index of what women of color (or any grouping of women) would "naturally" elect.

Moreover, for every poor, pregnant Alpha patient who "wants" a medically managed pregnancy, there may be a woman like Summer, who was pregnant with her first child when I met her. I was sitting behind the front desk when she approached me and explained she had just returned from an extended trip to visit her family in Israel. She said she had gone to the doctor while in Israel and he had given her and her fetus many tests. She asked if she would have to repeat those tests. I responded, "Probably. Alpha likes to do all the tests itself." Later on, while she waited for the midwife to call her, I asked if she wanted to be interviewed more formally for my research. I learned she was one of many women who preferred prenatal care far away from the extreme end of the medicalization continuum at which Medicaid recipients at Alpha are situated:

SUMMER: Here it is different because in America, they are so fanatic. So, here you have to do all the tests. So, I kind of go with it. If I was in Israel, I wouldn't know if it was a boy or girl. I would just go into labor and that is it. Here it is impossible. That is why I told you in the beginning that I did some tests in Israel and didn't want to do it again. I am probably going to have to do everything again.

KHIARA: So, in Israel, your doctor has a different approach?

SUMMER: It is very alternative. You can do whatever you want. You can refuse. I went to the doctor, but the only thing I did was give blood and [listen to the fetal] heart[beat]. No sugar test or ultrasound. She told me if I wanted to do it, I can; but, it is not mandatory.

KHIARA: You feel that they compelled you to the do ultrasound here?

SUMMER: Yeah. Otherwise, I wouldn't have done it.

KHIARA: So, I know that every time you come, you have to do the urine testing. . . .

SUMMER: Yeah. But, I wouldn't do that if I didn't have to.

KHIARA: Then why don't you refuse?

SUMMER: To me it is not a choice. . . . [It is] unnecessary. But what can we do? I guess saying nothing is better than having somebody come to see your house and all that kind of stuff. I am just going to keep my mouth shut for now.

Interestingly, Summer understood the difference between the more "alternative" approach to prenatal care she enjoyed in Israel and the highly medicalized approach she received at Alpha in terms of the hospital's "American"-ness. She did not seem to realize that the absence of choice—that is, her inability to opt for an alternative approach to prenatal care—is a burden that only poor women in the United States are forced to bear. Also noteworthy, she believed the price for arguing against the medicalization of her pregnancy and refusing to submit to the myriad tests prescribed for her was state surveillance and possibly regulation—"having somebody come to see your house and all that kind of stuff." Concluding that such a price was too much, she opted to submit to the medicalization of her pregnancy and "keep [her] mouth shut for now."

Insofar as the model of prenatal care enacted at and by Alpha Hospital is one premised on the monitoring of a body that is always capable of failing at a moment's notice, one may argue that the foundation of this prenatal regime is the *unruly body*. I suggest the construction of the pregnant body as an unruly one occurs whenever it is intensively medically managed; consequently, the pregnant bodies of the non-poor may be thus constructed and treated accordingly. Thus, the unruly pregnant body is not specific to the Medicaid poor, but is characteristic of the body of any pregnant woman who elects (insofar as any woman, living within a society in which the medicalization of pregnancy is the norm, can conceive of there being a choice) to be treated within and subjected by the standard biomedical paradigm. But, as discussed above, therein lies the fundamental difference between the unruly bodies of the poor and the non-poor. Although the non-poor may elect to have their bodies administered in such a fashion, to the extent Medicaid coverage of prenatal expenses is, in practice, concomitant with a pregnancy administered squarely within the biomedical paradigm, poor, uninsured women do not choose to have their bodies constructed as unruly. Moreover, to the extent Medicaid's medicalization of pregnancy is in excess of the medicalization done to the pregnancies of the non-poor, the bodies of the poor might be understood as exceedingly unruly.

Furthermore, the unruly bodies constructed by Alpha rarely disappoint. That is, anomalies, disorders, abnormalities, and malfunctions are regularly and relentlessly found within them. Yet many of these "resolve themselves" or otherwise have no effect on the health of the fetus or the mother. For instance, on several occasions, I have translated to Spanish-speaking patients the ultrasound technicians' explanations that placenta previa was detected during their sonograms. This is a condition in which the placenta partially or completely covers the cervical opening, or os. Patients with placenta previa are advised to undergo a C-section as they are at risk for massive hemorrhaging if the placenta covers the cervix when it begins to dilate in preparation for the birth of the baby (American Congress of Obstetricians and Gynecologists 2007). However, after the ultrasound technicians give the women the disheartening news that if the condition persists, the women will have to endure a C- section, the technicians usually assure the women they should not worry because the placenta usually moves away from the cervix over the course of the woman's pregnancy; thus, the potential issue is resolved without the necessity of a radical medical intervention. I imagine the effect of a diagnosis of placenta previa merely serves to remind the woman that she occupies an unruly body that may fail at any given moment. She is thereby warned that her submission to the biomedical paradigm and the physicians that perform it is required if she hopes her baby to be healthy. That patients are frequently diagnosed with conditions that proceed to no effect might be explained as a success of a medical technology that "sees too much." Or, it might just be the effect of screens, tests, and examinations that speak in terms of probability, risk, and likelihood: all patients are rendered at risk for *something*, even if that risk is a miniscule one.

Women I interviewed told countless stories concerning the plethora of diagnoses made by Alpha providers that served little purpose beyond reiterating the fact of patients' unruly bodies. I offer only one: I recall having a long in-depth interview with one delightful patient while she waited over two hours for an ultrasound scan. After she was finally called and had completed her scan, I asked one of the nurses if the patient had left for home yet, as I wanted to exchange contact information with her. The nurse replied, "No, she's talking to a doctor. They saw something with the baby's heart in the ultrasound." I became distraught, imagining the patient's own distress at receiving news of a problem with her fetus. In response, the nurse said, "No, no, no. Don't worry. It's no big deal. They see this all the time. It usually goes away." I looked at her skeptically. She laughed and said, "It's nothing to worry about. Really. It usually goes away." Indeed, when I talked to the patient after her meeting with the doctor, she said, "They want to run some sort of blood test. If it comes back negative, then there really is nothing there. But, if it comes back positive, then they would just have to monitor me to make sure that the heart thing goes away." Again: such an anxiety-producing diagnosis for a "heart thing" that would go away with or without a medical intervention probably did little more than to produce anxiety and reiterate the unruliness of this patient's body. This might be understood as a different iteration of the same problematic: the life of the fetus is fragile and requires medical supervision against the opacity of the woman's body as an imperfect incubator.

In essence, poor, uninsured women in the state of New York—with the exception of only the savviest—are compelled to inhabit unruly bodies and the medically managed pregnancies that are both their cause and effect.

This is significant because in the absence of an effective choice of a low-intervention prenatal care program, Medicaid (and the state that administers it) enacts the poor, pregnant body as one that can and should only be treated medically, scientifically, and clinically. Prenatal care within the Medicaid regime proceeds from the assumption that the errors and risks within the poor, pregnant body (which are invariably "there" and must be detected via constant screens and tests) can only be remedied by medical science. The poor body, then, is one exposed to bacteria and viruses; hence, antibiotics, antiviral medications, and vaccinations are administered. The poor body is one that is malnourished; hence, WIC (and the concomitant prescription of prenatal vitamins and recommended consumption of meat and dairy) are provided. The poor body is one whose reproduction is dangerously unrestrained and, yes, unruly; hence, the parade of contraceptives placed in front of the postpartum body—ranging from the lower-intervention condoms to the intensely high-intervention Depo-Provera injection. (Expectedly, the Depo-Provera injection—which consists of a high dose of progesterone, thereby preventing the woman from ovulating for three months at a time—is the birth control method that comes most highly recommended by Alpha providers and staff.) The consequence is a medicalization of poverty, which is treated as a condition that produces ailments and disorders all rectifiable (or at least managed) via medical science. In these ways, the poor are treated as biological dangers—to themselves, to their fetuses, and to the society within which they exist.

SOME CONCLUDING THOUGHTS

Medicaid's profoundly medicalized management of pregnancy, and the simultaneous production of poor, pregnant women as biological dangers, might be understood as an admission by the state of the unjust nature of capitalism and the class structure that is its sine qua non. Essentially, the state assumes the poor, pregnant body that presents itself to the obstetrics clinic is one that has not had the benefit of regular (or, even irregular) medical checkups—an assumption especially true for the "undocumented" women who come to Alpha. The battery of tests to which patients must submit themselves might be understood as a corrective to the years of medical inattention that poverty and the absence of health insurance compel. The function of every organ and every system is assessed because class inequality dictates their health would not have been established previously via periodic evaluations—a comfort the insured enjoy. Indeed, it is not entirely unreasonable to assume an aggressive medical gaze is appropriate for the uninsured. Consider a report that showed the higher rates of maternal mortality among the poor, uninsured women served in New York City public hospitals:

> Women who gave birth in New York City hospitals are dying of obstetrical problems at almost two-and-a-half times the national rate of 8.9 deaths per 100,000, according to 2002 figures. . . . Researchers say the problem is linked to the high number of pregnant women with underlying risk factors, including obesity and diabetes—particularly common in recent immigrants and those living in underserved communities who may not get prenatal care. "Many of our hospitals deal with women who are already in poor health, and their bodies have no reserves," says . . . [the] chairman of obstetrics and gynecology at [a Brooklyn public hospital]. Bearing out his observation, preliminary statistics show that of 28 such deaths in New York City in 2004, 13 occurred in public Health and Hospital Corp. facilities, which shoulder the heaviest burden of caring for the poor and uninsured. (Scott 2006)

And so, there might be something entirely appropriate about the excesses of the prenatal care given as a matter of course to the Medicaid-insured poor. These are women who do not have the benefit of annual Pap smears to detect abnormal cervical cell growth. These are women who do not have the luxury of having a urinary tract infection diagnosed before it becomes asymptomatic and manifests itself as a problem with the kidney. These are the women who do not have the advantage of being told whether a lump in the breast really is nothing to worry about.

All of this is to say that Medicaid's tenacious management of pregnancy performs a confession: it confesses that capitalism and the poverty that is its effect create a state of affairs that allow common and curable ailments within the poor body to go undetected. The insistent medical manipulation of the pregnant body mandated by Medicaid is a limited attempt to temporarily rectify that situation; hence, within that attempt is an implicit acknowledgement of the unjust nature of the class structure of capitalist society.

Yet, the admission dissembles and dissimulates precisely to the extent it renders the poor woman's body itself to be inherently suspect, problematic, and unruly. It discloses its confession only to then disguise it anew: by blaming the victim as being sickly, uncared for, and dangerous. This is the paradigmatic gesture that moves from an indictment of poverty to a castigation of the "culture of poverty" the poor are imagined to create and inhabit.

Moreover, it becomes easier, perhaps, to blame the poor for their poverty when they are disproportionately people of color; long-circulating racial and racist discourses intersect with class discourses and provide additional fodder for pathologizing the racialized poor.

The next chapter begins to fold the analytic of race into a question that has been apprehended, up until this point, as one of class. In essence, it grounds the less-overt medical disenfranchisement, marginalization, and exploitation of poor women of color discussed throughout the book with a robust discussion of its plainer predecessor.

PART TWO

Race

FOUR

The *"Primitive Pelvis,"* *Racial Folklore, and Atavism* *in Contemporary Forms* *of Medical Disenfranchisement*

I FIRST MET SHAUNTAY JOHNSON in the Alpha WHC as she waited for her appointment in the High Risk Clinic. In those first few minutes of meeting her, she struck me as a nice, pleasant woman with a great sense of humor. I immediately asked her if she would like to participate in my study by sitting down with me for an in-depth interview. She seemed happy to agree, and we talked for the next hour-and-a-half about everything that came to mind.

Shauntay, a pretty, twenty-four-year-old Black woman who had lived in Harlem all of her life, was twenty-nine weeks pregnant with twins: two baby boys. Her sons would join Shauntay's already full family: unmarried, she had a set of four-year-old twin girls (whose father had only recently begun to give Shauntay $175 per month in child support) and a three-year-old son (with whose father she was romantically uninvolved, but who remained a friend and active co-parent). While the pregnancy was unplanned, and although she had no intention or desire to involve the father of her unborn twins in their lives, she was more than optimistic about the future: she had the support of her mother, brother, and her three-year-old son's father—who, although biologically unrelated to Shauntay's twin girls, helped to raise them as well as their son. "We were friends before I got pregnant [with our son]. And we are friends now." Indeed, when Shauntay informed him she was newly pregnant, he was disappointed at first. "He said, 'How can you do this to me? You already have the twins. You got Junior. And now you're going to have twins again?" But, he quickly changed his tune and reassured her that he would be a presence in all of her children's lives. "He said, 'I'm still here. My number hasn't changed. If you need me to change diapers, I'll change diapers. If you need me knock [the new babies' father] out, I'll knock him out.'"

Shauntay had been receiving prenatal care at Delta Hospital, a smaller public hospital close to her home, but her obstetrician there had recommended that she be seen at Alpha because it had superior ultrasound equipment. I asked her why the ultrasound technology at Delta—where she had delivered her twin girls and younger son—was insufficient. She explained:

SHAUNTAY: Yeah—one of the babies has some type of kidney problem—they couldn't tell the difference at the other clinic. They didn't know what it was. First, they were like, "Maybe you have another kid." The lady was just seeing something different with that machine. So, they sent me here. I guess, I don't know—I didn't get to . . . I guess they will see something more, or—maybe it isn't what they thought it was at the other hospital. Because they thought it was something worse than what it really is. But, still, I have to come here every week.

KHIARA: Now, were you worried when they told you that the baby might have a kidney problem?

SHAUNTAY: No, because they told me that it appears to be hereditary. And I know that it's from the father's side—it's not my side. I mean, it's not nothing you go home and say, "Oh Lord." [laughs] I mean, as long as it could be fixed and you catch it at an earlier time than later. . . . I mean, I don't worry myself about a lot of stuff. Because I have other kids. I don't have that kind of time to be worrying about everything. . . . It's better for me to come here because they see more and they are a little more effective. But, the other place, I just couldn't go.

Shauntay assured me the twin's condition was "no big deal," even though the obstetrician at the other hospital informed her that he would have advised her to terminate the pregnancy had he known about the twin's condition earlier.

It was a big deal at the other hospital because the doctor, he's not—how do I say this?—sensitive in any way. He was like, "Well, if I would have known this way before, I could have gave you the shot and you could have gotten rid of that one. This kid is going to have a life of going to the hospital. You don't want that—but it's already too late."

She told me that had she had a more vulnerable personality, the doctor's callous prognosis of her twin's condition would have troubled her.

If I was that type, he would have just—I would have been so sick [upset]. I would have been going through depression. You know what I'm saying? He would have really had my head somewhere. But, like I said, you don't let it faze you. He made me mad, but I wasn't ready to cry or nothing like that. I wanted to fight him, though. [laughs]

When she was called into her appointment with the physician, ending our interview, Shauntay gave me a hug and told me she would see me soon—which pleased me, as I was looking forward to following her throughout the remainder of her pregnancy and meeting her twin boys when they arrived. But, I never saw Shauntay again. Realizing her absence in the clinic one day, I checked her medical records to see if I could track her down. The notes in her chart told a tragic story.

Shauntay had been referred to Alpha from Delta because Delta was unequipped to handle the severity of the condition from which Shauntay's baby suffered. The Delta ultrasound had revealed that one of her twins (referred to as Twin B in her medical records) had anechoic structures overlying both of his kidneys—an ominous finding. Moreover, the ultrasound detected hydronephrosis (a swelling of the kidneys that occurs when the flow of urine is obstructed) as well as hydroureter (a swelling of the ureter). Both conditions imply that the ureter and the connection of the ureter to the kidney have been overfilled with urine. The severity of this condition was exacerbated by Twin B's growth having shown restriction (a condition called IUGR, or intrauterine growth restriction). Moreover, Shauntay's physicians also noted that Twin B suffered from AEDF, or absent end-diastolic flow, indicating that the placenta was not working properly and the fetal heart was struggling. A diagnosis of IUGR with AEDF is a dire one, and most fetuses with the condition do not survive absent immediate delivery.

On the same day I talked to an upbeat, laughing, and joking Shauntay, she was admitted to the hospital for the monitoring of Twin B's condition and given a course of dexamethasone to promote fetal lung maturity in anticipation of a potential preterm delivery. The medical records indicate that because Twin B was only being monitored daily, as opposed to continuously, Shauntay requested to be discharged the following day—most likely because she had three children at home for whom she needed to care. She agreed to return to the hospital daily for her physicians to check on Twin B's status. As planned, Shauntay returned the next day. A sonographic assessment of Twin B revealed his condition had worsened; moreover, although a fetal heartbeat was found, there was no spontaneous movement or breathing. Shauntay was counseled that Twin B would die if he was not delivered immediately. Complicating the matter was the fact that Twin A was completely healthy. If Twin B was delivered, Twin A would have to be delivered also—at only twenty-nine-weeks gestational age. A physician noted in the medical records, "The patient was counseled that if she desired to intervene for the sake of twin B, that intervention should be via immediate cesarean delivery. If she did not desire to intervene for the sake of allowing twin A to have more time to grow in utero, that was an acceptable alternative, but that likely twin B would not survive until a time when twin A could safely deliver."

Faced with such an unthinkable choice, the records indicate that Shauntay "opted to leave to speak with [her] pastor regarding the religious implications of this decision." She was advised against leaving, as the possibility of intervention at that point was still open, but might have closed by the time she returned. She nonetheless insisted on it, promising to come back when she had reached a decision. (Interestingly, a nurse who had cared for Shauntay in the labor and delivery ward told me Shauntay had left that day because "she said someone had been rude to her. I don't know who it was—a nurse or PCA or someone. But, she said that someone was rude and she wanted to leave.")

Shauntay returned the next day, having decided to undergo a C-section delivery of both twins. After delivery, Twin A was placed in the neonatal intensive care unit. Twin B, however, died shortly after being removed from the womb. The records sanitize the horror of the event: "[Patient] was told of Twin B's demise and patient requested time to herself."

At present in the United States, the infant mortality rate for Black babies is nearly two-and-a-half times higher than for white babies. This disparity has persisted despite the overall decline in infant mortality rates over the years. There has not been even a narrowing of the racial gap; although fewer infants died last year, the rate at which Black babies died remained twice that of white babies.

Perhaps it is easy to disconnect these shameful statistics from the experience they quantify and describe. Perhaps the estrangement that numbers produce dulls the senses and prevents outrage. Perhaps this explains the relative lack of public outcry and protest over what can dispassionately be called "racial disparities in infant mortality." But, Shauntay puts a face on the otherwise disembodied numbers and rates. Instead of carrying home two babies wrapped in blue blankets, Shauntay brought home one baby and planned a funeral for the other. An empty crib in her apartment would remind her of the baby who did not live, until she managed to—not quickly enough—give the unused crib to a pregnant friend. She would have to think of a story to tell all her neighbors who knew she was expecting twins; until word got around that one of her infants had died, how would she respond to the inquiry, "Where's the other baby?" Would she ever tell the baby who lived that he had a twin? Would she ever be able to look at her son and not be reminded of the other son who died?

Infant mortality among African Americans in 2000 occurred at a rate of 14.1 deaths per 1,000 live births—more than twice the national average of 6.9 deaths per 1,000 live births. Perhaps these facts and figures alienate those reading them from the human tragedy they condense. Black women experience Shauntay's ineffable pain at twice the rate of their white counterparts. Black women are twice more likely to know what it feels like to give birth, but have no child to mother.

Racial disparities in maternal mortality in the United States are equally lamentable. Black women die from causes linked to pregnancy and childbirth at more than three times the rate of white women. In New York City, the maternal mortality rate for Black women was more than five times that of white women. "In fact, 1 of every 2,500 black women in New York City who becomes pregnant dies. The similar figure for white women is 1 in 14,000" (Fang, Jing, Shantha Madhavan, and Michael H. Alderman 2000, 742). And although New York City's maternal mortality rate exceeded that of the nation as a whole, this excess is due to the elevated maternal mortality rate experienced by Black women. "Indeed, if all New Yorkers experienced the mortality of its white women, the rates for the city would be indistinguishable from the country as a whole" (743).

Fortunately, during my fieldwork I never met a pregnant woman who died during or shortly after her pregnancy; consequently, I cannot provide an ethnographic story that can help to personify the abstract figures. But, "maternal mortality" means a child will grow up never knowing the mother who gave birth to her. Maternal mortality means a husband, boyfriend, or partner somehow will have to balance the joy of welcoming a new life with the devastation of encountering death. Maternal mortality is an event that, despite a cause of death being noted on the death certificate, remains inexplicable to those it affects. And so, when one understands maternal mortality as such—as a personal, indefinable disaster—it seems manifestly unfair that this burden is imposed disproportionately on Black women, Black families, Black people.

The leading causes of maternal death have been identified as hemorrhage, pulmonary embolism, pregnancy-induced hypertension (leading to preeclampsia and eclampsia), puerperal infection, and ectopic pregnancy. That these conditions affect Black women with a disproportionate frequency and are more fatal has been attributed to the higher rates among Black women of high blood pressure, preexisting and gestational diabetes, and obesity. Indeed, one study reported that 54 percent of women who died from pregnancy-related causes had a history of chronic disease—among them hypertension, cardiac disease, diabetes, schleroderma, and sickle cell. Obesity was the most commonly identified condition (Campbell 2007). These are all conditions, in addition to decreased health care access (due to poverty), which affect Black women at disproportionate rates. Such information has led some researchers to conclude that to bring white and Black maternal mortality rates to parity, we ought to "eliminate socioeconomic disadvantage" by increasing Black women's access to early prenatal care, then monitoring them more closely for hypertension and diabetes while attempting to control the effects of obesity. This increasingly popular view explains racial health disparities as wholly a function of class and preexisting medical conditions while saying nothing about the individuals under whose care Black women are disproportionately dying.

However, at least one study challenges the conclusion that it is class that is the problem, disputing the claim that Black women are dying because they are poor and not because they are Black. Fang et al. (2000) released a study showing that although socioeconomic factors (such as marital status and educational achievement) were strongly correlated to maternal mortality for non-Black women, such factors had relatively little impact on the incidence of maternal mortality for Black women. The authors report "unmarried non-black women had a maternal mortality ratio more than twice that for married women, and non-black women with less than a high school education had more than six times the mortality ratio that did those with high school education and above." Meanwhile, a relationship between these socioeconomic factors and maternal mortality was not readily apparent for Black women: "[T]he mortality ratio of unmarried black women was indistinguishable from that of married black mothers, and black mothers with less than a high school education had 1.5 times the mortality of blacks with at least a high school education" (739). Similarly, for non-Black women, there was an association between residence in a low income community and higher maternal mortality rates. No comparable association was found for Black women; they were as likely to die from a pregnancy-related cause without regard to the affluence of the neighborhood within which they lived. Accordingly, Fang's study suggests referring to the phenomenon as "racial disparities in maternal mortality" is not a red herring. That is, race has everything to do with why Black women are more likely to die in the path toward motherhood— and not simply because race follows class closely in the United States.

Racial disparities in infant and maternal mortality are part of a larger phenomenon of racial health disparities experienced by Black people in the United States. That Black persons suffer from certain diseases at higher rates and die younger than their white counterparts has been well-documented in the literature (Institute of Medicine 2005; Office of Minority Health and Health Disparities 2009; National Center for Health Statistics 2007). Again, that Black people are disproportionately poorer than white people in the United States—and therefore more likely to be uninsured and lack access to regular health care—does not entirely explain away these disturbing statistics. The Institute of Medicine (IOM), a not-for-profit, nongovernmental organization that is part of the Academy of Sciences, released a report arguing that the poverty in which Black people disproportionately live cannot account for their being sicker and dying younger than their white complements. The IOM found "racial and ethnic minorities receive lower-quality health care than white people— even when insurance status, income, age, and severity of conditions are comparable" (Institute of Medicine 2005). "Lower quality health care" is not an amorphous, intangible concept; instead, it signifies the concrete, inferior care physicians give their Black patients. The IOM reported minority persons are less likely than white persons to be given appropriate cardiac care, to receive kidney dialysis or transplants, and to receive the best treatments for stroke, cancer, or AIDS (6–7). Mincing few words, the IOM described an "uncomfortable reality": "some people in the United States were more likely to die from cancer, heart disease, and diabetes simply because of their race or ethnicity, not just because they lack access to health care" (3).

The IOM gestures toward a phenomenon that, although going unnamed in the literature, could do much to explain racial disparities in health: physician racism. That is, perhaps the racist beliefs of physicians explain why Black persons do not receive the most effective and desirable tests, treatments, and therapies for their conditions. Perhaps physicians' devaluation of Black bodies—for no reason other than the fact that that they are *Black* bodies—explains why Black women die from pregnancy-related causes at three to four times the rate of white women. Perhaps the lesser regard with which physicians hold Black lives explains why Black infants die at more than twice the rate of white infants. Indeed, perhaps racism practiced by the persons who are empowered to care for them partially explains Black people's status as the sickest racial group in the United States.

Other factors named in the literature also contribute to racial health disparities—such as the disproportionate levels of poverty among Black people, which increases the likelihood they will also suffer from poor nutrition and obesity. Moreover, disproportionate levels of poverty increase the likelihood Black people will lack access to regular medical care, which, in turn, decreases the likelihood that medical problems will be caught at an earlier, treatable stage. But, these facts should not be used to argue that physician racism should be dismissed as an impossibility or irrelevancy—as if physician racism exists only in thought experiments (or, if it actually does exist, has no relationship at all to the racial disparities in health that shorten the lives of Black people across the nation).

A caveat: the discussion contained in this chapter may be accused of lapsing into individualism while losing sight of structures of racism. That is, it may be taken to argue that bad, racist behaviors of individual physicians—as opposed to more macro, institutional forces—produce the racial disparities in health that are so well-documented. If racist behaviors are the cause of the phenomenon, the way to eliminate racial disparities in health would be to rid the medical establishment of its bad actors. Once the guilty parties no longer practice medicine in the United States, we can expect parity among the races in all indexes of health. However, the ensuing discussion of physician racism should not at all be taken to advocate this position. Instead, individual racism exists simultaneously to and alongside structures of racism. Accordingly, bad, racist behaviors of individual physicians—in addition to more macro, institutional forces—produce the racial disparities in health. Physicians harboring racist beliefs (and physicians not harboring racist beliefs) practice medicine within institutions that function to both reiterate racial and racist discourses and to maintain racial inequality. Ridding the medical establishment of individual bad actors will not eradicate the large and small structures that are also responsible for racial disparities in health—structures that range from population discourse (which I explore in the following chapter) to a two-tiered system of health care in which people of color are disproportionately relegated to the inferior tier. And so, it is imperative that this chapter's exclusive focus on individual racism is not taken as an argument that it is exclusively responsible for racial health disparities.

NAMING PHYSICIAN RACISM

Cultural critic and race theorist John Hoberman (2005, 2007) has done illuminating work in this area, casting light on the ways in which the phenomenon of physician racism has been denied altogether or capably hidden in research regarding health disparities. Hoberman argues that racism—defined as "racially discriminatory rationing by physicians and health care institutions"—plays at least some role in the health gap between the races. Indeed, there is no reason to believe that a person's decision to become a physician somehow immunizes him or her from the racism, race-thinking, and race-consciousness that pervade the United States. It may be overly optimistic to think physicians' extensive training in the biological sciences in some way cleanses them of the biases and prejudices that run rampant in the social milieu in which that training takes place. Certainly, there is nothing intrinsic about medicine or medical training that should counsel us to believe physicians, as a class, are free from "deep-seated attitudinal biases that parallel those of the general public and the media and [could] confuse [their] best clinical intentions" (Hoberman 2007, 512).

Hoberman argues that when physician racism is invoked in studies of racial disparities, it is never by that name, and it is usually done through a "rhetoric of exculpation" and with "euphemizing vocabulary" in which physicians are excused for the racial biases they may harbor and put into practice. He notes the above-referenced IOM report—in which the authors damningly concluded that a person's ascribed race, independent of class, made it more likely he or she will die from cancer, heart disease, and diabetes—nevertheless expertly uses the "rhetoric of exculpation" when describing its findings: "Survey research suggests that among white Americans, prejudicial attitudes toward minorities remain more common than not, as over half to three-quarters believe that relative to whites, minorities—particularly African Americans—are less intelligent, more prone to violence, and prefer to live off of welfare. It is reasonable to assume, however, that the vast majority of health care providers find prejudice morally abhorrent and at odds with their professional values. But, health care providers, like other members of society, may not recognize manifestations of prejudice in their own behavior" (Institute of Medicine 2005, 10). Here, as throughout the literature, physicians are given "the benefit of the doubt" and presented "as the passive receptacles of powerful stereotypes" (Hoberman 2007, 511–12). When not representing physicians as the unfortunate victims of overpowering racist ideas, the literature presents physicians' racism as a "cognitive shortcut" upon which they rely because of time constraints. "[T]he physician who practices a racially biased form of medicine is not himself a racist, but is simply too busy to behave more carefully. He is distracted rather than negligent or hostile or indifferent" (Hoberman 2007, 511–12).

Hoberman's findings—that the literature has largely denied the possibility that physician racism may contribute to health disparities—hold true in the reports of racial disparities in infant and maternal mortality. Consider an explanation offered by the authors of a study finding that African-American pregnant women were less likely to receive surgical intervention for pregnancy-related hemorrhage, even though the severity of hemorrhage was equivalent between the racial groups studied: "In the case of postpartum hemorrhage, reluctance to report or under-reporting on the part of the patient or difference in history taking on the part of the physician could lead to differences in treatment for the same degree of hemorrhage" (Harper et al. 2007, 184–85). Oddly, the authors partially attribute the disparity between the rates at which physicians surgically intervene in Black women's hemorrhaging episodes to the Black women who are bleeding to death. It seems a bit peculiar to believe that a woman will not inform her physician or caretaker of her massive blood loss. The hypothesis that Black women will silently endure such frightening episodes probably says less about Black women's actions under such circumstances and more about discourses of Black women's fantastical stoicism and strength. Moreover, the authors also partly attributed the disparity to "difference in history taking on the part of the physician"—an obscure phrase explaining very little. It is unclear what the authors perceive as the "difference" in the histories taken of Black and white women. Is it that physicians are not quite as thorough or careful when they take Black women's histories? Why exactly would physicians take different histories of Black women? The authors could be gesturing toward the unnamable—that the personally held racist beliefs of physicians prevent them from providing the same quality of care to their Black patients as they do to their white patients—but the authors are careful to hide such a suggestion behind euphemism.

This same study also found that African-American women delivering preterm were less likely to receive antenatal steroids that could improve perinatal outcomes—a disparity the authors found "disturbing." They explained it as follows: "[D]ifferences in reporting contractions or accurately assessing risk for preterm birth from history could lead to differences in administering antenatal steroids" (Harper et al. 2007, 185). Again, the authors partly attribute the fact that preterm Black infants are more likely to be denied steroids necessary to develop their premature lungs to Black women's silence. Again, Black women are fantasized to be uncannily durable (or daft) women, bearing the pain of contractions without thinking to inform their physicians or caretakers of their premature labors. The other explanation the authors provide for the disparity in the administration of antenatal steroids—that physicians do not "accurately assess[] risk for preterm birth" in Black women—requires much elaboration. What is it about Black women that causes physicians to fail to accurately assess their risks? Could racism be partly to blame for physicians' inability to hear the histories Black women tell them?

The Harper study concludes by offering several ways to reduce the racial gap in pregnancy-related death. Among them, the authors propose that Black and white maternal mortality rates can be brought to parity by "eliminating unequal treatment." Here, the authors might be using "unequal" as a synonym for "racist." Or, they might not. It is unclear, and because of that lack of clarity, physicians who provide racially discriminatory care are absolved from responsibility.

The Harper report is far from the only study denying the role physician racism may play in the persistent disparity in rates of infant and maternal mortality and morbidity among Black and white people. Yet, there are notable exceptions to this practice of obfuscating or denying altogether the operation of physician racism in creating and maintaining racial disparities in maternal and infant mortality rates. One of the most overt namings of racism as an actor in this phenomenon comes, ironically, from a physician who appears to accept some notion of biological race. He argues that investigations that "show the persistence of high African American infant mortality[,] even when African American women enroll in early prenatal care at high rates[,] and that show that college-educated, middle-class African American women still have higher rates of low birthweight and infant mortality than poorly educated, impoverished whites" are "suggestive of genetics being a more powerful determinant" (Parker 2003, 336). Yet, this doctors' belief in biological race does not prevent him from also believing racism plays an indispensable role in creating health disparities:

> Efforts to study infant mortality have continued to trend toward studying the problem at the molecular level: the missing or defective gene, the environmental toxin. Such efforts, while personally rewarding to investigators, risk irrelevancy and unethical indictment when existing solutions operate at the macroscopic level. Group empowerment socioeconomically, health education, and abolition of racism have no gene markers, but they do raise a different issue. When infant mortality and disparity are examined in these contexts, there is no question that we know enough. The question is: as a resource-rich society facing significant health disparities that can potentially be resolved, are we "good" enough? (337)

Although Parker is candid in his articulation of racism as an actor, he notably does not name its perpetrator; he also does not name the physician as being the someone who treats patients differently on the basis of race. Parker's silence allows the subject of racism to be anything and anyone from physicians (in their interpersonal interactions with patients) to more diffuse institutional, cultural, and discursive practices. The hush that surrounds the naming of the physician as the person responsible for racism is echoed in other studies that dare to identify racism as a force in racial disparities in health.[1]

I met the newly pregnant Rhonda at her first prenatal care visit to the Alpha WHC. Rhonda, a native New Yorker, was a woman of Puerto Rican and African-American heritage who self-identified as Black. Because she appeared to be a friendly, talkative, and open person, I asked her if she would be interested in speaking to me more extensively about her prenatal care experiences. She agreed, and we made plans to talk during her next appointment. She warned me: "We're going to need a lot of time. I have a lot to talk about." Her current pregnancy was her fourth—she had twin sons who were thirteen, a daughter who was twelve, and another son who was seven. She then told me her youngest son was a "survivor": when she had given birth to him at twenty-six weeks, he weighed a little less than two pounds. She spoke about him with so much love that, throughout our interview, I found tears coming to my eyes. Although the medical conditions he would face for the rest of his life were daunting, she described him as a "happy kid":

> It takes him a minute to get it out, but he talks. That doctor said he'd be a vegetable—said he'd never do anything. Said he'd probably have hydroencephaly, he'd be institutionalized. But, he talks—too much, in fact! He doesn't walk—he has some issues. He's a quadriplegic. But, the only way I can describe him is "awesome." He smiles all day where you would be miserable in his condition. Some people say, "I don't understand your son because, if it were me, I'd be miserable—in a chair all day, can't do anything. We literally do everything for him and he still says, "Hi, how are you?" all day. He's a happy kid—happy kid. He loves school, loves his friends, loves his teachers. And they all love him.

It was not until we had a chance to talk again that she revealed the true extent of her choice to call her son a "survivor": he was one of a set of twins, but the other boy had died shortly after birth.

When I met Rhonda, she had just finished settling a lawsuit with the hospital that had delivered her sons—one she says she filed seven years earlier to get the answers the hospital had refused to give her: "Somebody had to tell me why my child was the way he was and why my son died. To be honest with you, I was prepared to lose. But, they still would have had to say something. They would have been forced to say, 'This is what happened.' That was my whole purpose." Over the course of the litigation, she learned she had had a Group B streptococcal infection during her pregnancy—something her physicians knew about, as it was documented in her medical records, but for which she never received treatment.[2] Although she now had the answers she had needed so desperately, they did not dull the pain of having to bury her child.

> When I first gave birth to my sons—when I had them. . . . First, [my husband] came to me. When I first woke up, he was the first person I saw. He said that Yusef, my surviving baby, needed a blood transfusion. Yusef needed a blood transfusion, but Xavier, my son who died, was okay. Um, he needed help breathing, but he was going to be all right. And I'm like, "OK." You know, because my only question was, "Are they okay? I want to see my babies." That was the first and only thing on my mind: "I want to see my babies." And my husband, he said that they need blood. And I said, "OK. Well, call everybody." And he was like, "I called everybody already." He let me know that he called everybody in the family, and my family was coming to donate blood. That was Friday . . . and then my son took a turn for the worse. Just a day later, Xavier died. [pause] I went to the nursery to see Yusef. I just had to be with Yusef. [pause]
>
> So, after I left, I came upstairs very emotional. I'm automatically blaming myself, you know—thinking "I killed my son." I was in my room—they gave me my own—I had my own room. Two beds. I'm in my room—hysterical. It was Saturday. It was quiet. And I was hysterical.

She described the death of her son as a heartbreak that threatened her mental health even after the initial shock. In the months after his death, she began collecting stray animals, stopped eating, stopped bathing, and stopped caring for her other children. In fact, she checked herself into the psychiatric ward at Alpha Hospital because she thought she was "crazy." "Losing my son was such a tragedy for me. It was just like . . . that's my baby. That's my son. I wanted those kids so much. . . . I never got over it. I probably never will get over it."

SOME CONTEXT: A LONG HISTORY OF MEDICAL RACISM

I do not tell the stories of Rhonda and Shauntay in order to make an argument that because they are Black women, physician racism contributed to their babies' deaths. This is an argument I am radically incapable of making. Rather, I include their stories to give a human face to a trauma that occurs disproportionately to Black women.

Even if one cannot argue that racism on the part of their physicians played some role in the experiences of Rhonda and Shauntay, those experiences ought to be put in context—embedded in a history in which race had everything to do with Black women's encounters with their physicians. Rhonda and Shauntay's experiences are, in fact, moments in a long history of Black women's contact with medicalized obstetrical and gynecological services. Indeed, one can argue that any ethnography of a clinic that provides obstetrical and gynecological services to large numbers of Black women—and any ethnography that is critical of the services provided—ought to be put in this context. This is important for two reasons: first, with this background, one can ground the present, less overt (yet effective) medical disenfranchisement of women of color that I discuss throughout this book in its more blatant predecessor. Second, this history should not be reified as a snapshot of a distant past that has no effect on the present, but rather can be appreciated as a practice that persists and can inform our understanding of the contemporary. That is, rather than grasping current demonstrations of racism, race-thinking, and disenfranchisement on the basis of race as anomalies, we can appreciate their consistency with the long history of medical racism in the United States.

One of the most salient aspects of the history of Black women's contact with medicalized obstetrics and gynecology is exploitation, unfortunately. In her history of nontherapeutic medical experimentation on Black Americans, journalist and medical ethicist Harriet Washington (2007) recounts numerous occasions of Black women being subjected to horrific experimental gynecological and obstetrical surgeries without their consent, ranging from vaginal surgeries, nontherapeutic hysterectomies, and contraceptive abuses. Another salient aspect of Black women's history with obstetrics and gynecology is the construction of the Black pregnant woman within the discipline as remarkably resilient. Hoberman describes this fantasized trait as "obstetrical hardiness," defined as the belief that Black (and other socially and politically disempowered) women are relatively unaffected by the expected pains of labor and childbirth. "Obstetrical hardiness" is part of a broader philosophy about the primal nature of Black people, who were thought to represent a "primitive human type that is biologically and psychologically different from civilized man" (Hoberman 2005, 87). Variations on the theme of the Black reproductive body as a hardy, primordial type include beliefs in: Black hyperfertility attributed to the truism that "[t]he simpler the organism, the simpler the genesis and the greater the prolific-ness"; the Black "primitive pelvis," which was thought to be narrower and deeper than the presumably more "civilized" pelvises of white women, and invariably enabled a complication-free passage of the infant during birth;

the absence among Black women of endometriosis, which was thought to be a "twentieth century disease" that only affected "civilized" persons within modernity; and the lessened sensitivity of Black women's vaginal tissues, which was thought to make Black women immune from injuries occasioned during birth.

History counsels us that the phrase "racial logic" is a misnomer, as the ways in which the concept of race has been deployed to make sense of human difference have not always been logically consistent. Therefore, it should come as no surprise that the belief in Black reproductive primitivity manifested itself in contradictory ways, with Black people being immune from certain types of disorders and diseases (such as endometriosis), yet ironically predisposed to other conditions (such as syphilis and pelvic inflammatory disease). Hoberman explains the incongruous logic of black racial hardiness:

> The discourse that distinguishes between "civilized" and "primitive" peoples has long been characterized by a deep ambivalence on the part of the "civilized" toward the "savage" type. The negative sides of primitive life are the ignorance and unsanitary conditions that threaten good health. In this context African-American women belong to the same "primitive" category as African women, so it is only natural for an American physician to assert that "the Negro's reaction to disease is primitive." On the positive side, the primitive is associated with a biological vitality and a hardiness that is finally indistinguishable from a profound harmony with nature and its mysterious processes. (2005, 94)

Hoberman goes on to argue that, although it has been discredited that people of African descent are a different, primitive type of human (certainly such views no longer appear in medical journals and mainstream media), ideas of black racial hardiness, "adapted to modern circumstances" of course, live on in medical schools, hospital wards, and operating rooms (2005, 97). Ideas endure about the ease of certain racialized women's labors and childbirths, the naturally healthy gynecological and obstetrical lives of other racialized women, and the resistance to infection and disease biologically possessed by other racially gifted women. Hoberman argues that these ideas persist through an oral tradition whereby attending physicians tell racial tales to their students, who pass the tales on to their colleagues, who eventually pass them on to their students, etc. He quotes one academic physician: "There are lots of little stories that physicians believe that are neither scientifically based nor are proven. That's the problem" (97). Hoberman argues that racial folklore may explain racial disparities in health, as "[m]edical personnel who believe in black hardiness may restrict access to certain kinds of surgery on the assumption that black patients have a less urgent need for such procedures. Conversely, the same belief in black hardiness might help to account for the disproportionate frequency with which black patients are subjected to more radical and damaging surgeries than whites: hysterectomies, lower-limb amputations, and bilateral orchidectomies (castration), since medical personnel may assume they are better able to tolerate such trauma" (96).

Consider statements made by one of the most senior attending physicians in the Alpha WHC, Dr. Veronica Rose. Dr. Rose had worked for thirty years in her own private practice in Long Island; after retiring, she was hired by the Omega University School of Medicine as a Professor of Obstetrics and Gynecology—a job she insisted upon calling a post-retirement "hobby." At the time of my fieldwork in the clinic, she had been teaching and practicing in Alpha for three years. About halfway through my interview with her, I remarked that the patients at Alpha experienced extremely long waits for appointments that seemed excessive in their frequency. She responded with her perception that Alpha patients were not scheduled for more appointments than their counterparts in private practice:

ROSE: That's standard. It's once a month from the first visit to twenty-eight weeks. From twenty-eight to thirty-six [weeks], it's every two weeks. And it's every week thereafter. That's standard stuff. And keep in mind that the people here have a lot more pathology than the people in a private setting. In a private setting, you're not going to see all of the hepatitis. You're not going to see the sickle-cell anemia. You're not going to see the . . . you name it. You're not going to see it.

KHIARA: Now, the increased pathology that you see here, what is that based on?

ROSE: It's cultural.

KHIARA: It's cultural?

ROSE: Oh yeah—it's cultural. And it's ethnic. Meaning that if you're coming from a private setting, where 92 percent of your population is white, you're not going to have a lot of sickle cell. You're not going to see a lot of hepatitis in people who live in upscale Long Island. Yeah, I actually had to go back and look some things up when I first got here. Because I hadn't seen them in years. People in a private setting are basically healthy. People here are not so healthy. They have a lot of issues that we're not going to see on a regular basis in a private setting.

KHIARA: Is some of that nutritional also?

ROSE: I'm sure it is. I think it's cultural. Somebody coming from the middle of Africa someplace is going to have a lot more issues than somebody coming from eastern Long Island is going to have. Plus, you're going to have issues of indigency, lack of education, the whole. . . . It's just poor people. Poor people don't have the same level of education obviously. They don't eat as well. They have a lot of obesity because they eat a lot of fast food and things of that nature. These are all things that are built into a clinic setting that you're not going to see elsewhere. But, they [the patients seen in the Alpha WHC] are not seen more often, generally speaking.

There is much to unpack in Dr. Rose's complex declaration. What is most clear is that she believes the "Alpha patient population" differs from the patients to whom she attended in her private practice because of the "increased pathology" present within the former group. Understanding Dr. Rose's philosophy of why the "Alpha patient population" has "increased pathology" is more challenging, however. To begin, she posits the cause as being in part "cultural." Although there is a lot vapidity in Dr. Rose's use of "culture," one can distill that it is not "indigency," lack of education, and nutrition. Rather, "culture" is *in addition* to those things: "I think it's cultural . . . *Plus*, you're going to have issues of indigency, lack of education. . . ." Moreover, place appears to inform culture: "Somebody coming from the middle of Africa someplace is going to have a lot more issues than somebody coming from eastern Long Island is going to have." Although the place of "eastern Long Island" corresponds with the "92 percent white" "private setting," its antipode is the presumably non-white "middle of Africa" represented in public clinics. Which is to say: race informs Dr. Rose's notion of "culture." And it is this notion of culture-qua-race that she views as the cause of the increased pathology among Alpha patients. For Dr. Rose, one will not find sickle cell or hepatitis among white people. Indeed, among white people, one will not find the plethora of diseases Dr. Rose had to "look up" when she was called upon to treat non-white people.

In sum, Dr. Rose explains the higher rates of pathology in public settings as being due in part to the race—the non-whiteness—of the patients managed there. Culture-qua-race also explains the lower rates of pathology in the private setting, which indeed is characterized by its lack: it is a place where the physician is not going to see hepatitis, will not see sickle cell anemia, will not "see the . . . you name it. You're not going to see it." This lack of pathology and "issues" mimics the lack of presumed racial and ethnic particularity—the normativity—in "eastern Long Island," as Dr. Rose is careful to articulate. Although Dr. Rose names neither racial biology nor some notion of the Black human type's primitivity as foundations for her theory of culture, it is not difficult to see that the "culture" she believes is found in the "middle of Africa" is congruent with the "image of the sickly and biologically deficient black person" that is paradigmatic of biological notions of race.

However, many physicians I interviewed disagreed with Dr. Rose's conceptualization of Alpha patients as being sicker than their privately insured counterparts. Indeed, many obstetricians considered Alpha patients, on the whole, to be a healthy group of people. As one resident explained, "We see a lot of young, healthy women. So, I don't find that [the assumption that poor, uninsured people are sicker than their insured counterparts] to be true, necessarily. Because I think a lot of—just by nature of our job— we see a lot of young, healthy, pregnant people." Another physician, Dr. Steven Shander, offered a similar opinion, and in the process, disputed Dr. Rose's construction of the "private population" as the absence of risk, disease, and pathology. I asked him if he found his Alpha patients to be sicker on the whole than their Omega counterparts. He responded:

SHANDER: I think it depends on your specialty, too. We're OB/GYN. We don't see a lot of—I mean, we have a lot of patients that come in for GYN exams with multiple medical problems that we don't primarily manage. Hypertension, diabetes— they are smokers. A lot of things that get taken care of in their medicine clinic. Whereas we primarily do a pap smear and a routine GYN evaluation. And then, of course, obstetrics: you are dealing with generally a young and healthy population. The advantage that we have here at Alpha is that we are the referral center for truly high risk patients. All [New York City public] hospitals have high risk obstetrical service—at least most of them. But, if they are too big to handle . . . for some of these other hospitals, they get sent to Alpha. And so we get to see some of the more interesting, more difficult cases.

KHIARA: And so these are issues that you wouldn't see in the Omega population?

SHANDER: Not necessarily. We have a lot of subspecialties at Omega as well. And so they develop a consultation pool as well. High risk situations. They have oncologists. They have Maternal Fetal Medicine doctors.

It would seem, then, that Dr. Rose's belief in the figures of the pathology-ridden racial minority and the constitutionally durable white person may have made it impossible for her to recognize the actual health states of the persons she attends.

Moreover, Dr. Rose's complex beliefs regarding "culture" speak to the argument I have been developing in this chapter. The scholar interested in locating conduits for the transmission of racial folklore may point to Dr. Rose as a concrete example. Indeed, Dr. Rose told me that she took up the "hobby" of working in the Alpha WHC because she wanted to share with future generations of doctors her accumulated wisdom and passion for gynecological practice. It may be overly optimistic to hope that Dr. Rose did not pass on to her constant coterie of medical students her "knowledge" of the relationship between culture-as-race and pathology. When one considers the danger such racial folklore historically has been to Black patients who have been both subjected to unnecessarily harsh medical treatments and denied essential therapies due to misdiagnosis, Dr. Rose's articulation of the power she has as an attending over her students sounds ominous. I had asked her if her students found the clinic's banal chaos a little unusual. She responded:

> You can't find something bizarre [when] you have nothing to compare it to. [The medical students] are a *tabula rasa*; they have no background against which to make any kind of comparisons at all. To them, they are coming in and they are learning something brand new. . . . They're so busy trying to figure out what's going on and trying to learn how to do stuff. . . . They are happy souls. And they're happy if they walk out of here learning how to do a couple of things.

Again, it may be overly optimistic to hope that Dr. Rose spared her "tabula rasa" the folklore that white people tend to be pathology-free while non-whites tend to be sites of disease, disorder, and "issues."

It is racial biology that unites lore regarding Black women's obstetrical and gynecological hardiness, predisposition toward pathology, primitive pelvises, and hyperfertility. Moreover, it is racial biology that counsels that the "Black race" is a concept referring to a biological entity—one possessing biological processes distinct from the "white race" or the "Asian race." It is racial biology that has created dangerous consequences, providing justifications for treating differently racialized people differently. Arguably, theories of racial biology were enervated by social constructionists who argued convincingly that "races" are the products of *social*, not biological, processes. Sociocultural anthropologist Kamala Visweswaran offers a particularly poignant formulation of this argument: "The middle passage, slavery and the experience of racial terror produce a race of African Americans out of subjects drawn from different cultures. Genocide, forced removal to reservations, and the experience of racial terror make Native American subjects drawn from different linguistic and tribal affiliations: a race. . . ." (1998, 78). However, despite the persuasiveness of Visweswaran's argument and the wide acceptance of the concept of race as a social construction, racial biology has experienced a reinvigoration in recent years.

In 2005, BiDil—a combination of hydralazine and isosorbide dinitrate that, among other things, widens blood vessels in the heart and could prevent death in people suffering from congestive heart failure—was the first drug approved by the FDA for the treatment of persons belonging to a specific race. The manufacturers and marketers of BiDil argued that clinical trials had proven the drug could successfully treat heart failure in Black persons, but could not produce similar results in non-Black patients.[3] However, the clinical trials forming the basis for these claims of BiDil's race-specific efficacy were poorly constructed, arguably proving only that BiDil was an effective drug, not that its effectiveness was unique to Black persons. In the clinical trials, BiDil reduced the mortality of persons with heart failure from 10 percent to 6 percent, giving those taking the medication a 43 percent survival advantage. However, all of the persons who enrolled in the clinical trials were self-identified African Americans. Accordingly, the trials could not and did not demonstrate BiDil would not produce similar results for members of other racial groups. Nevertheless, the FDA approved BiDil's race-based labeling. Consequently, if a physician prescribes it to a non-Black person, insurers do not have to cover the cost of its "off-label" use (Washington 2007, 322).

Biological race in the form of "genetic factors" was offered to explain the efficacy of BiDil for self-identified Black persons. BiDil's patent holder produced scholarship hypothesizing that heart failure in Black persons was primarily due to a genetic cause, excluding the plethora of nongenetic contributors. For these racial scientists, genes that were unique or restricted to Black people produced "a pathophysiology . . . that may involve nitric oxide insufficiency." One cardiologist explicitly disputed the relevance of nonbiological causes of the increased rates of heart failure among Black persons, arguing that data "do not support socioeconomic factors as important contributors to the excess mortality rate seen in African Americans affected with heart failure." This cardiologist avowed "[h]eart failure in blacks is likely to be a different disease." Moreover, the difference was all in the genes: "[T]he emerging field of genomic medicine has provided insight into potential mechanisms to explain racial variability in disease expression" (Washington 2007, 322).

The reaction to BiDil was complex. Supporters of the drug ranged from the politically conservative to the politically liberal. BiDil worked well with conservative political ideology because it offered a genetic, not social, explanation for racial inequalities (Roberts 2008). BiDil also worked well with liberal political ideology, as it is consistent with identity politics and demands for inclusion by historically disadvantaged groups (Roberts 2008). However, other progressives reacted with horror to the arrival of BiDil and the resurgence of racial biology that it heralded. They feared BiDil would encourage people to conceptualize race as a biological entity, undoing decades of progress made by scholars and activists who had argued (and persuaded many) that race was a social construction. Many were concerned that the nuance involved in using race in biomedical research—that is, race as a simultaneously overinclusive and underinclusive concept allowing researchers to get an imperfect hold on genetic variation among human beings—would be lost with the advent of BiDil. A contingent of scholars who have thought extensively about BiDil's problems (and benefits, inasmuch as BiDil represents a concerted effort to confront the racial disparity in mortality from heart failure) wrote hopefully, anticipating that, in the future, physicians will be able to easily divine the genetic makeup of any individual who presents herself for treatment (Tutton et al. 2008, 466). In an era of pharmacogenomics, the use of a social construct such as race in a biomedical research would be obsolete, as "it will be possible to treat every patient based on her specific genetic traits rather than on the genetic traits she is presumed to have on the basis of her affiliation to a particular racial/ethnic group" (466). In the present, however, using race may be an important interim measure as it allows "geneticists and biomedical scientists [to get] some purchase, however crude, on genetic variation amongst different human populations" (466). It is worth noting, however, that BiDil can not be understood as a step towards pharmacogenomics because "the mechanism of action by which it appears to have a beneficial effect on heart failure patients is unknown" (Kahn 2008, 742).

Unfortunately, the nuance the use of race in biomedical research involves is frequently lost, as "biomedical differences between racial groups are routinely misinterpreted as evidence of innate genetic differences" (Ellison et al. 2008, 449). Moreover, the marketers of BiDil, as well as the FDA committee that recommended approval of the drug, disavowed the relevance of nuance—making the stark claim that a *biological* difference in white and Black persons explained BiDil's unique efficacy for the latter group. The committee's chairman, Steven Nissen, contended that African-Americans have inherited genes from African forefathers that affect salt retention and the ability to coagulate blood. For Nissen, the difference was genetic and, literally, all in the blood of Black people: "Respecting biological differences, based on selective evolution, is not racial bias" (Reverby 2008, 481). Nissen articulated his sentiment that "there were enough differences in self-identified African Americans' responses to this and other drugs to satisfy what he called 'biological plausibility'" (482).

In the end, BiDil was approved and marketed as a drug tailored to the unique physiology of Black persons. Accordingly, every advertisement of BiDil that features a smiling Black woman—smiling because, as an African-American woman who has been prescribed BiDil, she is confident that she enjoys a greater chance of surviving a diagnosis of congestive heart failure—makes the argument that Black people possess a distinct genetic composition. Every pamphlet distributed that shows a concerned Black man, who, clearly, wants to learn more about how BiDil could help him, makes the case that races are biological categories and all arguments to the contrary are fallacies. Moreover, these problematic, potentially dangerous arguments are likely to become more ubiquitous: since the FDA approved BiDil, there has been a dramatic upsurge in the number of race-based patent submissions to the Patent and Trademark Office (Dorr and Jones 2008).

Although BiDil makes a strident case about the biological reality of race and racially specific responses to pathogens and disease, these arguments have been heard throughout history. "In this country physicians have long assumed that different races . . . experienced diseases differently and required distinctive therapeutics. As recently as the 1940s, physicians debated whether or not treatments for tuberculosis would work as well in American Indians as they did in whites" (Dorr and Jones 2008, 443). Racial biology formed the foundation for the "Study of Syphilis in the Untreated Negro Male" at the Tuskegee Institute, as physicians sought to finally answer the question of just how differently syphilis coursed through Black bodies as compared to white ones (Duster 2006, 491). Although syphilis was thought to do most of its damage to the neurological systems of its white victims, for Blacks the cardiovascular systems were thought to be the principal targets of its ravages. Indeed, one Johns Hopkins physician asserted "syphilis in the negro is in many respects almost a different disease than syphilis in the white" (Reverby 2008, 480)—a statement that echoes the BiDil proponent's assertion that "heart failure in blacks is likely to be a different disease."

Even after Nazi Germany took racial biology to the most horrific of its logical conclusions, theories of racial biology and investigations into racial therapeutics did not completely fall into disfavor. "In the 1940s and 1950s, medical researchers described a series of racial variations in drug response, most famously the increased incidence of hemolytic anemia seen in black soldiers given malaria prophylaxis during World War II" (Dorr and Jones 2008, 443). Indeed, the Tuskegee syphilis study did not end until the 1970s, representing forty years of applied racial science. Which is to say: BiDil is no anomaly, but rather a consistency—in harmony with the history of medical racism and biological notions of race.[4]

Most importantly, at the very crux of theories of biological race is the belief in fundamental difference. When difference is at the molecular level—that is, when it is the product of simple genetic expression—it becomes insurmountable. Biological race argues that dissimilarity is intractable and undefeatable. When the difference is in the chemistry, there is nothing one can posit that can negotiate the divide. There is also nothing one can do to avoid the construction of the divide; its construction is predetermined. Indeed, the form the divide will assume is determined by molecules and genes. Accordingly, someone from a "different" race represents radical alterity. When faced with a racial Other, one is looking at another who is, at his or her most basic, *not like* oneself.

Accordingly, biological race Others racialized people and groups, and radically so. However, recent scholarship has demonstrated biological race does not have a monopoly on the process of Othering. Indeed, the concept that had been proffered and developed as an antipode to race and biological determinism has come to represent insurmountable basic difference. I am speaking about culture, a topic I will return to later in the chapter.

RACIALIZED OBJECTS OF CONTEMPT

Thus far, I have proposed that racial health disparities may also be explained by physician racism, and I have proffered physicians' faith in enduring theories of racial biology as the substance of that racism. However, I would like to push the argument a step further by contending that racial health disparities may also be explained by looking to a more crude form of physician racism: the plain, deep-rooted contempt for a racialized group harbored by a medical provider. As Hoberman writes, "[T]here is no reason to believe that medical personnel enjoy any sort of immunity to societal ideas about race" (2005, 86). And there is no reason to believe physicians are immune from making certain racialized groups and persons the objects of race-based derision. Hoberman recounts an incident at the University of Alabama at Birmingham where three medical students wore blackface to a Halloween party, making themselves caricatures of Stevie Wonder, Fat Albert, and an unspecified black woman. It is not unreasonable to argue that some form of contempt—some disdain—for Black people had to have informed their decisions to make Black bodies into objects of entertainment and mockery. And it is not unreasonable to have little faith that people (including doctors) who feel this way could bracket it when called upon to provide care for the subjects of their contempt. Health disparities between Black and other racial groups may also be explained by looking to physicians' simple devaluation of the lives of their Black patients.

Consider another portion of my interview with Dr. Rose. After she had spoken fondly of her medical students (who observed her intimate examinations of her patients as part of their instruction), I asked if her patients ever objected to having students in the room during their gynecological examinations. She responded:

ROSE: Yes. They do consistently.

KHIARA: Really? How do you feel when that happens?

ROSE: My feeling is . . . I have a number of feelings. I think there should be a sign out there that says, "Turn your cell phone off"—just like there is in a movie theater. [pause] There should be a sign out front that says: "This is a teaching institution. You are getting world-class care for nothing. Suck it up." And that's it. And that's an ethnic thing also. Spanish, the Hispanic crowd are much more compliant to that kind of thing. Whether they like it or they don't like it, they seem to be okay with it. The Bangladeshi crowd, they're not—if there's a male involved, he has a big problem with that. That's a cultural thing. You can't do much about it. Interestingly enough, the biggest ones that complain the most and refuse are the African-Americans.

KHIARA: Really?

ROSE: Absolutely. I can't—I don't know why. I just think it's sort of an entitlement thing that comes with being a New York Medicaid recipient. They sort of figure that they're special. I don't know. I can't figure it out. And that's not a racist remark; it's an observation. They are the ones that most likely say, "No. I prefer not." You have a certain number of people in the older age groups who are very modest. They are going to say no. Your best bet is a young Hispanic girl who has a bunch a boyfriends and who doesn't care. If you get one of those, you're in pretty good shape.

Here, Dr. Rose articulates her contempt for three racialized groups: the "Hispanic crowd," the "Bangladeshi crowd," and African Americans. Within Dr. Rose's schematization, Latinas are a sexually dissolute bunch whose promiscuity—their sexual availability—informs their willingness to have student onlookers observe their gynecological examinations. History counsels us that the stereotype articulated by Dr. Rose is a particularly insidious one, as the belief in the sexual licentiousness of racially minoritized women (specifically Black women) made it more likely that physicians would attribute any pelvic pain or gynecological discomfort these women experienced to sexually transmitted infections. Writes Hoberman, "Socially conditioned to regard all black women as promiscuous, 'gynecologists would almost automatically diagnose a black woman with symptoms of endometriosis as having pelvic inflammatory disease' as a consequence of her sexual behavior" (2005, 92). He cites the work of Dorothy Roberts, who has argued that "rather than think of black women as vulnerable to endometriosis, 'gynecologists are more likely to diagnose

Black women as having pelvic inflammatory disease, which they often treat with sterilization'" (quoted in Hoberman 2005, 92). Accordingly, if history is a teacher, Dr. Rose's conception of her Latina patients' sexual lives may have led to misdiagnoses of gynecological conditions, willful blindness to others, and demonstrations of tactlessness to those Latina women actually saddled with a sexually transmitted infection.

Bangladeshis are also articulated as subjects of Dr. Rose's contempt. Although it is probably true that any patient who refuses to allow Dr. Rose's students to observe her examination incurs Dr. Rose's wrath (in the form of rudeness, insensitivity, or a disturbing lack of "bedside manner"), the woman presenting the phenotype or other characteristics of what Dr. Rose believes to be "Bangladeshi" probably incurs that wrath to a greater degree as her refusal would be based on an "irrational" "cultural" belief and not a perceived more legitimate personal circumstance. That Dr. Rose does not think highly of "Bangladeshis" was made apparent in another portion of our interview. Lamenting the transformation of the practice of medicine from one grounded in interpersonal relationships to a less relationship-focused, profit-driven enterprise, Dr. Rose spoke about the inability of patients with private insurance to enjoy continuity with their physicians throughout their pregnancies:

> When I did my private practice, I was solo. But, there are no more solo practitioners. They don't exist anymore. Just financially. You now have groups of three, four, and five. But, they're starting to be towards six, seven, eight, nine, and ten. And they're adding another concept, which has been called a "hospitalist": a lot of hospitals are hiring someone to work the labor room 24/7—[someone] who has nothing to do with the patients that we're seeing in prenatal care. So, you walk in [to deliver] and it will be Dr. Gupta from Bangladesh who is moonlighting at the hospital; you've never seen this person. All that is changing.

In Dr. Rose's race fantasy, the figure of "Dr. Gupta from Bangladesh" stands for all that is wrong with the current, rapidly altering practice of medicine. "Dr. Gupta's" parasitic opportunism operates to the "detriment of the patient—both physically and emotionally . . . because pregnant women like to bond" with their caretakers. Moreover, because it is reasonable to doubt Dr. Rose's ability to accurately identify someone from Bangladesh (or to identify others who are *not* from Bangladesh), her uncomplimentary opinion of "Bangladeshis" as unfortunate interlopers in the "American" system of health care who are, in another circumstance, revealed to posses regrettable, fixed, "cultural" ideas is apt to work to the detriment of all South Asian women who find themselves in the unlucky circumstance of being one of Dr. Rose's patients.

Finally, it appears transparent that Dr. Rose's unflattering description of her African-American patients, who are most likely to "complain the most and refuse," is informed by discourses of the "welfare queen"—the always Black woman whose receipt of government assistance as an entitlement has corrupted her work ethic, values, and sense of responsibility. Reminiscent of the welfare queen who believes she should not have to engage in labor outside of the home in order to support herself (as those making up hard-working America must do), Dr. Rose believes that the African-American New York Medicaid recipient thinks she is "special" and her body is not the stuff on which professors should teach and students should learn. In Chapter 6, I will explore more expansively the dangers and consequences of suspecting that entire groups of people are welfare queens; it should suf-fice to observe at this point that the low regard with which Dr. Rose holds her Black patients might not translate into the provision of quality health care for them. In sum, Dr. Rose allows us to see what plain racial contempt looks like and how it may lead to racial disparities in health.

Unfortunately, Dr. Rose was not the only physician I met who demon-strated some contempt toward her racialized patients. Another attending lamented to me "Spanish-speaking patients take it for granted that every-one will speak their language. They expect you to speak Spanish with them. That's the problem: they come here and expect everything to be given to them." It was unclear whether the "here" to which this attending referred was Alpha Hospital or the United States more generally, but what was clear was the disgust that provided the texture for understanding her comments. This attending, like Dr. Rose, also had a reputation among the staff for be-ing tactless, impatient, and occasionally rude to her patients. Such data may lead us to wonder about the way her beliefs about race may influence the quality of the health care she provides.

RADICAL OTHERNESS: THE CORE OF RACIAL BIOLOGY, RACE CONTEMPT, AND CULTURE

I have argued above that racial biology is an idea about the fundamen-tal *dissimilarity* of racialized persons. Furthermore, what is racist contempt for other racialized persons but a hatred for those who are thought to be deeply and basically unlike the racial group to which the racist belongs? When one distills that ideas of radical difference are the foundations of all of these concepts that have operated to shorten (and diminish the quality of) the lives of racially dominated persons, one can see that the danger lies not in the specifics of the concepts but in perceptions of insurmountable difference. Now, although Dr. Rose's conception of "culture" is nothing more than a euphemistic turn of phrase for traditional notions of "biological race," I now argue that more conventional usages of the culture concept are just as deterministic as biological-race determinism. Accordingly, when "culture" is revealed to signify radical Otherness, one can see that cultural stereotypes and beliefs in the way people from certain cultures "just are" can be just as dangerous—and just as racist—as racism.

In a seminal article, "Race and the Culture of Anthropology," Visweswaran (1998) traces the deployment of the culture concept by Franz Boas, largely considered the father of modern anthropology. She writes that, due to his commitment to racial equality, Boas situated race and culture in an antipodal relationship. Indeed, culture was defined through a process of negation. "Culture was expressed through the medium of language but was not reducible to it; more importantly, it was not race. Culture became everything race was not, and race was seen to be what culture was not: given, unchangeable, biology" (Visweswaran 1998, 72). Although, progress-oriented scholars of today lament the biologization of race, Boas' argument for race as a biological category was part of a two-part case for racial equality: the second movement in the case was to argue that the biological nature of race made it value-neutral, having "nothing to do with the superiority and inferiority of given races," to quote his student, Ruth Benedict (73). Boas was arguing against a conception of race in which biology determined the lives and livelihood of people or groups of people. His intervention was to argue that biology-qua-race explained nothing about the potential of people or groups of people: it was simply an insignificant description or possession of a person, having no fundamental relationship to the life a person is capable of living.

Boas and his students contended that the stuff of human difference was not in the "biologically transmitted traits" that constituted race, but rather found in race's antonym—culture. "Culture, not race, was a more meaningful explanation of significant differences between groups of people" (Visweswaran 1998, 75). Race's consignment to the realm of irrelevance forced culture to become *all* that was relevant about a person or group of people. Moreover, because the problematic assumption that biology could determine a person's or a people's life was never questioned, this determinism lived on in the culture concept. Racial determinism simply became a rapidly more ubiquitous "cultural determinism," defined as "the emphasis upon cultural differences for determining outcomes to the 'neglect of normative and political aspects of a cultural process'" (76). And although the intent behind Boas' and his students' deployment of the culture concept was an anti-essentialist one, it has come to freeze "difference possessed by concepts like race" (76). That is, although culture is understood as something that "is learned and can change," as Abu-Lughod (1991) has written, very rarely in its myriad deployments has it been described as changing. A "culture" is static and rigid or, alternatively, it is destroyed and replaced by a new one.

This deterministic, unalterable notion of culture has become common currency. In this way, culture has come to do the work that race is no longer capable of doing; as a consequence, we witness more and more of what I call "culturalist racism," wherein culture is used to condemn persons or a group of people as effectively as did the race concept of yore.

> [B]ecause everyone "talks culture" (that is to say, has access to the concept of culture), its relativist outlines have been increasingly filled by racist content. But does that not illustrate how culture has come to stand in for race? Without a way of describing the sociocultural construction of race, culture is asked to do the work of race. This is perhaps what Walter Benn Michaels means by the title of his essay "Race as Culture." He writes, "Our sense of culture is characteristically meant to displace race, but . . . culture has turned out to be a way of continuing rather than repudiating racial thought." When race functions at all, "it works as a metonym for culture; and it does so only at the price of biologizing what is culture or ideology." (Visweswaran 1998, 76)

Now, culture need not acquire a biological connotation for it to operate as a deterministic concept, although examples of the biologizing of culture surface frequently. Consider an interview I had with a chief resident, Rhea Waxman, who expertly demonstrated the substitution of biological race for biological culture. Dr. Waxman, a white woman in her mid-twenties, spoke openly about her conviction that all patients should be screened for genetic conditions based on their racial background (and her consequent habit of encouraging her patients to test their fetuses for certain conditions depending on their race). Although she believed all patients "regardless of where they are from" should be tested to determine whether they are carriers of problematic genes, "African Americans" and "Asians" were the racial groups that raised the most red flags for her, as those were the only racial groups she named to justify her practice of interrogating her pregnant patients regarding their racial backgrounds: "African Americans are more associated with sickle cell disease [and] Asians with thalessemia." She explained, "Certain ethnicities have certain conditions that are kind of inherent to them due to old, old, old mating habits of people—where you don't mate outside your comfort zone. So, that's the reason why I ask." Although Dr. Waxman clearly subscribed to some notion of biological race, further elaboration revealed her to also subscribe to a notion of biological culture.

When I pressed Dr. Waxman about the fact that, due to centuries of slavery, colonialism, imperialism, global capitalism, and other macro processes, genes that may have been common to one region or group are likely to be found in people of various ascribed and self-identified races, she responded: "You can stand there and tell me that you're White. I'm going to argue a little with you. I'm going to say, 'Are you sure somewhere around there, somebody is not from Africa or the islands?' . . . There's been a lot of press about people's admixture. I'm probably part African somewhere around there. But, I don't associate with that culture or that way of life or anything. So, I don't say that I'm African American." Dr. Waxman appears to admit that a certain irrationality governs her practice of encouraging race-based genetic screening: although she avows that all African Americans ought to be screened for the sickle cell trait and sickle cell disease at birth, she personally would not be screened for the gene or condition, as she does not "say that [she's] African American"—although she is "probably part African somewhere around there." Yet, in Dr. Waxman's wrestling with the illogic of race-based genetic screening, she begins to articulate an interesting conception of "culture." For Dr. Waxman, there is an "African [American] culture" and an "African [American] way of life"—homogenous entities that, when an individual "associates" with them, allow that person to say he/she is "African American." Dr. Waxman appears to suggest that if she did associate with "that culture or that way of life," she could indeed say she is African American. So, at first blush, there appears to be electability to "culture"; one could choose to be or not to be a member of any given culture. Yet, Dr. Waxman's ability to elect membership in a culture is not similarly available to me, as I "cannot stand there and tell [her] that [I'm] white"; she would argue against such an avowal without having queried whether I "associate" with "white culture" or "the white way of life." Accordingly, for Dr. Waxman, it would appear culture is as much of a biological entity as her conception of race. Implicit in her reasoning is that the ability to "associate" with a culture depends upon one's genetic (that is, racial) constitution, buttressing Visweswaran's observation that because "the dominant view of race is a biological one, when this substitution of [culture for race] is effected, culture and ethnicity are themselves essentialized or biologized" (Visweswaran 1998, 76).

Visweswaran's article, first published before the turn of the century, was prescient, as demonstrations of cultural determinism and culturalist racism have multiplied dramatically in recent years. Even when culture is understood as learned (as opposed to biologically inherited) behavior, it still is thought to overdetermine outcomes. Culture has been offered as that which explains everything, including the centuries of violence between "the West" and "non-Westerners"—an argument the late Harvard professor Samuel Huntington parlayed into an influential, best-selling book, *The Clash of Civilizations and the Remaking of World Order* (1996). Huntington posited that cultural difference (i.e., fundamental, nonnegotiable difference) would be the origin of future conflict in the world arena. Civilizations, understood as culture-writ-large, would clash because of the radical alterity they posed to one another. Huntington hypothesized "the fundamental source of conflict in this new world will not be primarily ideological or primarily economic. The great divisions among humankind and the dominating source of conflict will be cultural" (1993, 22).

Nor should culture be understood as deterministic only in world politics; it determines the success and failure of racialized peoples within nations as well. Whereas race used to explain Black people's poverty and disenfranchisement in the United States, culture does so now, as when Harrison (1998) argues, "[H]ere in the United States, we find ourselves debating whether current political discourses on, in one instance, welfare reform and, in another, criminal justice encode race and reinforce racial domination by pathologizing what are being represented as irreconcilable sociocultural differences" (610). When exploring culture's role in explaining racial stratification in the United States, Chang (2002) echoes Visweswaran's findings: "While scientific racialism is generally not a defensible position, there remains what might be described as a social or cultural racialism that attributes certain characteristics to racial groups and explains racial differences as the natural outcome of meritocracy and the free play of the market." (88). Culture has become the entirely defensible position to which dispossession in a "post-racial America" can be ascribed. "This new racialism, which may not be so different from the old racialism, is necessary to maintain the widely held belief among Whites that race has little if any effect on one's life chances in a country where the average wealth of a White household in 1993 was more than $45,740 and the average wealth of a Black household was $4,418" (Chang 2002, 88).

I posit that physicians' belief in "culture" could contribute to racial disparities in health in the same way Hoberman believes physician racism (understood as physicians' beliefs in racial biology and/or the physicians' plain racist contempt) has contributed to racial health disparities. Interestingly, culture has already been offered by many scholars to explain racial disparities in health, as commentators relate the higher morbidity and mortality of Black people to African-Americans' (indelibly cultural) fear of the medical establishment (in the wake of the Tuskegee syphilis study) or Black people's eating habits (common to an entire "culture" and impossible to change). Here, however, instead of replicating this problematic scholarship by looking at how some notion of the "culture" of the victims of health disparities produces different rates of mortality and morbidity, I question how physicians' ideas about the "cultures" to which their patients belong may contribute to health disparities when "culture" is understood as a signifier of fixed alterity.

That is, if at the crux of biological notions of race and racial hatred is the perception of (or desire to believe in) insurmountable difference between racialized persons and groups, the modern concept of culture shares that foundation of radical, unchangeable, nonnegotiable, and deterministic alterity. When we understand that culture can be used to signify fundamental, insurmountable difference (i.e., radical Otherness), then cultural stereotypes and assumptions about the way people from/with certain cultures "just are" may produce the same effects produced by racial discrimination. Hoberman may be correct that physician racism has been an as-of-yet unnamed contributor to racial disparities in health, but he may appreciate only part of the phenomenon by excluding culturalist racism from the ambit of physician racism. When writing about the incident in which three University of Alabama medical students wore blackface to a Halloween party, Hoberman notes it "raises the question of where cultural stereotyping ends and biological race fantasies begin" (2007, 508). For Hoberman, the danger lies only in the physician's harboring of biological race fantasies. And so, I would enhance Hoberman's account of physician racism by including cultural stereotypes within the concept: physicians' beliefs in cultural stereotypes can do the work that beliefs in racial biology have done to shorten (and diminish the quality of) the lives of racially dominated persons.

Consider in this regard a quotation in the aforementioned report concerning racial disparities in health issued by the Institute of Medicine. The report quotes an "African American patient," who says:

> I've had both positive and negative experiences. I know the negative one was based on race. It was [with] a previous primary care physician when I discovered I had diabetes. He said, "I need to write this prescription for these pills, but you'll never take them and you'll come back and tell me you're still eating pig's feet and everything . . . Then why do I still need to write this prescription." And I'm like, "I don't eat pig's feet." (Institute of Medicine 2005, 6)

This physician need not have harbored any beliefs about Black people's biological inability to process sugar or genetic predisposition to retain salt. This physician's cultural assumptions were as total (because all Black people eat pig's feet, the Black person sitting in front of him eats pig's feet) and deterministic (Blackness causes a person to eat pig's feet and fail to fill prescriptions, despite having been diagnosed with diabetes) as is biological racism. Beliefs in Black "culture" could be as harmful as antiquated beliefs in Black primitive pelvises, obstetrical hardiness, or hyperfertility.

Accordingly, one need not look only for physicians' articulations of their beliefs in biological race, as one can look also for their ideas about the way people belonging to certain cultures think, feel, and behave. Such attitudes about culture can be appreciated as "data about individual racial thoughts and fantasies" insofar as culture and race have begun to proceed to the same effect. Indeed, one will find articulations of "cultural thoughts and fantasies" easier to find, as it is still quite acceptable to "talk culture," whereas "talking race" has fallen into disrepute.

My interviews with physicians underscore that culture is understood to be an indicator of difference that is both immutable and impossible to negotiate. It is a wall that—independent of and unrelated to language differences, which can be overcome—prevents communication and mutual understanding between cultural Others:

DR. CATHY ORVILLE, A WHITE SECOND-YEAR RESIDENT: There are
     cultural barriers. Like, I had a woman from Tibet the other
     day who was basically having a miscarriage. I spent 45 minutes
     on the phone with her being as direct as I could: "You're

having a miscarriage. The pregnancy is not growing. It's not living. That's why you're bleeding." But, at the end of the conversation, she said, "Oh, so the baby will be okay, though?" And I just don't think—her culture—she just couldn't understand because of her culture. Sometimes the difference is too big.

KHIARA: What did you do?

ORVILLE: I talked to her for another thirty minutes. I have no . . . you just do your best.

DR. PHILLIP VINCENT, A WHITE SECOND-YEAR RESIDENT: In terms of general health, definitely they are healthier at Omega than at Alpha. And a lot of that is a culture thing. It is just my own personal experience. [At Alpha,] I have had problems getting people off fatty diets and they are diabetics. It is very hard because that is what they eat and their whole family eats it and everyone in their neighborhood eats it. It's their culture. They can't cook any other way.

DR. SARA TRIPP, A WHITE THIRD-YEAR RESIDENT, REMARKING ABOUT THE LARGE NUMBERS OF CHINESE PATIENTS WHO RECEIVE PRENATAL CARE AT BETA HOSPITAL, A SMALLER PUBLIC HOSPITAL ON THE LOWER EAST SIDE: It would be interesting to do something down there, too. It's such a lot of Chinese women. For them, [childbirth education] classes really don't matter. Honestly, Chinese women and Bengali women have a very hard time sometimes, I feel like. I'm just not—even if I have the interpreter phone and somebody who speaks Bengali, I feel like sometimes, we're just not getting through to each other. There are some cultural difference that I just don't get, or they are unable to tell me about something. So, that would be an interesting place.

For these young physicians, culture is used to signify a radical, fixed Otherness; accordingly, the cultural Other comes to represent an alterity that is evocative of the racial Other. Cultural difference of today becomes akin to racial difference of yesterday.

On Chinese-ness

Consider another portion of my interview with Dr. Waxman, in which I asked her if her patients were receptive to her suggestion that they screen their fetuses for genetic conditions based on race. She responded in cultural terms:

> I've found that the Chinese population—they have a lower level of tolerance for difference and disability. So, they almost all test, and they almost all terminate if the results are abnormal. I think that just culturally, there's a lot of pressure. This is what I've experienced. . . . I don't have a lot of background, so much of this is just anecdotal. But, I've found that the women that [immigrate to the United States] have had one child and then two abortions. And when I take the family history, I always ask people, "Were your terminations personal or were there problems with the baby?" Because it's helpful for me to know that. And everyone is very free: "No, they were government [due to the One Child Policy in China]." So, people come here [to the United States] presumably because there are no government restrictions and it's a better life. But, they still want totally normal, healthy babies. So, even though no one is imposing that, they will still have an abortion even though they *had* to abort their last pregnancy. I would think that people would latch on to this pregnancy, like "I can have it. So, I will." But, I think that culturally, it's just acceptable—in that culture—to terminate the pregnancy. And disability is not widely accepted on a stereotypical level.

Dr. Waxman describes a highly durable conception of culture. To her, one result of governmental policy is that Chinese culture is averse to disability and difference while being amenable to abortion. Accordingly, Chinese people, who are bearers of the culture, are similarly averse to disability and difference and amenable to induced terminations of pregnancy. Chinese people's relationship to disability and difference is not contextual; it does not depend upon the social or political milieu in which they live. Rather, it is cultural. And as culture, it is static, unalterable; once formed, the bearers of it will carry it around with them. Their culture determines their beliefs and actions. Moreover, Chinese people and the culture they inhabit (and that inhabits them) are to be counterpoised to a figure that operates only implicitly in Dr. Waxman's narrative: the noncultural woman, historically racialized as white, whose relationship to abortion is based on noncultural reasons: financial, religious, or personal. In Dr. Waxman's narrative, Chinese women and Chinese culture are the Others to implicitly white women and their cultural lack.

What is the relationship between Dr. Waxman's confident views about Chinese-ness and physician racism—the anonymous and largely unacknowledged process that likely contributes to racial health disparities? I offer that Dr. Waxman's ideas about Chinese-ness are also the stuff of physician racism. Although Hoberman may concede only that her views raise "the question of where cultural stereotyping ends and biological race fantasies begin," Waxman's "culture" can have the same effects as biological race fantasies. That is, Dr. Waxman need not believe Chinese persons possess a distinct genetic or biological constitution for her to assume a Chinese patient sitting in front of her will tolerate an induced, or even spontaneous, abortion better than a non-Chinese patient. As beliefs in the biological hardiness of Black patients may cause physicians to recommend more invasive surgeries, beliefs in Chinese women's permissive attitude toward abortion may cause physicians to recommend abortion for difficult or high-risk pregnancies.

Moreover, Dr. Waxman's theory regarding the Chinese demonstrates just how easily beliefs in radical, fundamental difference inform plain (race-based or culture-based) hatred. If one despises laziness, violence, criminality, and materialism, then one would despise the racialized individuals (i.e., Black persons) whose "culture" ("Black culture," "culture of poverty") causes them to be lazy, violent, criminal, and materialistic. Similarly, one can see how contempt for abortion bleeds easily into contempt for the racialized individuals whose "culture" counsels them to conceive of abortion as an "acceptable" practice.

On Mexican-ness

Perhaps one of the most apparent and ubiquitous cultural stereotypes in the Alpha WHC was the assumption that Mexican origin corresponded with prenatal and postpartum health. In truth, there has been some research showing Mexican immigrants, in spite of poverty and a lack of access to regular health care, show relatively good health indicators (Gálvez 2007, 1). However, this consequence is a result of particular practices— "practices associated with diet, physical activity, social ties, and preparing for the arrival of a child" (2)—that are not intrinsic to Mexican origin, but the result of behaviors that are learned and mutable. The stereotype that Mexican women receiving health care from the Alpha WHC are in excellent health and have very few gynecological or obstetrical problems—and "that's just the way they are," with any nuance regarding the necessity of engaging in particular learned behaviors having been lost—was articulated frequently and shamelessly. Consider an interview I had with Hannah Ferguson, an amiable, talkative white woman in the second year of her residency. Dr. Ferguson was commenting on her desire to impress upon the "Alpha population" the importance of getting yearly gynecological screenings. She related a story of having done a Pap smear on a woman who was fifty, with the test being the woman's first. Dr. Ferguson elaborated:

> She had, like, never seen a gynecologist before. I mean, there was nothing big that I could see on her cervix. But God forbid that she had a really horrible strain of HPV. I could have found a really advanced cervical cancer that could have been treatable if only she had come earlier. So, that's one of those things I find to be frustrating because I feel like we do see more advanced GYN cancers sometimes. And if women had more education about that, then we could maybe help. But I feel like a lot of our other patients are really very healthy. Especially the little Mexican women that come in to deliver. I think they've never seen a doctor before they come in at like, you know, nine centimeters. And they're like—they're perfectly healthy and they look. . . . There was one woman who came in here who was—she was in her late nineties. And I was like okay well, so you know, do you want to come back in a couple of months. Because she had never had a colonoscopy and I was like, you know, maybe she should have a colonoscopy. . . . And I was like, "Do you want to come back and talk about having a colonoscopy?" And she says, "Well, I'm going to Mexico for a couple of months. . . ." Good for you, man! See the world! So, you know—I mean they're—she's seen precious few doctors in her life, but she's in perfect health.

Mexican-ness was thought to imbue Mexican women with an enviable and inexplicable level of health. This natural—almost preternatural—healthiness was usually accounted for in cultural terms, as when one resident remarked to me, "Mexicans just have this healthy culture; you can't explain it." The vitality that flows to Mexican women by virtue of their culture—a cultural vitality—is reminiscent of the construction of Black women as biologically sturdier than their white counterparts. As Blackness was thought to immunize Black women from endometriosis and to endow them with "tough" vaginal tissues that would not tear during birth, Mexican-ness is thought to make it less likely that Mexican women would suffer myriad gynecological and other medical problems. A midwife's remark to Gálvez, an anthropologist who conducted fieldwork research in the Alpha WHC with a specific focus on the experiences of Mexican immigrant women, accurately summarizes the general attitude toward Mexican culture and the people who bear it: "We love the Mexican patients. That's why we love working here. They're so healthy" (Gálvez 2007, 2).

As discussed earlier, the biological hardiness of Black women was thought to be manifested in the effortless and painless labors and births "primitive" Black women experienced. "The easy labors of primitive women' are made possible by the simplicity of their lives, while 'our present civilization with its artificial refinements and customs has made women less able nervously and physically to stand the strain of a hard, prolonged labor'" (Hoberman 2005, 95). Compare this narrative of Black women's simple and trouble-free labors with a story related to me by Gálvez. She had been in the delivery room with a Mexican woman during her extremely painful labor. When the woman lay in the hospital bed, the pain was intolerable; accordingly, she preferred to stand. However, because hospital policy was to maintain the patient in a prone position, the nurses and the woman's obstetrician insisted that she remain in bed. Thus, there began a dance wherein the woman would stand, furtively, when alone in the room with Gálvez and, when any of the staff or her physician entered, attempt to rapidly lie down in bed. After some time, the pain became unbearable, and the woman opted to have an epidural. Once the epidural had been placed and the woman's misery subsided, one of the nurses, perplexed, remarked to Gálvez, "This is so strange. The Mexican women usually don't have such a hard time." Although the nurse did not explain to Gálvez precisely why she believed Mexican women do not "have such a hard time" during their labors (i.e., whether biology or culture was at play), the assumption that Mexican women will have easy labors could have the same consequence for them as assumptions about Black women's immunity to pain: the denial of analgesia and anesthesia or delay in administering them, the insistence that women undergo vaginal deliveries when a C-section may be indicated, or the failure to take the precautions to prevent trauma and infection that the physician might take with other racialized patients. (Hoberman 2005).

Unfortunately, I was not privy to many physician ruminations about "Black culture" or "African-American culture," save for the aforementioned comments by Drs. Rose and Waxman. This could be for any number of reasons: physicians' discomfort with describing to a Black woman their beliefs about Black people, the care taken by most when making generalizations about Black people as a consequence of this country's long history of anti-Black racism, and/or the smaller numbers of Black patients (relative to Chinese and Mexican women) seen in the Alpha WHC. As a result, I am unable to track the function of the culture concept as it specifically relates to Black women. But, given the evidence that "culture" does a lot of work to legitimize the problematic assumptions physicians make about Chinese and Mexican women, there is little reason to doubt it has the same effect as it relates to Black women.

SOME CONCLUDING THOUGHTS

The Prenatal Care Assistance Program and sites such as Alpha Hospital are fairly understood as efforts to ameliorate the effects of this country's history of racism and racial inequality by ensuring that an individual's ascription as a racial "minority" or "Black" does not determine whether she lives or dies or whether she is healthy or sick. And so the program, and the hospital that effects it, should be celebrated for its laudable purposes. But, at the same time, it must be recognized that such programs and institutions are not self-effectuating; *people* give them life. Moreover, people who harbor problematic ideas about race and culture can undermine the goals of these programs and institutions. If we are really committed to ensuring that a person's racial identity does not overdetermine her health status, we must demand that the persons caring for them do not harbor dangerous beliefs. Accordingly, physicians and other health care providers ought to be interrogated about their ideas concerning race and culture.

This suggestion will be met with resistance, as it has become acceptable to conceptualize physicians' personal beliefs, harmful or otherwise, as somehow protected by notions of privacy. But, when we acknowledge that " 'doctors' 'private' moral dilemmas involving their patients are actually interpreted and resolved according to relationships of power in the larger society" (Roberts 1996, 118), we understand the relationship between the physician and her racialized patient is far from a "private matter." Because this relationship is informed by the problematic macro processes that we are ethically charged to investigate and scrutinize, we are, similarly, ethically charged to investigate and scrutinize the "private" thoughts that have helped to overdetermine the life chances of racial minorities in the United States. Literally it is a matter of life and death.

In this chapter I have explored medical disenfranchisement in its most evident and recognizable forms: racial disparities in health, physician racism, and theories of racial biology and culture-as-race. In the subsequent chapters, I turn to more discreet demonstrations of medical disenfranchisement—deprivations that begin at the level of discourse. Although I describe these discursive processes as discreet, they operate to devastating effect, functioning to reiterate race and racial inequalities in the United States. Accordingly, in no way should their subtlety—that is, their discursive nature—be used to argue against the profundity of their material impact. That said, I next examine the curiosity that is the phrase "Alpha patient population."

FIVE

The Curious Case of the "Alpha Patient Population"

INTRODUCTION

On one sunny day in the spring months, when I was rapidly finishing up my first year of conducting fieldwork at Alpha, I sat in a courtyard outside of the hospital and chatted at length with Odette Carter, a genetic counselor who had worked in Alpha's obstetrics clinic for close to two years. Odette told colorful stories about her Alpha patients and those at the private practice where she split her time. Her job at both locations was to provide information to women whose initial blood screenings had revealed the possibility of a genetic anomaly in their fetuses or whose advanced maternal age made them appropriate candidates for amniocentesis or further genetic screening. And so, as the ambulances and police cars whizzed by and into the emergency room located close to the patio where we sat, Odette compared her experiences with the "Alpha patient population" and the "private population."

ODETTE: The private population has a higher education level. Most of them have read one to two books about being pregnant. [laughs]. [Pregnancy] is definitely not as instinctive for the private population, whereas most of these women at Alpha are on their fourth or fifth kid by the time they are thirty-five or thirty-six. They've been having kids for a long time. Everybody

thirty-six. They've been having kids for a long time. Everybody in their family has had a lot of kids. It's just more natural. I get a lot more math questions from the private population. I think that people in this [Alpha] population, they don't get too hung up on the math. Whereas people in the private insurance world, they are very: "1 out of 56. Okay, what does that mean? And if this is a false positive, what does. . . . ?" And I'm like, "[exasperated noise]." . . . This population here doesn't have access to the Internet. So, I don't have to worry about people going home, doing all this research, and then calling me up later to drill me on the math again. . . . In the other, you get a lot of people who are like, "You know, I was reading the *Journal of Neurological Disabilities* the other day." And I'm like, "Really?"

KHIARA: Do you find that people tend to know the genetic history of their family?

ODETTE: In this population? No. There's a lot of family lore. So, if you have someone with mental retardation, they'll say, "Oh, he lost oxygen at birth." Or, "He fell as a child." Or, "My mother was walking down the street and laughed at someone with that problem. And there you go." And that's what they believe. . . . So, people, I think, don't know a lot about it. There are a lot more family stories here. High fevers. Falling. Mom was kicked by Dad when she was pregnant. Things like that.

At the time of my interview with Odette, I had been at Alpha long enough to know that, although many Alpha patients had several kids by the time they turned thirty-five, many other patients were experiencing their first pregnancies at that age. Many patients came from large families—with their parents, siblings, cousins, aunts, and uncles having several children apiece—but many others had small families, and the present pregnancy would provide their parents with their first grandchildren. At the time I interviewed Odette, I had conducted enough interviews to know that many women who received their prenatal care from Alpha were terrified of the possibility of carrying a fetus with a genetic anomaly and would go home, do research on the Internet, and "drill" Odette "on the math" if the results of their initial screenings made such behavior necessary. Indeed, one of my most memorable interviews was with a woman who had been informed that she had a nongenetic condition called vasa previa, in which a blood vessel completely covers the cervical opening. She had been told that she would need to have a C-section to avoid the possibility of hemorrhaging during a vaginal delivery. This patient returned for her next appointment with a stack of papers about two inches thick of research she had printed off of the Internet; the papers were shot through with highlighted paragraphs and notes scribbled in the margins. This woman, like the one who approached the front desk and asked how soon she could be scheduled for a nuchal translucency, would most certainly have "drilled Odette on the math again" had she been told her fetus possibly had a genetic anomaly.

On that sunny day, as I approached twelve months of ethnographic research in Alpha, I knew Odette was doing a great many Alpha patients a disservice by denying that they knew their families' histories. Although I could count several women who I believed would offer stories like "my mother was walking down the street and laughed at someone with that problem" as an explanation for a family member's mental or physical disability, just as many women would provide explanations in terms of genes and biology. And so, I recognized Odette was not describing the so-called "Alpha patient population" but *caricaturing* it. And I began to wonder the extent to which the concept of "population" was responsible for that caricature.

In a lecture given in 1978 at the Collège de France, philosopher Michel Foucault (1991) analyzed the trinity of "security, population, government." As to the second term of the triumvirate, population, Foucault remarked, "Interest considered as the interest of the population regardless of what the particular interests and aspirations may be of the individuals who compose it, this is the new target and the fundamental instrument of the government of population." (100) Foucault articulates the sense that, once constituted as such, a population dissolves the individuals who compose it. Once apprehended as a "population," it is the population that is acted upon; those who make up the entity become nothing more than the stuff through which the population can be touched, manipulated, and affected. The particular is dissolved in order to produce the universal.

Although Foucault speaks about population relatively neutrally, evidencing no clear normative judgment of the phenomenon, it becomes more difficult to remain agnostic about the question when one is confronted with its manifestation in the form of the "Alpha patient population." Foucault's instructions cited above suggest that when one can refer to a collectivity of persons as the "Alpha patient population," one is speaking of an instrument of government made possible by the effacement of individual interests, desires, and needs. Much is at stake, then, in "Alpha patient population."

The following is an attempt to understand the stakes of this population. I begin with a more exhaustive elaboration of Foucault's notion of population, then discuss its particular invocation in "Alpha patient population."

FOUCAULDIAN POPULATION(S)

Foucault's exegesis on the origin of population in the final chapter of *The History of Sexuality, Vol. 1: An Introduction*, is an apt place to begin an exploration of what is at issue in the demarcation of the women within the Alpha obstetrics clinic as a specific, bounded "population."

Foucault explains that "population" appears at the same time as does biopower, a modernity-specific form of power that is to be counterpoised to the "ancient and absolute form" that demonstrated itself in and through the taking of life. Quite conversely, power in its modern manifestation is one that is "bent on generating forces, making them grow, and ordering them, rather than one dedicated to impeding them, making them submit, or destroying them" (1978, 136); in contradistinction to the classical age's power over death, ours is a power over life. Further, Foucault describes this new mechanism of power as having evolved along complementary trajectories. One concerns itself with disciplining, optimizing, and cultivating the capacities of the individual human body; the other is involved with the human body writ large.

> The second, formed somewhat later, focused on the species body, the body imbued with the mechanics of life and serving as the basis of the biological processes: propagation, births and mortality, the level of health, life expectancy and longevity, with all the conditions that can cause these to vary. Their supervision was effected through an entire series of interventions and *regulatory controls: a biopolitics of the population*. (139)

Foucault can be read to describe "population" as both the object and the effect of power in its modern form. That is, Foucault explicitly articulates "population" as the analytic unit onto which biopower acts; yet, one can also understand him to describe "population" as concurrently constituted through these same acts of power. The state that yields and deploys biopower, then, *creative*-ly administers the population—submitting it to elaborate apparatuses of calculation, regulation, and management that, in turn, create the population through its calculation, regulation, and management. Once brought into being through the government's will to know it, population reveals itself as an entity that can be understood numerically—indeed, that demands to be quantified. Accordingly, modernity witnessed an "avalanche of printed numbers," to borrow Ian Hacking's (1982) apposite turn of phrase, as statistics functioned to complete the objectification of population. The measurement and quantification of population does not occur after the population has been constructed; rather, population is constructed simultaneously with its measurement and quantification. The thrust of the argument here is that population is always already problematized; it is always already an object of knowledge and a field of intervention. As Foucault (1980) writes, "The great eighteenth-century demographic upswing in Western Europe . . . and the urgency of controlling it with finer and more adequate power mechanisms cause 'population' . . . to emerge not only as a problem but as an object of surveillance, analysis, intervention, and modification" 171). To be sure, population emerges as a problematized object of knowledge.

In his elaborations on population, Foucault never expressly articulates how any given population comes to be delimited; he does not engage with the question of how a state comes to define the population it will take as its object. Accordingly, it is unclear whether Foucault imagines the constitution of any particular population to be axiomatic—that there is a self-evident nature to the selection and inclusion of those individuals who will come to be the stuff of a given population. Perhaps it is because Foucault did not contemplate how any specific population comes be populated that his use of the term is imprecise. At times, the borders of his population are contiguous with the nation such that "population" becomes synonymous with "citizenry," or, more expansively, the "residents" or "inhabitants" of any particular nation. Consider his discussion of the "explosion of numerous and diverse techniques for achieving the subjugation of bodies and the control of populations. . . . As for population controls, one notes the emergence of demography, the evaluation of the relationship between resources and inhabitants. . . ." (1978, 140). In this instance, "population" appears to be synonymous with the individuals in and of the nation. "Population" as "nation" is also deployed when Foucault writes about the nature of war in the nineteenth century versus that of the classical age: "[N]ever before did regimes visit such holocausts on their own populations. . . . Wars are no longer waged in the name of a sovereign who must be defended; they are waged on behalf of the existence of everyone; entire populations are mobilized for the purpose of wholesale slaughter in the name of life necessity: massacres have become vital" (1978, 137). Yet, further on in this same discussion, Foucault expands the limits of the population under consideration in such a way that it becomes coterminous with the human species: "The atomic situation is now at the end point of this process: the power to expose a whole population to death is the underside of the power to guarantee an individual's continued existence" (137). But still further on, Foucault redefines the boundaries of "population" once again such that it appears to be no longer coextensive with "species": "If genocide is indeed the dream of modern powers, this is not because of a recent return of the ancient right to kill; it is because power is situated and exercised at the level of life, the species, the race, and the large-scale phenomena of population" (137). Assuming Foucault does not offer "life, the species, the race, and . . . population" as an itemization of equivalent terms, then here, "population" is something that perhaps exceeds or perhaps is exceeded by "species."

The variability of that which is signified by "population" is what interests me. Simply stated, "population" possesses a certain ambiguity; what it refers to in any particular instance is not overdetermined by previous uses. Instead, "population" derives its content from the context of its immediate usage. It may be invoked as a benign classification in one instance while acquiring more invidious undertones in the next. David Horn (1994) issued an admonishment about this capaciousness of "population"—that it could be, and often is, much more than a dispassionate signifier. The present chapter attempts to defamiliarize "population" and to inquire into its utter failure as a neutral category when it is invoked to refer to the patients receiving care from the Alpha WHC: the "Alpha patient population." That an entire course of treatment (characterized by an excessive medical zeal, as argued in Chapter 3) is practiced upon the individual bodies of those within the "Alpha patient population", and that such an immoderate treatment course is justified because it is being given to the "Alpha patient population," suggests that the "population" being invoked in this instance is not a neutral signifier. It also suggests that "Alpha patient population" does not simply refer to a random grouping of bodies that, at some point in the time, have entered and will enter the Alpha WHC for the purpose of receiving prenatal care. Rather, the exceptional course of treatment practiced upon the individual bodies that form the "Alpha patient population" suggests that the population is not imagined to be contiguous with the "species" or the "nation," but rather composed of a smaller, more precarious element of the former categories.

MAKING THE "ALPHA PATIENT POPULATION"

The program of prenatal care provided to persons receiving Medicaid coverage of their prenatal health care expenses exists, in all of its specificity, prior to its implementation on any individual body. That is to say, the physicians, epidemiologists, and legislators who are the program's authors designed it for a woman who was only imaginary when the program was conceived; the embodied women to whom the program is presently provided are inheritors of a course of treatment that is suited to satisfy not their particular needs, but rather their generically anticipated needs. The fact that an elaborate apparatus of quantifications, examinations, screenings, and preventive efforts was erected for a theoretical, disembodied subject does not necessarily threaten the ability of the apparatus to successfully deal with material women's actual needs, but what is required is a high degree of similarity between the imagined woman and her embodied heir. When we consider that the architects of the prenatal course of treatment knew only that the women for whom they designed the program were 1) uninsured, 2) pregnant, and 3) sufficiently impoverished such that their incomes did not exceed the limitations set for Medicaid, we might be skeptical about the likelihood of similarity between the hypothesized subject and her actual successors. Accordingly, the program of prenatal care for Medicaid recipients may say relatively little about the needs of the women who have come to compose the "Alpha patient population," yet speak volumes about what the authors of the program believe about poor, uninsured, pregnant women. In essence, one can understand the course of prenatal care provided by Alpha Hospital as a representation of the poor, uninsured pregnant woman through the eyes of the persons and institutions empowered to construct programs to suit her needs.

Moreover, although Alpha providers, administrators, and staff members use "Alpha patient population" as if the term is self-evident and determinate, there nevertheless is great indeterminacy in the phrase. Although "Alpha patient population" refers to the considerable numbers of actual women who bring themselves within the physical space of the clinic to receive prenatal and postpartum care, it also refers to women who have never set foot within the hospital, women who are not presently pregnant, and even women who may not yet be born. Indeed, like the imaginary woman for whom the Medicaid architects designed the prenatal care program, there is a certain, disembodied, hypothetical and imagined quality to "Alpha patient population." The parlor trick of the Medicaid apparatus is that, however the specific constellation of the "Alpha patient population" may be in any particular moment, it is always already anticipated with an elaborate apparatus specifically "designed" to meet its needs.

The most salient characteristic of the course of medical treatment designed for the "Alpha patient population" is its excess: a distortion of the prenatal care program offered to women with private insurance is provided to Medicaid-insured patients insofar as certain aspects of the private program are distended and bloated (such as the screenings provided for sexually transmitted diseases and infections), while others are slimmed down or altogether nonexistent (such as the ability to elect a C-section, schedule an induction of labor, or select a provider). The balance of this section explores how the excess of technology practiced upon the Alpha obstetrics clinic's patients becomes justified on the grounds that it is being dispensed to the "Alpha patient population"—a population that is supposedly at "high risk" for various pathologies due to an assumed shared history, environment, and set of behaviors. As one resident, Cathy Orville, succinctly explained to me:

> We do things a certain way [at Alpha]. But, I think we do things in a certain structured way because of our population. . . . For example, every single person that comes here gets a diabetes screening in the first part of their pregnancy. Other patients out in the world don't get that. Private patients don't get that. But, our population is at such a high risk that everyone gets screened. That's why we are much more aggressive about doing testing for certain infections.

As Dr. Orville's syllogism makes clear, pathological conditions and undesirable health states are found within the Alpha "population" at elevated rates. This is what makes it "high risk." Aggressive testing is done as a result. However, these pathological conditions and undesirable health states are precisely what constitute the "Alpha patient population"; pathology, and the risk thereof, justifies referring to the individuals who seek care from Alpha as a coherent entity. However, as pathology and the risk of pathology constitute the "population," the "population," dialectically, constitutes the pathology and its risk.

The Dialectical Formation of the "Alpha Patient Population"

Prior to beginning fieldwork at Alpha Hospital, I was asked to do a formal presentation about my project at a conference during which Alpha OB/GYNs and others could present their research (and findings, if any) to their Alpha colleagues. I had the distinction (and the difficulty) of being the only presenter whose primary training lay outside of the "hard sciences." I remember sitting in the audience and becoming more and more anxious as physician after physician stood behind the podium and displayed charts that graphically illustrated the disproportionate incidences of sundry gynecologic diseases and obstetric conditions among "Blacks," "Hispanics," and other racialized groups; to my growing distress, many offered biological race as the explanation for the higher rates of pathology among the racially minoritized. Soon, it was my turn. It became obvious relatively quickly that the question-and-answer portion of my talk was going to be particularly painful after more than a few hands shot up when I projected my first PowerPoint slide on the screen; it read: "This project defines race as a biologically arbitrary, socially constructed ideology about physical differences among humans—a 'race' being a socially salient, hierarchically ordered category (American Anthropological Association 1998)." I remember, quite distinctly, an African-American resident (who I would eventually befriend and interview) approaching a microphone stand in the audience and saying, "I think your research is really interesting, but. . . . You say that race is a social construction, but, all day, we've been hearing evidence that suggests otherwise." I could only reiterate that the literatures my audience and I had read disagreed on this point.

My experience at this Alpha conference underscores that studies demonstrating the social origins of purportedly "race-related" medical conditions are long overdue: although race as a biological category has fallen into disrepute among many, I have found that even the most critical thinkers look to the fact that certain medical conditions occur disproportionately among Black persons as evidence there must be *some* truth to the claim that race has biological origins. (The most notorious "Black disease" is probably sickle cell anemia, but hypertension and diabetes also are widely renowned.)

Tapper's (1995) investigation of the sordid history through which sickle cell anemia came to be identified and conceptualized as a "black-related disease" is a helpful riposte to the positions held by the Alpha OB/GYNs who I encountered. It is also an entrée into a discussion of how pathology could come to constitute a "population" while the "population" makes coherent the pathology that is found within them.

Tapper's study suggests that sickle cell anemia could only be understood as a disease specific to "Blacks" or persons of "African descent" when the phenomena is filtered through a sieve of racial common sense. Tapper argues that the racialization of sickle cell anemia occurred as a product of a still-extant racial logic—that of "sociomedical racialism." This logic argues that the disproportionate rate of a disease's occurrence in a racial group is a function of inherited, biological racial features. Thus, Black persons contracted—and died from—tuberculosis at higher rates than their white counterparts "because they were 'natural carriers' of or 'naturally susceptible' to that disease" (80). Similarly, sickle cell anemia is a "black-related disease" because only Black persons naturally carried the sickle cell trait within their blood, making them naturally susceptible to development of the disease. Or so the logic goes. Once sickle cell anemia acquired its racial association, a persistent, tenacious racial logic ensured that association would remain. Thus, the abundance of evidence demonstrating that sickle cell anemia could, in fact, manifest in white persons did not threaten the status of sickle cell anemia as a "black-related disease," but rather threatened the "non-Black" status of the person manifesting the disease.[1] Sickle cell anemia remained a "black-related disease" by "making Black" all persons who had it.

However, the Blackening of sickle cell anemia sufferers was just one method of ensuring that the condition persisted in being understood as a "black-related disease." Another method of maintaining the condition's racialized status was to delegitimize symptoms of sickle cell anemia as symptoms of sickle cell anemia. If a thorough history of an individual apparently manifesting symptoms of sickle cell anemia produced no evidence of "negro blood" in the family, and if, consequently, the whiteness of the person was unassailable, the evidence purporting to indicate sickle cell anemia was discredited.[2] In effect, an adamant racial logic discounted evidence that threatened the status of the disease as "black-related." Thus, Blackness—or rather, to begin an analogy to the present concern with the "Alpha patient population," the "Black population"—helped to constitute sickle cell anemia: blood cells were only "truly" sickled (and, consequently, only "truly" indicated sickle cell anemia) when they occurred among the "Black population." Ostensibly sickled cells that manifested outside of the "Black population" could not belong to or indicate sickle cell anemia. On the other half of the unfortunate dialectic, sickle cell anemia helped to constitute the "Black population": the suffering of a body from this "black-related disease" ensured it would be embraced within the ambit of the "Black population."

A similar dialectic is at work within the Alpha WHC. Pathology and the risk thereof constitute the "Alpha patient population"; indeed, the "Alpha patient population" comes into being as a pathology-laden, "high-risk" grouping of individuals. At the same time, on the other side of the dialectic, the "Alpha patient population" constitutes the pathology and the risk that is presumed to be present within it; pathologies, and the risk of them, come into being by virtue of their location within this "population."

The First Term: How Pathology and Risk Constitute the "Alpha Patient Population" The bodies onto which the Alpha WHC delivers its program of hypervigilance and super-prophylaxis are, by virtue of their poverty and lack of insurance, deemed to be at risk for pathology that, if not discovered early and addressed promptly, may threaten the health of mother and/or child. The legislated PCAP/Medicaid guidelines dictate that upon beginning prenatal care, every pregnant, poor, uninsured woman must undergo a "risk assessment" inquiring into "individual characteristics affecting pregnancy, such as genetic, nutritional, psychosocial, and historical and emerging obstetrical and medical-surgical risk factors" (New York State Department of Health 2009). The mandate that all poor, pregnant, and uninsured individuals be "assessed" for "risk" may be understood as a mechanism that identifies the individuals who are at risk and those who are not. Yet, one can also reasonably interpret the mandate as articulating the sense that *all* poor, pregnant, uninsured women are at a not insignificant level of risk by virtue of their poverty, pregnancy, and lack of insurance; if so, the PCAP provider's duty is to determine the level of the risk extant and to provide prenatal care accordingly. Thus, no poor, pregnant, uninsured woman escapes the imputation of being at risk; instead, it is the degree of risk that is uncertain and subject to appraisal.

The latter interpretation is most consistent with poor women's experiences in the Alpha WHC. In the legislation establishing the Supplemental Food Program for Women, Infants, and Children (WIC), the program is proffered as a preventative measure designed to meet the dietary needs of women, infants, and children who are specifically at nutritional risk and, therefore, predisposed to having certain undesirable health outcomes. However, per the PCAP guidelines, PCAP providers must "ensure" that every pregnant woman they encounter is referred for WIC. Accordingly, it is not unreasonable to construe this as a presumption that all poor, pregnant, Medicaid-insured women are imagined to be at nutritional risk. These women become united by the nutritional risk they are imagined to bear— a risk that not only justifies their inclusion into yet another elaborate bureaucracy of the welfare state (i.e., the Food and Nutrition Service, the agency that administers the nutrition assistance programs run by the U.S. Department of Agriculture), but also makes it logical to refer to these individuals as a coherent group. The nutritional risk that unites them begins to make possible the frequent and naturalized references to poor, pregnant, Medicaid-insured women as a "population."

The relationship that "population" has to nutritional risk is subtle, but important: "population" presupposes some significant shared characteristic, and, by implication, a certain degree of homogeneity. The attribution of nutritional risk to all women seeking prenatal health care at Alpha provides a baseline level of homogeneity onto which a "population" can be built. Nutritional risk functions to blur distinctions within the group; in fact, it demands that healthy, sufficient diets be misrecognized and regarded as insufficient. This risk elides multiplicity. It expunges differentiation. The work that the concept of nutritional risk does is understated, but extensive. Moreover, it is just one element in an entire constellation of what can be termed "population"-producing pathology and risk.

Consider in this light the "health education" protocol demanded in the PCAP law. The "health education" provided to Alpha obstetrics patients in satisfaction of the legislative directive demonstrates how heterogeneity and diversity get ignored when pathology and risk are imputed to all— that is, when "population" is constituted. Pursuant to the PCAP mandate, "Health and childbirth education services shall be given to each pregnant woman based on an assessment of her individual needs" and taking into consideration any "language and cultural factors." The statute then offer an itemization of topics that "should be provided as needed," including "signs of complications of pregnancy," "physical activity, exercise and sexuality during pregnancy, and "family planning" (10 NYCRR S 85.40).

That information on these topics is dispensed as a matter of course to all women seeking prenatal care within the Alpha WHC reveals that differences within the group are not contemplated—or, rather, the group is imagined to be united by a shared lack of knowledge about these facts. Indeed, Alpha has constructed a standardized form itemizing each of the topics and providing a space next to each item where the "health educator" can indicate that she has "educated" the patient on the topic. Further, although I have carefully read many completed standardized forms in patient charts, I never observed any notations indicating that provision of information on a topic was "not needed" or "not applicable." Once again, a sound conclusion to draw is that the different "needs" of the individuals within the group are expunged in the face of their construction as a coherent "population." The "population," in its entirety, is imagined as needing education on all the topics; consequently, individual health education needs are figured outside of the legibility of hospital policies. Differences are suppressed, and it is through their suppression that the "population" garners its coherency.

Additionally, it is telling that the Medicaid law requires that Alpha patients be "educated" about "family planning." As articulated by the statute, information on family planning should be offered "as needed." However, as I have discussed in earlier chapters and will discuss in more detail later in the next section, Alpha patients are "educated" about their contraceptive options without regard to whether they express an interest in preventing future conceptions; indeed, this is an "education" that is repeated several times over the course of their pregnancies and once again during their postpartum visit. Thus, contraceptive "advice and services" are provided to women without regard to their "individual needs." Again, we witness the suppression of individual particularities among women for the purpose of realizing an intelligible "population"; moreover, based on the zeal with which information on contraceptive options is submitted to women, this is a "population" desperately in "need" of the handicapping of their fertility: this "population" is at especially "high risk" for the repetition of unplanned, government-subsidized pregnancies.

And this represents just a fragment of the pathology imagined to be present within the "Alpha patient population." Providers I have interviewed cite the "Alpha patient population" as one that has increased incidences of diabetes, anemia, chronic pelvic pain, hepatitis, and high blood pressure (although, as I have discussed in the previous chapter, the sickliness of Alpha patients relative to their privately insured counterparts was something thoroughly disputed among the healthcare providers). These pathologies tended to be cited rather matter-of-factly, as if their presence within the "population"—composed, as it is, of poor people—is to be expected. In light of the hypothetical nature of the woman for whom the PCAP program was authored, one might be suspicious whether these pathologies are real. Do they exist on the level of unrealized expectation, or do the bodies of the material women seeking health care within the clinic actualize them? The answer to the question ultimately may be unimportant, as the mere imagination of shared pathology does the work of producing a recognizable, apprehensible "population" out of individual women.

Nutritional risk, a lack of basic knowledge (about pregnancy, childbirth, and infant care), a fertility that is realized in its excess, a predisposition to diabetes (an issue I will discuss in depth in the following section) and anemia, an increased incidence of chronic pelvic pain, high rates of hepatitis, a heightened prevalence of hypertension: all these elements become the stuff from which the "Alpha patient population" is built. One could analogize this constellation of pathology with the sickle cell anemia that could only be found within the "Black population". Indexing the racial common sense of the early twentieth century, Tapper cites the notion that "populations and races can indeed be categorized by the difference in the rate by which they possess any given anemia" (1995, 81). The construction of a "population" out of the individual women who seek prenatal health care at Alpha borrows and adapts this notion; like the "Black population" that gains coherence (or whose coherence is reiterated) by the increased rate by which it possess sickle cell anemia, the "Alpha patient population" gains coherence by the elevated rate at which it possesses the constellation of pathology noted above. Essentially, the "Alpha patient population" becomes legible through its amplified pathology. When a "population" is defined by its pathology, and when differences between the individuals who compose the totality of the "population" become elided, the "population" can be acted upon with all the force required to address the pathology that defines them. Individual bodies become the means to an all-important end: facilitating the health of the "population." Thus, medicating individual bodies without regard to their individual needs is justified. The overmedicated, hypervisible patients within the Alpha WHC are testaments to this.

The Second Term: How the "Alpha Patient Population" Constitutes Pathology and Its Risk   On the other side of the dialectic, the "Alpha patient population" constitutes the pathology and risk that function to delimit it.

At first blush, it appears somewhat counterintuitive that pathology—a presumably material entity—could be constituted by the socially constructed phenomena that is "population." However, the British historian of medicine, Karl Figlio, long ago suggested that pathologies are not "natural" entities awaiting discovery, but rather are socially constructed by the medicine that perceives them: "[D]isease as a clinical object structures a cluster of social relations, and . . . at the same time . . . is itself socially constructed." (quoted in Tapper 1995, 78). If diseases may be socially constructed, we have the provocative possibility that the "Alpha patient population" could construct the pathologies found within them. Differently stated, a body that meets the conditions of inclusion into that nebulous, fluid entity referred to as the "Alpha patient population" will be found to demonstrate that pathology and its attending risk. Yet, someone who does not come within the ambit of the "Alpha patient population" will not likely be seen as demonstrating pathology and risk. Thus, in a vicious tautology, the "Alpha patient population" comes to constitute the pathologies and risks that inhabit them, as the fact of a body's inclusion within the "population" informs the interpretation of pathology and risk.

The most obvious example of this process at work is the issue of contraception. As discussed above, the unambiguous message communicated by the verve with which contraceptive options are presented to patients receiving prenatal care within the clinic is the government's desire to curb the women's fertility. The assumption appears to be that if the women were left without guidance—in the absence of regular, recurrent reminders by clinic staff that they ought to decide upon a method of contraception—a repetition of their (assumed) unplanned, state-supported pregnancy will occur; thus, the government-qua-clinic interjects itself into the narrative and compels the women to avoid the otherwise inevitable result. The woman's body, as informed by its inclusion within the "Alpha patient population", becomes a sign of the intractability of its procreative facilities. That very body indicates that she is at risk for the recurrence of pregnancy. The presence of risk in the body, or rather, the riskiness *of* the body, justifies subjecting it to an abundance of caution and prophylaxis—in this case, in the form of encouragement to medically control its fertility. Significantly, this interpretation of the body is reserved for those who compose the "Alpha patient population"; private insurance and/or the economic wherewithal to pay out-of-pocket for medical care not only rescues women from actual and discursive inclusion within this "population", but frees their bodies from being construed as signs of reproductive unruliness. Thus liberated from the imputation of procreative risk, the woman inhabiting the body is left to determine her reproductive future and the desirability of additional children in the absence of the state's implicit condemnation of a future pregnancy. As a body's inclusion within the "Black population" helped to determine whether sickled cells were truly a sign of sickle cell anemia, a body's inclusion within the "Alpha patient population" helps to determine whether that body is a sign of its own disruptive and lamentable fecundity.

Another example of the process whereby "population" constitutes the pathologies that are thought to be present within it is the government-qua-clinic's policy regarding screening patients for sexually transmitted diseases and infections. As discussed in Chapter 3, although all pregnant women (with or without private insurance) should expect a test for gonorrhea, chlamydia, and syphilis during the Pap smear they receive during their initial prenatal care visit, only the Medicaid-insured are tested for these diseases again during their third trimester, and once again during their postpartum visit. Repetition of the test for gonorrhea, chlamydia, and syphilis during a woman's third trimester is based on the assumption that she may have exposed herself to sexually transmitted pathogens by having unprotected sexual intercourse after discovering her pregnancy and beginning prenatal care, an assumption that is not altogether offensive. However, obliging a woman to submit to testing during her postpartum visit assumes that she may have engaged in unprotected sexual intercourse in the days and weeks immediately after she has given birth—an outrageous assumption.

This policy may be the product of a recognition that indigent women are more likely to engage in prostitution than non-indigent women. As such, the policy may not be informed by an assumption that indigent women are simply predisposed to ill-informed sexual choices and behaviors, but rather that poverty frequently creates the conditions within which the exchange of sex for money appears to be a sensible trade. If the treble testing of women for STDs and STIs is informed by the evidence that economic inequalities push women to prostitution, then the policy essentially assumes that every woman within the "Alpha patient population" could be a prostitute—and thus the policy treats every woman within the "Alpha patient population" as if she is likely to engage in prostitution. This is a rather odious assumption. What one must ask, then, is why the authors of the prenatal care program fail to attempt to tailor this policy of otherwise excessive preventive medicine by identifying those women who do, in fact, engage in prostitution? Why do they not simply require PCAP providers to pose to women the question, "Have you ever exchanged money for sex?" I asked Dr. Trisha Valencia, an attending physician, why Alpha subjected every pregnant woman who walked through its doors to such an extreme course of screening for sexually transmitted diseases and infections, and why the hospital did not give its providers the flexibility to provide individualized care to women based on their particular needs. She responded that health care was provided by Alpha in that manner

> because [Alpha is] an epidemic institution and we're actually following the guidelines of [the American Congress of Obstetricians and Gynecologists]. They say that you need to do this, this, this, and this. If not. . . . They give you leeway. But, it's up to your individual practice. But, this here—everybody comes in here. So, it's very difficult to say, "We will test you and you, but for some reason, I will not test you."

However, Dr. Valencia's explanation is not entirely convincing, as the question "Have you ever exchanged money for sex?" may rather effortlessly sort the women who have engaged in prostitution and may require an aggressive course of screening for STDs from their differently situated counterparts. Moreover, in addition to the easy availability of this question, its posing has precedence, as it is asked as a precursor to the HIV test. Accordingly, Dr. Valencia's justification for the universality of the aggressive STD screening policy at Alpha—because "epidemic institutions" cannot identify those who require testing and those who do not—is not persuasive. As such, why then does the STD screening policy (if it is, indeed, informed by an acknowledgment of the relationship between poverty and prostitution) choose not to identify subpopulations of women who have engaged in prostitution within the larger "Alpha patient population" and tailor a program of testing to meet their specific, unique needs? Why insist upon the present, heavy-handed program, which discursively constructs the poor, pregnant woman as sexually irresponsible and materially enacts the discourse by submitting her body to repetitive STD screenings? The answer may lie in the inability of the PCAP/Medicaid authors to recognize the program's caricaturing of the poor.

Trebly screening women for STDs assumes a sexual gluttony on the part of the "Alpha patient population." The bodies that, in aggregate, compose this population are assumed to be sexualy avid. The authors of the prenatal care program provided by Alpha Hospital read these bodies as pathologically promiscuous, irresponsible, and, consequently, at risk for disease and infection. The risk that is ascribed to the bodies is used to justify a regime of STD surveillance and prophylaxis that is superfluous at best. That women with private insurance, safely disqualified from the "Alpha patient population", need not submit to STD-testing in triplicate suggests that their bodies are not interpreted as having a tendency to overindulge sexually.[3]

The final example of how the "Alpha patient population" constitutes the pathology and risks attributed to them concerns the testing of patients' blood for glucose levels. Although all women, with or without private insurance, should expect to be screened in their twenty-eighth week of pregnancy for heightened levels of glucose in their blood (the presence of which would indicate gestational diabetes), only Medicaid-insured women will also receive the screening at their initial visit for prenatal care—usually during their first trimester. Initially, one could read this double screening for gestational diabetes together with the emphasis that the prenatal care program places on the dietary habits of the patients as seeing the poor, pregnant body as being at nutritional risk and thus predisposed to the resulting pathologies. However, the gestational diabetes double-screening at Alpha is more complex than this initial reading—namely because any pathology revealed by the early glucose assessment would fail to adhere to the categories of diabetes posited by biomedicine.

As explained to me by one of the most senior attending physicians in the Alpha WHC, there are several types of diabetes: Type 1, Type 2, and gestational. The onset of Type I usually occurs during childhood, and the onset of Type 2 usually occurs during adulthood. Although Type 2 diabetes is commonly associated with obesity and a poor diet, Type 1 is not similarly associated. Both Type 1 and Type 2 diabetes are conditions that, once manifested, endure for the rest of the individual's life. However, distinct from Type 1 and Type 2 diabetes is gestational diabetes, which only presents itself in the later stages of pregnancy—never before the twenty-eighth week. Yet, the women who comprise the "Alpha patient population" are given their first screening for gestational diabetes early in their pregnancies. As a consequence, if the result of the glucose testing—proffered as a screening for gestational diabetes—is positive, it cannot indicate actual gestational diabetes because the woman will not be far enough along in her pregnancy for this pathology to qualify as such as it is commonly understood. This attending physician suggested that the screening was done because "a lot of people [here] are borderline diabetic before their pregnancies." Thus, although the glucose testing may identify those who have heightened glucose levels in their blood, and therefore diabetes, ironically it would fail to identify those with the type of diabetes from which the "gestational diabetes" screening garners its name. However, the final twist is that the pathology discovered by the early screening cannot be properly understood as Type I or Type II diabetes because, like gestational diabetes and unlike Type I and II diabetes, the condition detected by the "gestational diabetes" screening would be expected to resolve itself after pregnancy. We are left with a hybrid pathology—with an onset like that of Type II diabetes, but the ability to resolve itself like that of gestational diabetes. For that reason, it is not clear what exactly the providers are detecting when they "find" gestational diabetes with the early glucose challenge. Nonetheless, the belief that something is being "found" justifies continuing the policy. I had asked Dr. Valencia to help me make sense of the gestational diabetes screening that found a pathology that disobeyed the parameters of gestational diabetes:

> KHIARA: Do you find—like, with the glucose challenge—are you finding gestational diabetes that early?
>
> VALENICA: Yes. Yes. Because our patients are high risk for it. So, for this population, it's actually very good that we're able to be very aggressive because we are finding it. Our own residents— they did a research study comparing our practice and what would happen if this was just a regular practice. And we would miss people.
>
> KHIARA: Is that published somewhere?
>
> VALENCIA: No—it was just a poster. At an ACOG conference, one of our residents presented it.

Dr. Valencia's final comments reveal the particular singularity of the "gestational diabetes" found at Alpha: this is a pathology that is mysteriously locatable within the "Alpha patient population," yet unlocatable within the biomedical literature. As one resident explained to me, "The former chair of the obstetrics department [at Alpha] . . . thought that there were two different forms of gestational diabetes. And it's not published anywhere in the literature, to the best of my knowledge. They still haven't published it anywhere. But it seems to be true because a lot of these women, we test them after their pregnancies and they test that they're not diabetic in their real life. Outside of pregnancy, they're not diabetic at all. So, it's interesting." Indeed, it is interesting: not only are women's bodies taken as a sign of their own pathologies, but at least some of the pathologies signified are revealed to be exotic and population-specific. A relevant query is whether the pathology and risk of pathology found at Alpha would be understood as such if they were not exhibited within the "Alpha patient population." And, in this way, the unfortunate dialectic proceeds— the pathologies (and the risks thereof) make intelligible the "Alpha patient population," which, in turn, makes intelligible the pathologies (and the risks thereof), which makes intelligible the "Alpha patient population," yet again, ad nauseum, ad infinitum.

The dialectic of pathology and population may be understood as yet another illustration of what Tapper aimed to illustrate in his investigation of how sickle cell anemia became a "black-related disease"—that is, how "medicine is implicated in the social" (91), or, more forcefully, in Nikolas Rose's formulation, how "[m]edicine . . . has played a formative role in the *invention of the social*" (55).[4] In both Tapper's study and the present one, medicine is deployed in such a way that it invents knowable "populations" that serve to stratify society—or rather, rearticulate, reinscribe, and/or reify existing stratifications. Medicine and medical science function to naturalize distinctions that have been socially produced and justify the differential treatment of the persons so distinguished.

A Defense of the "Alpha Patient Population"

The most obvious critique at this point would be to insist upon recognizing that the authors of the PCAP protocol (and the ACOG recommendations that the PCAP protocol closely follows) did not legislate in a vacuum. More explicitly, although the protocol itself does not cite its sources or the evidence from which it bases its unarticulated assumptions about the relationship between poverty and the pathologies discussed above, surely the protocol is informed by an abundance of such epidemiological data. Even more explicitly, there must be a statistically significant relationship between the poverty that characterizes the "Alpha patient population" and the pathologies that are more likely to manifest there. Given the data, the treatment course would be appropriate. Or so the argument goes. But, as Fogel (1996) admonishes us, "stories about 'populations' . . . are as important as the words and statistics found for them" (1). Which is to say: one ought not to assume that it was an objective, neutral, dispassionate science that produced correlations between poverty and pathology. (Indeed, one might query the very possibility of an objective, neutral, dispassionate science.) What I articulate here is the necessity of considering how the term *poverty* operates when epidemiological scientists seek— and find—correlations between poverty and poor health states. Poverty unavoidably carries the history of its significations within it—an ironic wealth of images of the poor alongside sundry ideas of how the impoverished behave. Even when poverty is operationalized as a designated income level, a level of education, or some relationship between the two, and even when it appears as a disinterested variable that one correlates with another, its ability to tell the time-worn stories about "the poor" (and their deviance, their lack, their excess, their Otherness) persists.

This uneasy relationship between science and class has many a precedent; indeed, this relationship has all too often manifested as a kind of "science of the *under*class." Many of the techniques presently used to scientifically "know" contemporary populations are the products of efforts to know the so-called underclass. Writes Procacci (1991) in her brilliant political economic genealogy of the modern state, "We are the heirs of [the poor's] vagrancy, their insanitary slums, their illegalities, as of all the sociotechnical inventiveness that has been at once demanded and produced by the need for their socialization" (152).[5] Accordingly, contemporary population science is the heir of attempts to control the deviance and social malaise the poor represented and threatened.

The most spectacular demonstration of the unfortunate relationship between science and class is probably eugenical science. As Nye (1993) writes of the rise of eugenics, the science was far from objective, neutral, and dispassionate. "[I]t was the politics—an ideology of class bias—that drove the science, not the other way around" (688).

Although the logic of PCAP and the Alpha prenatal care program cannot fairly be described as eugenical—indeed, the cause of the "Alpha patient population's" pathology is imagined to be environmental or behavioral, not biological or genetic—there is a remarkable similarity insofar as both eugenics and PCAP take as its target the poor and attribute to them risk, pathology, and social disrepair.[6] The similarities between the two uses of science should not be ignored. Tellingly, Nye (1993) writes, "A passionate concern with race hygiene and the identification of dangerous human pathologies did not, accordingly, end in 1945, but has been subsumed into the logic and practices of the modern welfare state, though in forms more compatible with contemporary sensibility on these matters" (687). Nye's guidance helps us see that PCAP is a technique with which a "modern welfare state" manages "dangerous human pathologies." As a program that articulates its purpose as that of providing prenatal care to the most marginalized, most vulnerable element of society, PCAP can be taken as a method of managing a constellation of "dangerous human pathologies" in a form most compatible with contemporary sensibilities. I am not arguing that PCAP is the result of eugenical politics, but only that PCAP shares a logic with that of past eugenic campaigns by which the state attempted to "improve" the health of the nation by problematizing the reproduction of the poor.[7]

It is in this sense that "Alpha patient population" exceeds class; indeed, "Alpha patient population" should not be understood as a mere synonym for "poor, pregnant women." Rather, it carries connotations of danger, moral failure, pathology, and instability that are in excess of that indexed by class. Adopting Procacci's (1991) reading of that "class of men injured by society who consequently rebel against it" (158), one might understand the individuals who compose the "Alpha patient population" as analogues of the "paupers" of yesterday. "The definition of pauperism . . . does not work essentially through economic categories; rather than a certain level of poverty, images of pauperism put the stress principally on feelings of fluidity and indefiniteness, on the impression, at once massive and vague, conveyed by the city crowd, accounting for all its menacing character" (158–59). "Alpha patient population" does not simply index a group of poor women; it indexes a group of pauperized women. The packaging of the pauper into the statistical form of a variable, calling that variable "poverty," and correlating it with other variables within ostensibly neutral, dispassionate, objective scientific discourses does not wash the pauper of its connotations. The result is a prenatal care program provided to poor women, but designed for the pauper.

The treatment of the discursively pauperized poor within the Alpha WHC—as a "population" that is best managed by excess—is not the inevitable effect of a science that is able to locate disease and pathology in individual bodies; that is, the PCAP protocol is not the overdetermined result of a technology capable of seeing illness. As Paul Rabinow (1992) writes, "Specific projects themselves did not emerge from within scientific practice" (241). PCAP is not simply a scientific project: it is a state project. The excess of technology that is brought to bear on the poor en masse is a *decision*; the discursive construction and the material manipulation of individual poor women as a pathology-defined group, as "biological dangers" within the body politic, could be avoided. Once acknowledged, our aim should be to contemplate why this construction is embraced. What kind of work does the imagination of a pathologized population—indeed, an underclass—perform for the national psyche? I am reminded of Kathleen Stewart's (1996) poetic ethnography of a West Virginian coal mining community. It was a community that a social worker in the area advised Stewart to avoid. Stewart writes:

> For her it was an imagined landscape beyond the pale—a place given over to dirt and violence, lack and excess. In the landscape of lack there was not enough money, not enough schooling, no lawns, no police, no fire stations, no paint on houses, no city water, no cable TV, bad plumbing. It was unsanitary. There would be no one for me to talk to. There was nothing out there. In the landscape of excess there was the insanity of ecstatic fundamentalism, the danger of wild bars where drunken men cut each other with knives, the filth of pigs and chickens, the smell of wildness and dirty bodies and unwashed hair, the piles of junk on the porches and in the yards. . . . (67)

For the social worker, the mining community that was located just five miles from her suburban enclave (but into which she had never stepped) was the Other against which she could define her middle-class Self. The more the marginalized people who called the community home could be imagined to ricochet between lack and excess in quotidian fits of bipolarity, the more the middle class could come to occupy the even-tempered space of moderation and restraint. Stewart reads the social worker's imagination of the community as "encas[ing] in it the prefabricated code of a class defending itself against the contamination of a surrounding 'Other' through the class-conscious phantasm of a life that would somehow contain itself in coded norms of order, cleanliness, propriety, safety, and self-control." I believe this is the work performed by the imagination of a pathologized "population" created out of the women who seek prenatal care from Alpha. In this "diacritical construction of self," the more sexually promiscuous, uneducated, and diseased the "Alpha patient population" becomes, the more sexually responsible, educated, and healthy the nation can become. The volatility of the Othered "Alpha patient population" can be matched by the stability of the Self-as-nation.

What I also want to underscore here is the violence that the logic of "population" can do to the individuals who come to compose one. As Haggerty (2002) succinctly notes, "Statistical institutions must treat people as members of abstract groups rather than as individuals with unique histories and motivations" (100).[8] Thus, when a statistical institution that creates something such as the "Alpha patient population" acts on the individual poor, pregnant woman as a member, the woman is forced to part with her unique history and motivations. This particular objectification compels her to become a medium through which the government can act on an identified "at-risk" "population" of which she is imagined to be a part. Indeed, the woman vanishes; the outline of her individual form becomes indecipherable as she is swallowed by the population whose production is facilitated by her evanescence. "What we witness here is a shift in the clinical gaze from the individual patient, his or her complaints, and biography (name, age, race, gender, occupation, marital status, and geographical location) to . . . populations" (82). So erased, efforts of individual women to differentiate themselves from other Alpha patients become recognizable as attempts to reclaim a sense of their individuality. We may reasonably understand them as endeavors to reverse the violence performed by the logic of "populations." Moreover, we may also understand the ubiquitous attempts by ancillary staff members to differentiate themselves from the Alpha patients that they are employed to serve—by reiterating, in various forms, the fundamental Otherness of the pregnant patients—as efforts to prevent their inclusion within a problematized, pathologized "population."

THE WORK OF RISK

At Alpha, as we have seen, the women who enter the clinic in search of prenatal health care are presumed to be "at risk" for a plethora of social and biological ills. Their "risk" status is thought to be substantiated by their search for state-subsidized health care. Presumptions of the "riskiness" of their bodies and lives are confirmed by their very presence at the clinic. Moreover, the clinic demonstrates its agential nature as it ascribes risks to the pregnant women who seek health care there. Thus, the women's presence within the clinic facilitates the projection of risk onto and into their bodies. The women on the supplicant side of the Alpha obstetrics clinic front desk find themselves overwhelmingly embedded in a discourse of risk—as risk is projected onto their bodies in the same moment that their bodies are interpreted as possessing it.

The attribution of risk to every woman who enters the Alpha obstetrics clinic for the purpose of receiving prenatal care works to produce an apprehensible, and homogenous, population. As an insurance term of art, "risk" presupposes a population. Thus, when a woman is interpellated as being "at risk" or "high risk," the very description of that woman as such presupposes the existence of a similarly situated population of women—all at a similar degree of risk, and all with the same relationship to the risk they are thought to embody (Ewald 1991). As it relates to the Alpha WHC, the population presupposed by each hailing of a woman as "at risk" or "high risk"—a population that need not be physically encountered in order for its existence to be assumed—is that which is signified by "Alpha patient population." Further, population discourse generally demands the elision of individual particularity in the service of producing a homogenous whole. The imputation of risk erases much of that particularity. "A risk is first of all a characteristic of the population it concerns. No one can claim to evade it, to differ from the others like someone who escapes an accident" (203). And thus risk amputates difference: "The idea of risk assumes that all the individuals who compose a population are on the same footing" (203). In this way, risk *produces* the individual who has been hailed as a member of a population as "an average sociological individuality"; moreover, this "average sociological individuality" is a distant relative to the embodied, unique woman that the "average" purports to represent.

Shared risk makes poor, pregnant, uninsured women into a coherent population. Shared risk erases the vast diversity—of health states, of relationships to biomedical discourse, of desire for the medicalization of their bodies and pregnancies, etc.—within this sizable and dissimilar group of individuals. In her analysis of the "pauper" as a dangerously antisocial threat to capitalist society and the concomitant need of the capitalist state to contain that threat, Procacci describes a process remarkably similar to that of creating the "Alpha patient population": "The homogeneous consistency of the category of pauperism, used without any concern to break it down into a distinct conception of the various micropopulations it brackets together, indicates its fictitious character: what is really designated by the term is . . . the ensemble of adversities/adversaries which confront the project of social order" (1991, 163). Analogously, the homogenous consistency of the "Alpha patient population," used without any concern to index the various particularities, relationships, desires, and needs it brackets together, indicates its fictitious character. Indeed, "Alpha patient population" indexes not real people, but "the ensemble of adversities/adversaries which confront the project of social order." This pornography of risk is in no way specific to Alpha. One could reasonably argue (as does Rabinow) that the projection and pursuit of risk defines the modern practice of medicine: "Modern prevention is, above all, the tracking down of risks—not in the sense of the result of specific dangers posed by the immediate presence of a person or a group, but rather, the composition of impersonal 'factors' that make a risk probable. Prevention then, is surveillance not of the individual but of likely occurrence of diseases, anomalies, deviant behavior to be minimized and health behavior to be maximized" (1992, 242).

In the balance of this section, I am interested in how risk inflects on the subjectivity of the risk-bearer. More specifically, I ask about the significance to women of the abundant message that is communicated by the care provided by the Alpha obstetrics clinic: "You, the unsafe bearer of risks, must be subjected to a series of quantifications, examinations, and investigations in order to avoid the dangerous manifestation of the risk that you embody." What is the effect of the imputation of risk on identity? How might there be a recognition of a shared identity? What might be the relationship of such a recognition to race and racial logic(s)?

Risk and Biosociality

An apt place to begin this inquiry is with the observation that medicine and medical discourses can—and frequently do—have powerful effects on an individual's self-perception. Although Lupton (1997) aims to problematize the view in her appraisal of what she calls the "medicalization critique," it is reasonable to assert that "individuals' lives are profoundly experienced and understood through the discourses and practices of medicine and its allied professions" (93). The imputation and projection of risk is just one medical discourse, just one medical practice, that deeply affects the individuals it encounters and who encounter it. This is to say that individuals' lives can be "profoundly experienced and understood" through their risk factors; indeed, the risk an individual is thought to bear may become the substance around which she forms an identity. Clarke (2003) has made such an argument: through the application of science and technology to bodies, "[b]iomedical technosciences create new categories of health-related identities and redefine old ones. For example, through use of a risk-assessment technique, one's identity can shift from being 'healthy' to 'sick,' or to 'low risk' or 'high risk.'" (182–83). Clarke refers to such identities as "technoscientific identities," and underscores that—like many other identities that we acquire, including racial ones—the acquisition of these subjectivities ought to be understood as coercive processes: "These new genres of identities are frequently inscribed upon us, whether we like them or not" (182).

Whether they like it or not, the individuals attended to within the Alpha obstetrics clinic have an identity of "high risk" inscribed upon them, and, whether they like it or not, their bodies are managed accordingly, pursuant to the dictates of a bureaucratically prescribed regime of care. By virtue of the intersection of their pregnancy, poverty, and lack of insurance, they become enlisted into a high risk population—a "social form" that is, importantly, made possible through "'dividing practices' that specify population segments such as risk groups" (Clarke 2003, 165). The interpellation of an individual as "high risk" enables—indeed, demands—the individual to begin to conceptualize herself as "high risk." The conscription of the individual into an "at risk population" and the inscription of her body as one that is "high risk" enables—indeed, demands—the woman to acquire a technoscientific subjectivity in line with her risk. Evidence that such technoscientifc subjectivities were acquired in the clinic was provided in the frequently heard statement, "I am high risk." As when I asked one patient why she had been given several appointments during the course of the week, and she replied, "Because I'm high risk"; as when I asked one patient why she received her prenatal care from Alpha as opposed to a hospital closer to her apartment, and she replied, "I am high risk, and so they transferred me here"; as when I asked one patient why she was compelled to have a consultation with the social worker, and she responded, quizzically, "I don't know; maybe because I'm high risk?" In the statement, "I am high risk," the woman speaks of herself *as* the relationship she is forced to have with biomedical discourse and the biomedical establishment. She confirms that the interpellation of herself as "high risk" has been successful and that a technoscientific subjectivity has been effectively obtained. The Alpha WHC demonstrates the truth of the observation that "statistical classifications can become incorporated as a part of a person's self-identity"(Haggerty 2002, 101).[9]

That a discourse of "high risk" can be formed, and that a woman could come to conceptualize herself in the terms of that discourse, demonstrates the productivity of population discourse generally. Ian Hacking (1982) argues that the technology of counting—which, itself, is a condition of possibility for "population"—"creates new categories of people,"[10] and, in turn, "creates new ways for people to be" (223). Thus, the creation of a population of women who are defined in terms of the risk they are thought to possess creates the possibility that those women will think of *themselves* in terms of that risk. Because "[p]eople spontaneously come to fit their categories" (223), the poor, uninsured, pregnant woman comes to fit the volatility, marginalization, and problematization that "high risk" presupposes.

What is the significance of the manufacture of a group through the inscription of risk onto individual bodies? What is the significance of the formation of a collectivity through their shared volatility, marginalization, and problematization? In his exploration of a related question, Rabinow (1992) has given the term *biosociality* to the formation of collectivities around medically and scientifically ascertained facts. He writes about the "certain formation of new group and individual identities and practices arising out of these new [scientific] truths. There will be, for example, neurofibromatosis groups who will meet to share their experiences, lobby for their disease, educate their children, redo their home environment, and so on" (244). "Risk" becomes the stuff around which identities may be formed and shared identities may be recognized. In such recognition, group identities may coalesce.

Bear in mind that we should not assume all group identities that coalesce as a result of medicine, science, and technology will have equivalent moral salience. A group identity that coalesces around, for example, neurofibromatosis, or Rabinow's example of "chromosome 17, locus 16,256, site 654,376 allele variant with a guanine substitution" will likely be given a qualitatively different moral judgment than one that forms around the constellation of increased risk for sexually transmitted disease, diabetes, heart disease, and obesity. A moral condemnation would likely trace the borders of this latter group in a way not expected for the group suffering from a disorder produced by the unhappy switch of a gene. And so, there is the (im)morality of certain pathologies and categories of disease and risk.

However, there is also the (im)morality of the fact of sickness: illness, as deviance from health, has at times been an occasion for censure or the attribution of blame. Turner (1997) writes of "disease categories as elements of the moral control of individuals and populations" (ix); accordingly, coming within a disease category—that is, having disease and deviating from a preferred state of health—can be read to indicate some moral failure on the part of the sick individual or population.[11]

Thus, the always already "high risk" individuals within the Alpha obstetrics clinic are doubly culpable: first, they are deviant insofar as the level of risk they embody exceeds the acceptable level of the "average" or "normal" person; in the simple fact of their elevated risk, in their deviance from health as a preferred, lower level of risk, they might be regarded as morally culpable.[12] On top of this baseline culpability, they are subjected to the additional blame attributed to those who come within, or who are at risk of coming within, disease categories—such as diabetes, heart disease, some lung cancers, HIV/AIDS, etc.—for which a moral failure is ascribed to the sufferer *because of* the disease from which she suffers. When this analysis is applied to the "Alpha patient population," it reveals the manifest injustice of the easy and indiscriminate imputation of risk to the women who compose the group. Inclusion within a morally denounced group is another avenue through which the pregnant poor can be conceptualized as immoral. Indeed, it is another justification for the moral condemnation of the woman whose pregnancy intersects with her poverty.

Although Rabinow's concept of biosociality is helpful to my analysis, it veers away at a very important point from the argument I make about the "Alpha patient population." Rabinow envisions the possibility of the creation of "desubjectified" subjectivities from biomedical science and discourse; he imagines that identities and group identities will form from fragmented, isolated and isolatable, scientifically ascertained truths. "Through the use of computers, individuals sharing certain traits or sets of traits can be grouped together in a way that not only decontextualizes them from their social environment but also is nonsubjective in a double sense: it is objectively arrived at and does not apply to a subject in anything like the older sense of the word (that is, the suffering, meaningfully situated integrator of social, historical, and bodily experience" (1992, 243). And it is at that point that my analysis diverges: The creation of the collectivity signified by "Alpha patient population" fundamentally rests upon assumptions about the social environments and social relations of the individuals who compose the group. The (imagined) social, cultural, and environmental context in which individuals are located is built into the very fabric of their biomedically facilitated and ascribed identity; decontextualization, even when computers are used to collate and sort the traits they are thought to have, becomes impossible. Tellingly, Rabinow writes of the individual's ability to avoid anything like moral condemnation due to these scientifically ascertained truths: "It is not who one is but what one does that puts one at risk. One's practices are not totalizing, although they may be mortal (243). Indeed, the focus of my inquiry is the presumption that Alpha's prenatal care program functions as though a totalizing knowledge about an individual—the "truth" of her physical environment, nutritional intake, education, and sexual practices—can be ascertained (and subjected to an elaborate apparatus of medical surveillance and treatment) by virtue of her status as pregnant and poor. The prenatal program at Alpha is paradigmatically totalizing.

And what about race? Will the coalescence of group identities around biomedicalized subjectivities work to undermine race? More specifically, does the formation of an "Alpha patient population" undermine race and racial inequalities insofar as that which is of greatest consequence about this group—that which defines them as a group—is not their racial truths as such, but rather the class-inflected biomedical truths within the individuals who compose the group? Consider Rabinow's contemplation of the effects of the "new genetics" in this light:

> In complicated and often insidious new ways, the older categories may even take on a renewed force as the new genetics begins to spread not only in the obvious racism so rampant today but more subtly in studies of blacks' alleged higher susceptibility to tuberculosis. My argument is simply that these older classifications will be joined by a vast array of new ones, which will cross-cut, partially supersede and eventually redefine the older categories in ways that are well worth mentioning." (1992, 245)

Rabinow's conclusion is compelling, as it seems that "Alpha patient population" cross-cuts racial categories in ways that do not threaten to supersede them, but rather work to reiterate them: "Alpha patient population" is embedded within and informed by discourses of class; indeed, "poor" is one of the most salient descriptors of the women who compose the group. Given the mutual constitutive nature of race and class in the United States, it seems that the racial salience of "Alpha patient population"—and for that matter, any group within the United States that is composed exclusively of the poor—is inevitable. In this way, "Alpha patient population" reiterates the significance of race while recognizing, nevertheless, that the form of that reiteration is not overdetermined. Within a racializing logic of class attributes, the unprivileged class positioning of Alpha patients serves to locate them as members of a racially disempowered group—a point I will elaborate on in Chapter 6. And so, racial categories may in one instance be reaffirmed by "Alpha patient population"—as, for example, when the population works to reaffirm the relationship between poverty and racial Otherness through its ability to index poverty and the racially marked individuals who compose the group. Yet, in a concurrent instance, "Alpha patient population" may work to diminish other racial categories (as I will also argue in Chapter 6) when phenotypic expressions of race become disarticulated from social understandings of race. Other rearticulations, redefinitions, and supersedings of race—unpredicted and unforeseen as of yet—are not only possible but likely. We, who are interested in justice, must not solely fight antiquated forms of racial injustice, but must be prepared to recognize race's irruption in evolved guises. "Alpha patient population" ought to be understood as both an agent and a form of the evolution of race.

In a later section of this chapter, I will investigate the relationship between race and population more expansively. But, first, I turn to an investigation of the work of risk and population in a larger project of governance.

Risk and Governmentality

What is the significance to a project of governance that the "Alpha patient population" is defined by the (high) risk(s) they are thought to embody? How might "Alpha patient population" be understood as a mechanism of governmentality? And also, how might we appreciate *as a technique of governance* the production of an apprehensible "population" out of poor, uninsured, pregnant women?

We could begin to answer these questions with an articulation of the basic relationship between population and state power in that they frequently presuppose one another. Often, they appear to exist dialectically. The (at times, coercive) recruitment of individuals to compose a population comes subsequent to a state being empowered to do so; yet, the formation of a population through the enlistment of individuals simultaneously empowers the enlisting state. State power as the cause and effect of population derives from the fact that in an era of biopolitics, a population is always an already-known and knowable collectivity; population, always problematized, presupposes that it will be the object of knowledge production. The constitution of a population assumes a biopolitical state prepared to gather knowledge about it; concurrently, the gathering of knowledge about its population facilitates aggrandizements of state (bio) power.

Thus, population and its accoutrements—counting, numbers, demography, and importantly, statistics[13]—should be recognized for the (biopolitical) state power whose existence they assume (Rose 1994, 60). Although the motivations for compiling statistics may be "genuinely philanthropic," they also may be fairly understood as a means to preserve the state that compiles them (Hacking 1982, 281). And should the relationship between population, statistics, and state power be doubted, one need only be reminded that the means of establishing the breadth and depth of the population has been explicitly articulated in that (purported) apotheosis of democratic intention and possibility, the U.S. Constitution. Indeed, it is categorically unconstitutional for the U.S. government to fail to count, to *know*, the population it endeavors to govern. (See Article 1, Section 2.)[14]

Moreover, should it ever be doubted that "population" also facilitates social inequality, domination, and subjugation, one need only be reminded also that the same apotheosis of democratic intention and possibility contains the formula for valuing some subjects above others. (See the Three-Fifths Clause in that same paragraph of the Constitution.)[15] I do not cite this to argue that population and population discourse is always despotic and illiberal but to indicate that population, statistics, demography, numbers, and counting, as techniques of knowledge and governance, can easily shade (and have easily shaded) into techniques of repression. Indeed, the line between repression and governance is highly negotiable, respected in one instance, traversed in the next. And so the challenge is to understand where along the governance/repression continuum lies that bounded (yet aspirational) entity signified by "Alpha patient population."

Entangled within the question of "Alpha patient population" is the question of risk. It bears repeating that the individuals who compose the "Alpha patient population" are interpellated as being risk-bearers of an exaggerated degree at the same time that they are interpellated as members of a bounded population. Although the hyperbolic nature of the risk Alpha patients are thought to embody is significant, risk need not be amplified for it to promote the cause of self-regulation: because of the logic of risk, self-regulation and self-surveillance follow every instantiation of risk, however minute. Indeed, risk and self-subjection are complementary terms in a self-sustaining dialectic: "Risk and surveillance mutually construct one another. Risks are calculated and assessed in order to rationalize surveillance, and through surveillance risks are conceptualized and standardized into ever more precise calculations and algorithms" (Clarke 2003, 172). Furthermore, because risk possesses an inherent latency—that is, contained within the concept of risk, there exists the notion of the small becoming big, the few becoming many, the insignificant becoming substantial—every occasion of risk demands the most expansive of self-surveillance. Because what a risk will ultimately refer to is unknown, every risk demands the greatest preventive measures. "A risk does not arise from the presence of particular precise danger embodied in a concrete individual or group" (Castel 1991, 287). It is the absence of a "particular precise danger" that makes any conservation of prophylaxis unreasonable.

Now, if governmentality is only truly realized when self-regulation is linked to state regulation, as Turner (1997) suggests,[16] the ubiquity of discourses of risk and the quotidian quality that has come to characterize their invocation intimates the prescience of Foucault. In a singular fashion, the possibility of risk (and the management thereof) tends to persuade those so affected to assume behaviors and ways of thinking that coincide with the behaviors and ways of thinking the state seeks to inculcate in its subjects.

> The act of governing involves efforts to direct a population toward certain prescribed ends. The political dimension of such processes derive from the fact that human decisions, rationality and behavior are manipulated to accord with the aims of authorities. Contemporary liberal forms of governance generally operate through a calculative logic that seeks to align the rational interests and limited freedoms of subjects so that individuals become involved in their own self-regulation."
> (Haggerty 2002, 98)

Risk is revealed to be quite an effective liberal form of governance when the self-regulation of the risk-bearer becomes the only behavior in which the rational actor can defensibly engage and it is aligned simultaneously with state interests.

This demands some elaboration: when and why would the state be interested in the self-regulatory behaviors in which the risk-bearer, interested in her own health, engages? That is, if the risk-bearer self-regulates by monitoring her diet, exercising, using condoms, getting yearly gynecological examinations, and allowing at least two years to elapse between pregnancies, what is the state's interest in these particular behaviors? To begin a response: on the most materialist, Marxian level, the state has an interest in the health of the individual, as the individual is the paradigmatic source of labor. "[H]ealth is a form of policing which is specifically concerned with the quality of the labor force" (Turner 1997, xv). Accordingly, if dieting, exercising, using condoms, receiving Pap smears, and spacing pregnancies—in concert—ensure the availability of a robust collectivity of present and future laborers, the state has an interest in encouraging those behaviors. In this sense, individual health becomes a material resource of the state—and all the more so if an individual's viability in the labor market also precludes her dependency on state-sponsored welfare. From a more Foucauldian perspective, in the era of biopolitics, the health of the people (and even more specifically, the health of the reproductive woman) has been read as a sign of the health of the nation. Indeed, the health of the population-as-nation is that which demonstrates and foments the state's (bio)power. Thus, modern subjects find the government promoting healthy behaviors for the subject's (read: state's) own good.

Now, consider Clarke's proposition that "[r]isk technologies are . . . 'normalizing,' not in the sense that they produce bodies or objects that conform to a particular type, but more that they create standard models against which objects and actions are judged" (1993, 172). When the discourse of risk is understood as a project of normalization, the application of a discourse of "high-risk" to the uninsured, poor, pregnant women who seek their prenatal care from the Alpha obstetrics clinic appears more loathsome. When "risk" is contemplated as a normalizing discourse, the "high risk" that describes the bodies and environments of Alpha patients can be interpreted as denoting the desperation that characterizes society's need for their normalization. One might say that norms have replaced the classical-era police and military as the ideal tool with which to control the (modern) population. The "high risk"—that is, the exceeding abnormality—that describes and defines Alpha patients indicates the population's estrangement from state regulation, and, therefore, the state's need to (re)establish authority over their lives. Alpha patients' "high risk" status denotes that they lie farther away from the norm than does the average (read: non-poor, non-pregnant, privately insured) person. As such, their risk is "high," as "high" indicates both the expanse that separates their social location from the norm/control, as well as the enormity of the need to bring these women away from the margins and within state authority. The intensity of their marginalization renders them pathological and, by implication, dangerous: Alpha patients are embodiments of "poverty intensified to the level of social danger" (Procacci 1991, 158). Accordingly, should there be any doubt that their pregnant bodies would reflect that danger through manifestation of disease and pathology?

Procacci's reading of the "pauper" is again helpful here. Insofar as poverty is assumed to be an inescapable feature of capitalism, efforts to eliminate it are futile. (Additionally, efforts to eliminate poverty within capitalism are, in fact, undesirable, as poverty is the condition of possibility for wealth and its accumulation.) Pauperism, however, must be contained. As such, programs of "poor relief," of which PCAP/Medicaid and the services provided by public hospitals such as Alpha Hospital are paradigmatic, might be understood as normalizing techniques that alleviate difference, not inequality. Explains Procacci, "By the term 'difference' I want to underline that the essential significance of the term 'pauperism' consists in indicating a series of *different forms of conduct*, namely those which are not amenable to the project of socialization being elaborated: 'Indigence is a set of physical and moral habits' " (1991, 160). The provision of health insurance during pregnancy will not purge inequality from society, as such could never be an attainable goal of PCAP/Medicaid or Alpha Hospital. However, feasible aims of such programs are educating the pauperized poor as to the folly and treacherousness of their "difference" (in conduct and ways of thinking), as well as reeducating them toward proper ways of thinking of and being in the world. Discourses of risk do that work. The successful interpellation of the woman as "high risk" enables the process of normalization to begin. It hails her to a state institution for repeated educations, surveillances, and opportunities for discipline. However, pauperism must be produced before it is formally denounced. The PCAP program does not eliminate pauperism; on the contrary, the program conjures it into existence so that its exorcism may be perennially performed, but never achieved.

Furthermore, I do not believe that the amplified risk that is imagined to follow the woman interpellated as such escapes her. To be precise, Alpha patients self-regulate in quantities that correspond with the risk they come to believe they embody. It is irrelevant that their bodies rarely give evidence of the "high risks" they are imagined to carry, as "[i]t is no longer necessary to manifest symptoms to be considered ill or 'at risk' " (Clarke 1993, 172). The power of biomedical discourse is such that it requires only the pronouncement of "high risk" upon a woman—by the social worker, the nutritionist, the health educator, or the nurse (and usually in collaboration)—for her to accept the augmented "riskiness" of her body. And so, for the most part, the individuals who compose the "Alpha patient population" dutifully meet with the social worker, the nutritionist, and the health educator, the latter reiterating the precariousness of the women's pregnant bodies by didactically reading a list to them of the "warning signs" of labor. Understanding their "high risk," Alpha patients call the clinic telephones with anxious questions about the health of their bodies and the fetuses they carry; moreover, they dutifully go to the labor and delivery emergency room when advised to do so by the nonmedical staff who answers their calls.[17] They come to most of the appointments made for them. They submit to the myriad tests prescribed for them. In essence, they *hyper*-self-regulate, as the "high risk" are expected to do.

THE MIMETIC LOGICS OF RACE AND POPULATION

"Population" is mimetic of "race" insofar as both concepts share a logic of differentiation. Population works by constructing what appears to be a self-evident group around a selected characteristic, feature, or attribute. The groups enacted by population conceal their social construction insofar as, once constructed, the populations appear to be "natural"; that is, they appear to be natural ways to refer to social phenomenon. Obscured are the motivations—social, political, economic, and otherwise—behind the selection of the attribute around which any population is organized; moreover, each reference to the grouping as a population reiterates the "naturalness" of the assemblage. As I have discussed above, the attribute around which many populations have been constructed has been "nation." However, nation as an organizing principle is only one of sundry possibilities; "Alpha patient population" demonstrates that class, pathology, disease, imagined risk (or some combination of the four) may function as the stuff around which a population can be organized and that can make coherent the use of a lone signifier to refer to a disparate combination of individuals.

Like population, race functions to differentiate clusters of people. For race, the characteristic upon which the differentiation has been based has transformed over the years—from purported phenotypic expressions of biological facts to socially recognized affiliations, identifications, and/or ascriptions. Despite the organizing principle employed in any particular invocation of race, racial logic insists, as with population, on some reified notion of enduring difference.

The shared logic of race and population goes some way toward explaining why "Alpha patient population" is frequently invoked in ways that reveal a restrained insistence upon the racial difference of the "population" referenced. Although "Alpha patient population" purports to refer to the simply uninsured, pregnant, indigent woman, folded up within it are notions of the racial and ethnic difference of the individuals who compose the group. As such, I interpret population discourse within the Alpha obstetrics clinic as an example of a deracialized racialist discourse. "Alpha patient population" is deracialized insofar as it, ostensibly, does not reference race; its apparent purpose is to signify the group of individuals who receive care from the Alpha obstetrics clinic without explicit regard to their racial identifications and ascriptions. However, it is a racialist discourse because it is invoked in ways that foreground the racial particularity possessed by the individuals who form the population. The deracialized racialism of "Alpha patient population" explains the numerous slippages I observed during which the racial logic regarding "Alpha patient population" revealed itself.

The most exaggerated slippage to which I bore witness occurred during an interview with senior attending physician Dr. Veronica Rose. I have discussed Dr. Rose's comments in the previous chapter; in short, Dr. Rose conceptualized the "Alpha patient population" as a pathology-laden group of racial minorities; moreover, for Dr. Rose, the "Alpha patient population" could be productively compared to their healthy, white counterparts in the "private population." One of the most remarkable aspects of my interview with Dr. Rose was the ease with which she articulated outrageous racial stereotypes about her patients. Yet, it is important not to dismiss Dr. Rose and her remarks as "racist." Now, although I have no doubt that the tactlessness and impatience she demonstrated with her patients and the abrupt manner she reserved for the (non-white) ancillary staff who assisted her were, in large part, informed by her imputation of racial stereotypes to them and her consequent feeling of racial superiority, I do not believe her comments should be dismissed on that basis. Although Dr. Rose's racism perhaps enabled her to make readily apparent the racialist logic that undergirds the population discourse in operation within Alpha, this logic is not idiosyncratic or specific to the individual invoking the population. Instead, a racialist logic of differentiation structures the very concept of "Alpha patient population" itself.

That population shares a logic of differentiation with race, and that "Alpha patient population" could be understood as a deracialized racialist discourse explains the not-infrequent instances in the clinic where race appears to erupt from population. On these occasions, race and population demonstrate their simultaneity by blending into the other; a conversation about population transforms seamlessly into one about race. As an example: I interviewed a fourth-year resident, Gabriela Worth, who had also attended medical school in New York City prior to beginning her residency at the Omega University School of Medicine. Her medical school had been affiliated with a small public hospital in Brooklyn, Gamma Medical Center, and she had been able to do several rotations through a number of the Gamma clinics. She explained that part of the reason she had chosen the OUSOM residency program was that she had enjoyed working with her Gamma patients and "thought Alpha would be similar to Gamma in terms of the patient population." I asked her in what ways were the two populations similar. She responded: "I think having a diverse ethnic and racial background, you know, population. And definitely having a good high-risk population. It is similar—in terms of the patient population." As shown by her comments, the characteristic around which Dr. Worth defined population was precisely the race/ethnicity of the patients; indeed, the race/ethnicity of the patients superseded competing definitional possibilities for population. Interestingly, Dr. Worth does not mention that the racial/ethnic composition of the population who seeks medical care from Gamma is, in fact, different from the racial/ethnic composition of the "Alpha patient population": because of the community within which Gamma is situated, the majority of the persons the hospital attends to are African-American and West African. Alpha, on the other hand, is remarkable for the sheer heterogeneity of the racial and ethnic backgrounds of its patients. In order for Dr. Worth to understand the Gamma patient population to be "like" the "Alpha patient population" in terms of racial and ethnic background, she had to dismiss the racial and ethnic particularities of the groups and understand them as simply *not white*. The generic racial and ethnic Otherness—that is, the non-whiteness—of the populations was paramount in Dr. Worth's reading of population.

Dr. Worth also mentions that Alpha, like Gamma, had a "good high risk population." Subsequent comments reveal that, for Dr. Worth, the risk possessed by the populations is but a function of the race/ethnicity that defines them. I posed the question of whether the high risk status of Alpha patients translated into an increased incidence of health problems among them. She responded:

WORTH: Yeah. I think we know that people of lower socioeconomic status have higher rates of diseases. People of certain ethnic backgrounds have higher rates of diabetes. Those people are the patients at Alpha.

KHIARA: They're represented. And the ethnic backgrounds with higher rates of diabetes are . . . ?

WORTH: I'm not sure. . . . I can't say off of the top of my head.

KHIARA: Well, for example, is "African-American" one of them?

WORTH: For diabetes particularly? It would be South Asians—or, as I should say, Indians. [pause] People from Mexico. [asks another resident in the room] Do African-Americans have higher rates of gestational diabetes? [to me] No—not African-Americans.

KHIARA: No?

WORTH: They have other problems.

Dr. Worth essentially responds to the question of high risk in a way demonstrating that to her it signifies (or is synonymous with) "higher rates of disease"—the latter to which she then affiliates two partially overlapping subsets: "lower socioeconomic status" and "certain ethnic backgrounds." She then posits Alpha's population as a demographic that captures these two "known" high risk categories. Moreover, although African-Americans initially escape pathologization as possessors of bodies that are more likely to fail in their ability to process sugars (thus causing them to become diabetic), their pathology is reinstated by the elusive condemnation "they have other problems." The race or ethnicity of these bodies gives them a presumption of the likelihood of failure.

Compare Dr. Worth's articulation of the causes of pathology and disease among the "Alpha patient population" with that proffered by Allison, a midwife who had worked in the Alpha obstetrics clinic for almost two years at the time of our interview. I asked her if she saw a higher rate of health problems among her patients due to their poverty. She responded:

You know, I've never worked in a private population, so I don't really know what to compare it to. I'm sure though that there is a higher rate of health issues. I think—one, just being in an urban environment is a huge problem. I think they are at a higher risk for certain types of cancers because they're in a big city. And, you know, poor nutrition and things like that lead to a lot of problems. So, it would seem that more of the people of a lower income are more at risk for problems. I just think the lack of continuous care also puts people at, you know. . . . That in and of itself maybe puts them at more risk for more health problems; but, definitely, once you catch something, it's a lot farther along.

For both Allison and Dr. Worth, the bodies against which the "Alpha patient population" are to be compared are those within the private population. However, although Dr. Worth figures the former poor bodies to be "raced" and "ethnic" and allows race/ethnicity to explain the comparatively higher incidence of disease and pathology among them, Allison does not explicitly racialize the bodies within the "Alpha patient population." Thus, although both population and race may share a logic of differentiation (as I suggest), Allison does not allow race to inform her articulation or definition of population in the case of the "Alpha patient population." The races and ethnicities of the women who compose the populations Allison compares appear to be irrelevant, as she submits environmental causes and estrangement from medical care as explanations for the differing rates of disease and pathology. Race and ethnicity are not built into the very fabric of her invocation of population, but rather are extraneous to it. That is, race and ethnicity are *in addition* to her "population," not *of* it. Consequently, one can understand the population discourse in which Allison engages as qualitatively and fundamentally different from that of Dr. Worth. Yet significantly, for both class is the differentiating factor between the two populations; in one instance, it gets ethnicized/racialized, while in the other, it is more meticulously deracialized.

Notably, the question of whether Alpha patients are, in fact, sicker than their privately insured counterparts is disputed. As discussed in the previous chapter, some providers believed that the patients seen at Alpha, for various reasons, were not quite as healthy as those seen at Omega. Like Allison, another nurse practitioner I interviewed offered a particularly poignant, structural explanation for the higher incidence of pathology she observed among her Alpha patients:

Chronic pelvic pain would probably be one of the more common problems. And it's very difficult to say whether that is because there is so much more stress involved in their daily lives, whether there is more infection, I don't know—because chronic pelvic pain may be caused by infection. And also I think for some of the population—especially this subset of the population—having a physical complaint is the one way that they can actually get attention in this world.

Still, other providers believed the patients seen at both hospitals did not differ greatly with respect to their levels of health.

Even when Alpha patients are perceived to be sicker than Omega patients or those in the private population more generally, they are sicker only in comparison. The bodies of the Alpha patients produce a greater incidence of pathology or disease only when they are compared to another grouping of bodies, as the prelude to Allison's response makes clear: "I've never worked in a private population, so I don't really know what to compare it to." The incidence of pathology the bodies of Alpha patients produce can only be understood as "high" when there is a "low" against which they are figured. For Dr. Worth, the explicitly ethnicized and racialized bodies of the Alpha patient population are figured against the bodies of women from presumably "non-ethnic, non-raced backgrounds"— that is, white women. These women, found in the private population, go unarticulated, but nevertheless function as the norm from which the bodies of Alpha patients deviate. The unarticulated, although undeniably normalizing, non-ethnic, non-raced, privately insured women against which Dr. Worth figures the ethnic and raced bodies of the "Alpha patient population" irrupt explicitly when Dr. Worth discusses the high(er) rate of C- sections performed at the private Omega hospital—a rate that is high when compared to the low(er) rate of these operations performed at Alpha:

WORTH: Yeah, and I also think this population [at Alpha]— they don't want C-sections. They are much less likely to want a C-section than the Omega population.

KHIARA: That's interesting.

WORTH: And that's a cultural thing. That's very much a cultural thing. I mean the perfect example: I think around a lot of the Chinese population, to have an induction of labor even seems unnatural—let alone a C-section. So, in fact, we had a woman—a Mandarin-speaking patient—who had a forceps delivery a couple of weeks ago. God forbid her mother-in-law found out! She couldn't tell her mother-in-law that she had an epidural. She couldn't tell her mother-in-law that she had forceps. So, it was very, kinda. . . . Then, I had another woman who I was calling—begging to come in for an induction. There were reasons to be concerned. And she just wouldn't come in for an induction of labor. So, there's a lot of resistance to *unnatural* deliveries among certain cultures. Whereas in the private population it's not necessarily the case.

Here, the private population is figured as being non-cultural and free (by virtue of their cultural lack) from misrecognitions of the presumptively curative potential of biomedicine. The obvious point to make is that, surely, there are Chinese patients among the privately insured at Omega. However, their "Chinese-ness" is rendered invisible by their class position. Any ethnic or cultural particularity they may otherwise have loses its explanatory power by virtue of their inclusion within the "private population." As such, the "private population" can remain the site of racial, ethnic, and cultural absence; it can remain antipodal to the "Alpha patient population," which, itself, remains the site of culturally produced misinformation and racially and ethnically produced pathology.

Another resident, Phillip Vincent, similarly described the patients who compose the "Alpha patient population" as possessors of cultures that blinded them to the benefits of biomedicine. I had asked Dr. Vincent to compare the levels of health between the patients he saw at Alpha and Omega. As I noted in the preceding chapter, he responded:

> In terms of general health, definitely they are healthier at Omega than at Alpha. And a lot of that is a culture thing. It is just my own personal experience. [At Alpha,] I have had problems getting people off fatty diets and they are diabetics. It is very hard because that is what they eat and their whole family eats it and everyone in their neighborhood eats it. It's their culture. They can't cook any other way.

For Dr. Vincent, the culture of his Alpha patients makes it impossible for them to follow his medical advice. Meanwhile, Dr. Vincent's private patients are either culture-free or their culture does not overdetermine their eating habits and diets.

Representing the "Alpha Patient Population": The Uneducated Immigrant

The racialist logic that structures the concept of "Alpha patient population" may be responsible for the frequency with which providers, staff, and administrators allowed the figure of the indigent, uneducated immigrant to represent that entire population. As I will discuss in more detail in the following chapter, the immigrant becomes a racialized figure when whiteness is made synonymous with the nation; those who are not of the nation become, by definition, non-white. One can begin to see the contours of the racialized figure of the immigrant emerge in an interview I had with a second-year resident, Dr. Patty Tyson. As with many of the residents—who, as part of the residency program, split their time between Alpha and Omega—Dr. Tyson professed to adore her Alpha patients in comparison to her purportedly arrogant, wealthy, and educated (to a fault) Omega patients. After being prompted by my question of whether she had been enjoying her residency at Alpha, Dr. Tyson asserted:

> TYSON: I love my Alpha patients.
>
> KHIARA: What is it about them?
>
> TYSON: I think it's like—you feel how much you're able to provide for them. I feel that most of the patients here, be it good or bad, come in with a completely clean slate. You say things to them, and then you have to explain everything that you're talking about. Because a lot of times they don't do what the private patients do: go online, look up everything on the Internet, and come in with their own knowledge. So, you're starting completely from scratch. And even if you're not, if you treat each patient that way, then you're educating them about everything that's going on in their body. And I think that they just really, really appreciate that.

Dr. Tyson appears to compress the entirety of the women for whom she provides prenatal care into the figure of the uneducated woman. The incredible range that characterizes the educational levels of the patients seen at Alpha becomes abbreviated into a "clean slate." Indeed, over the course of my fieldwork, I interviewed many women who were, for the most part, uneducated with regard to their bodies and otherwise; however, I also interviewed many women who had completed master's degrees in a range of subjects, many more who were college educated, and a wealth of women who lacked a formal education, but whose knowledge of pregnancy and their bodies rivaled their formally educated counterparts. For example, there was Julie, a soft-spoken Black woman who had been diagnosed by her Alpha obstetricians with vasa previa—which as previously mentioned, is a condition in which a blood vessel covers the cervical opening. Women diagnosed with vasa previa are advised to deliver their infants by C-section as they risk massive hemorrhage and death if the blood vessel ruptures when the cervix dilates in preparation for a vaginal delivery. Julie had sought a second opinion from another hospital, Lambda Medical Center; interestingly, the Lambda obstetricians had failed to see any obstructing blood vessel during the ultrasound they gave her. She had returned to Alpha on the day I interviewed her with a stack of information about vasa previa that she had obtained from Internet research. During her ultrasound that day, she wanted to confirm that she did, in fact, have it, and she wanted to learn whether any options other than a C-section were available to her.

KHIARA: So, they tell you that you have *vasa previa*. And the research that you found. . . .

JULIE: It could go either way. But, I need them to be sure that I need to have a C-section. Because the recovery time is so much longer. And I have things to do! [laughs] I know that sounds bad. I'm not going to tell them that. I'm just going to say, "Are you guys sure? And if so, please put it in writing." That's all. "My second opinion thought differently." And then I'm going to say, "I did some research." That's the thing. I want to do it today. I want to talk to them, and I want the doctors to come in and conference and talk amongst themselves before I see the High-Risk Clinic doctor next week. And I'm going to talk to her, too. I just want them to think "you don't want to mess with her. She's knows what's going on." You know what I mean? Instead of trying to pull the wool over my eyes and say, "Well this is what you *have* to do." Things don't *have* to necessarily go that way. Necessarily. I want to be sure.

KHIARA: Do you think that by demonstrating that you are intelligent, they are going to give you more options? Or that they are going to treat you differently?

JULIE: Yeah, I think that I want to show . . . It's worth a try.

KHIARA: Well, do you think that they are treating you a certain way now because they don't think . . .

JULIE: Yes! Especially when. . . . OK, how the machine is set up at Lambda is that while she is looking and checking and measuring and all that, I can watch. Here it's like [she indicates with her hand that the screen is not facing the patient]. So, you have to be like, "Oh, can I see?" And I asked her. And she was like,

"Oh, this is medical professional stuff, and you wouldn't be able to understand it." And that's where I want to be able to say, "I understand enough to know how many centimeters from the cervix the head is. I understand how the coloring on that Doppler machine works—it presents colors where there are vessels. And just show me! Show me what you're talking about! I'm an intelligent person; I can figure it out. And if not, explain it." But, they didn't want to do that. And she barely turned the screen. She said, "Well, you won't understand it." And then she went back to whatever she was doing. And it made me feel like, maybe my intelligence level wasn't up to par. So, maybe *I'll* educate myself and come back to her and say well, "What's up? Show me. You say this, but you can't show me." Even my Lambda doctor said that he was going to call and find out if he could get a picture of what they saw. Something. But, I don't think he did. I don't think he did.

Like Julie, Samantha, who was pregnant with her first child at the age of forty, was far from a "clean slate." Samantha described to me her amniocentesis and the meeting with the genetic counselor that preceded it:

SAMANTHA: They give you genetic counseling and just sort of tell you what the amnio is all about. They show you these pictures and all this stuff. It's very basic—for the general public. And then they schedule [the amnio] for you. I also had a book at home to tell me—so I knew what it was all about.

KHIARA: You said that there were pictures?

SAMANTHA: Yeah—there were these pictures of regular chromosomes. And then they had pictures of when you get your results back and the chromosomes are wrong. And then there were pictures of chromosomes if you have a Down's Syndrome baby. And another picture of something else—you know, of something missing the link. And so, she shows you each picture. And after each picture she says, "Do you understand what I'm talking about? Does this make sense?" And that's it.

KHIARA: Did you find the pictures very helpful?

SAMANTHA: Um—well, I don't know. For me, I understood it because originally, I wanted to be a scientist. I was a biology major in college. So, I understood what was going on.

KHIARA: So, was it a simplified version?

SAMANTHA: Yeah—it was. It was kind of like that. But, I think it was probably good for people that don't understand that or don't get it. So, it was a very simple sort of picture. Like, "This is your proper line of chromosomes—all connected. And this is what happens when one is missing." And then there's a break. And then she's like, "If this happens, it means your baby could have this." Simple. Designed for the general public.

I also met several patients who could not be accurately described as "clean slates" although they did not have extensive knowledge about medicine or science. I asked Nancy, pregnant with her second child, why she believed that she had not experienced morning sickness during either of her pregnancies:

NANCY: Okay, I can answer this question rather matter of factly, but I don't want to come off sounding arrogant. I'm. . . . I'm steeped in certain beliefs from my studies in diet and nutrition since I was in my twenties. And I really did do a lot of studies of these things. And I'm a firm believer in the idea that if you eat sugar and you have a lot of medication or toxicity in your body, that is what causes morning sickness.

KHIARA: OK. So, when you say sugar, is it even like fructose—like sugar in fruit? Or. . . .

NANCY: No, no, no. I'm talking about white, refined sugar. I'm talking molasses, refined sugar, artificial sweeteners. And it's a build-up—it's not about what you've done over the past year. It's about what you've eaten as a child.

KHIARA: And when did you start—studying, or reading about the diet?

NANCY: When I was twenty-one. My father was into this kind of thing. So, I was brought up pretty naturally anyway, in terms of food. And I had to stay away from food items and stuff. It sounds weird, but we didn't drink soda or things like that. And um, preservatives—not even, I mean, loaves of bread; they have to be just like wheat or something. Nothing artificial. Because in the '70s, that was when they were just starting to introduce all the artificial colors and preservatives in the food. My father was older—an old time person remembering when that wasn't the case. And he really believed that saccharin and Sweet & Low and all these preservatives were dangerous. He didn't know how, but he was concerned about it. He was born in 1914. So, he was aware of changes that were happening in society and the food supply. And he was into theosophy when he was younger. And like, when he was a teenager, he was taking cod liver oil and all these health type things in the 1920s. Which was kind of unusual.

KHIARA: So, he was like a man ahead of his time.

NANCY: But, a lot of people back then were into that Back to Nature movement with Emerson and Thoreau, and the theosophists. Like, kind of from the Victorian era—and Frederick Law Olmstead believing in patches of nature for the urbanites to make sure that children would grow up normal and stable. You have to have grass and air and a little bit of green—that was the philosophy behind Central Park. The Emerald Chain up in Boston.

KHIARA: Yeah, that's really interesting. And you've continued—you did the same with your first pregnancy, with your diet and everything?

NANCY: Yes. And that's—that's what I attribute to [my daughter] never having gotten sick. And I haven't had any morning sickness with this pregnancy either. And it's not—like I said, it's not about what you do for a year preceding it. It's about what you've done for a decade. You can't be toxic for a decade and then switch over to having a healthy lifestyle. Things are still in the system.

What is most unfortunate about Dr. Tyson's easy abridgement of her patients into a "clean slate" was that it rendered her unable to recognize their differing requirements and to tailor the short amount of time she had with each to meet their specific needs.

Compare Dr. Tyson's "clean slate" with a description of Alpha patients offered by another second-year resident, Dr. Steven Shander.

SHANDER: I think that they're probably more—our population is more trusting than a private population. They haven't gotten that wave of criticism of the medical profession than the [pause] more educated population has gotten.

KHIARA: I see. I see. So, you get a lot more. . . .

SHANDER: "Oh, OK. Thank you, doctor."

Dr. Shander expunges the diversity of educational levels achieved by Alpha patients and reduces them to obsequious recipients of the medical expertise supplied by their doctors. This is not to deny Dr. Shander's portrayal accurately reflects the behavior of many patients seen within the Alpha WHC. Rather, I wish to underscore that Dr. Shander's portrayal accurately reflects the behavior of only some of the Alpha patients; moreover, I suggest the figure of the uneducated, recent immigrant is she who is reflected in Dr. Shander's depiction. That figure comes to stand in for the whole of the "Alpha patient population"; a description of her behavior comes to be a description of the behavior of the entire population. Notably, Dr. Shander speaks of a trust of, and acquiescence to, the biomedical establishment that is wholly at odds with the distrust many scholars argue characterizes the relationship African-American persons have with it (Washington 2007). Dr. Shander's description of the "Alpha patient population's" compliance with medical orders does not account for African-American cynicism toward the palliative and therapeutic intentions of medicine, although African-American women were among the many women generally treated in the clinic and among the many Dr. Shander personally attended. The erasure of this narrative of African-American skepticism is required to reduce the complex whole to a singular population. Curious as to whether Dr. Shander would recognize the violence his facile description of patient compliance did to the vast array of relationships to medicine represented in the clinic, I asked him to elaborate on this point during a second, follow-up interview:

KHIARA: You said last time that the Alpha population tends to ask fewer questions than your Omega population. And you attributed that to the fact that some of them are not familiar with the critique of medicine. . . .

SHANDER: So, certainly, there has been a big change in the public's view of medicine. It used to be whatever the doctor said went; and, people just trusted blindly. But, because physicians have abused it—I mean, we really do have a lot of power in our position. People trust you with a lot—their lives, at times. Physicians have certainly abused that. And patients have become more savvy about that—challenge that; they don't just take what the doctor says at face value. But, that comes partly from education, and exposure to the media, and things. Which people who are of lower socio-economic status, and particularly immigrants, don't have much access to.

I do not take the irruption of the immigrant woman at the conclusion of Dr. Shander's statement as an offer of a specific instantiation of a "[person] who [is] of lower socioeconomic status" who has not had access to the critique of medicine. Instead, I take Dr. Shander's reference to the immigrant woman as that which motivates his analysis; she is the figure on whom he bases his entire understanding of the "Alpha patient population"; she is the figure to which the entire group can be comfortably reduced. Moreover, she is evidence of the shared logic of race and population as used within the Alpha WHC.

Compare Dr. Tyson's "clean slate" and Dr. Shander's obsequious patient with a description of Alpha patients offered by Dr. Janice Riley, another second-year resident:

I think a lot our patients here are not in a position to have as much involvement as other patients. I mean, I think when you have someone who has come to this country, doesn't speak English, maybe comes from a country where medicine was much more paternalistic, they don't—they don't know—I think, they don't—they just are starting at a different level in terms of what they're capable of understanding or having access to. Um, I definitely think there's definitely more people coming in, saying, "Whatever you think, doctor. Whatever you think."

Dr. Riley's comments closely parallel those of Dr. Shander. Dr. Riley, once again, comfortably reduces the entirety of the "Alpha patient population" to the uneducated immigrant.

In several other interviews, the identity of the uneducated immigrant became more specific, as many providers described her as emigrating from Latin America. For example, at the very beginning of an interview with a midwife, Paula, I asked her an ostensibly innocuous question about "the patients that [she] see[s]." After she affirmed that most of her patients were "low-income," I asked her if she had the occasion to observe health problems that were attributable to poverty. She responded:

> I feel that we have a special population—here and at Beta [the smaller public hospital where she also worked and where I also conducted fieldwork]—of women who, uh, probably are recent immigrants. . . . I think we see almost—a huge amount of Hispanic women, most of them recent immigrants. And I have actually found that most women are in very good health. . . . In general, I feel, people are very well-nourished. But, probably, nutritionally—that would be the biggest issue that I've come across. I'm not sure where it comes from—a
> lack of knowledge about nutrition, or a lack of resources to get good food in their communities or whatever. But, obesity and poor nutrition.

What is remarkable about Paula's description is that although it is undoubtedly true that Alpha and Beta hospitals count as patients many women from Latin America, it is also undeniably true the hospitals attend to large numbers of women who do not fit that description. Again, one of the most remarkable aspects of the Alpha WHC was the incredible ethnic, racial, and national diversity of the women who receive their prenatal care there. Moreover, because of Beta's location in the heart of Chinatown, the hospital attends to a large number of Chinese women. The elision of this diversity in such a way that the recently immigrated "Hispanic" woman can stand for the whole is a result of the analogous logics of race and population. Indeed, that a question about the relationship between health states and the poverty of the "Alpha patient population" could be answered by speaking about the health states of the recently immigrated woman from Latin America is telling.

On yet another occasion, which I discussed in the previous chapter, the "Alpha patient population" was similarly condensed to the figure of the Latin American immigrant when second-year resident Hannah Ferguson said, "I feel like a lot of our other patients are really not—they live like very healthy lives. Especially the little Mexican women that come in to deliver. I think they've never seen a doctor before they come in at, you know, nine centimeters. And they're like—they're perfectly healthy."

The explanation that race and population share similar logics of differentiation may explain why the "Alpha patient population" is a racialized notion, but it does not explain why it is that the Latin American immigrant emerged as the figure who stood for the whole of that population. Why not the figure of the immigrant woman from Europe—having acquired her undocumented status after overstaying her student's visa? Why not the U.S.-born white, African-American, or Puerto Rican woman—uninsured because the part-time college program in which she is enrolled does not offer health insurance? I encountered several women with these stories during my fieldwork. Why was not the Alpha patient population reduced to figures of these women? Again, why the uneducated, Latin American immigrant?

I offer two interpretations: First, "illegal immigrants" from Latin America—Mexico, most specifically—have been vilified endlessly in political discourse and the media. The undocumented have been held responsible for making the nation vulnerable through acts of terrorism as well as the leaching of state coffers. As conveyed in these discourses, the undocumented, parasitically and excessively (the excess being a function of the parasitic), make abundant demands on the goods and services provided by the U.S. government for its citizens; the overburdening of public hospitals by "illegal immigrants" is offered as an example of how this particular subgroup of the "undeserving poor" overwhelms state resources. Such discourses inform the perceptions of the Alpha providers I interviewed. They are affected, viscerally, by a demand for clinic services that far outstrips the supply. Indeed, these providers are those whose bodies enact the inadequate supply.

Consider an interview I had with midwife Carol, during which I asked her about her work conditions. She said:

> It's a depressing environment to work in because I think, at the end of the day, the provider and the patient both suffer a lot. It's not fair. And I don't really think that it should be that way. . . . Sometimes you feel like you're doing this at the expense of your life.
>
> I knew that it would be this way. It's the way it is everywhere. The problem is that I just get frustrated with it anyway because we are legally held responsible for any mistakes we make when we have three or four patients booked in a fifteen-minute slot. You have to rush. And it's just an unfair position to be put in—for both the provider and the patient. And sadly, it's the norm for public health. And probably will soon be the norm for private also.
>
> I have been here until 7:30 at night. The entire clinic's closed. There is no one here to book appointments. [The patients are] irate. You're hungry. I think patients absolutely notice it.

Consider comments made by a second-year resident, Cathy Orville, who described what she felt was the unique exploitation of doctors who do their residency in public hospitals:

> It's really frustrating. We're the cheapest labor in the hospital. Per hour, we earn less than the people who clean the floors. So, it's frustrating to be abused in that way. But, on the other hand, there is clearly not enough money to hire enough people to do those things. So, it's very frustrating when you've been up all night, it's 5 a.m., you haven't had any sleep, you have a medical degree and 100,000 dollars in loans, and you're pushing a patient down the hall because there's no one else to do it. It's frustrating. But, if you really expected something different than that at Alpha, then you really weren't paying attention.

The Alpha WHC is a hectic space, and the persons who work there are assaulted daily with often unrealistic demands upon their senses, physical bodies, and emotions. The already maligned figure of the uneducated, undocumented Latin American immigrant, then, is an easy and almost obvious surface onto which providers can project their exhaustion, frustration, and contempt for stressful working conditions. This does not mean that the providers "really" feel contempt for their patients; on the contrary, I believe that the providers I interviewed spoke truthfully when they claimed to "like" and "love" their Alpha patients. Rather, the trope of the uneducated, Latin American immigrant functions as a vehicle through which these providers can comprehend the exorbitant demands that are made of them on a daily basis as persons engaged in the public health industry.

Second, I interpret the Latin American immigrant as being a reflection of the staff's appreciation of the precarious nature of the lives of their patients. The uneducated Latin American immigrant is, perhaps, the most marginalized of the possible figures that might stand in for the "Alpha patient population." Her lack of education limits her potential to escape poverty, debasement, and exploitation—and her frequently undocumented status almost guarantees its persistence, as it renders her incapable of making claims on the state, except when she is pregnant in the state of New York. Indeed her undocumented status produces an intransigent vulnerability that is not shared by the "welfare queen," who has the privilege of citizenship and the concomitant substantive entitlements. The uneducated Latin American immigrant becomes a vehicle for the staff to vocalize their understanding of, and sympathy for, the plights of their patients. As Dr.

Shander stated, "The Alpha patient has a different attitude about the world, because the world shits on her everyday." The uneducated Latin American immigrant embodies the staff's appreciation of the injustices that describe and define many of the lives of Alpha patients.

ALTERNATIVE DEPLOYMENTS OF POPULATION

Although racialized population discourse was highly prevalent in the Alpha obstetrics clinic, there were also observable instances of resistance to it. However, these episodes and articulations were so infrequent and dispersed that it would be overly optimistic to refer to them as a counter-discourse. The most memorable alternative deployment of population occurred during an interview I had with a midwife, Sheila, a middle-aged white woman. I had been eager to interview her because she seemed to exude a definite hostility toward my project and my presence as an observer within the WHC. Indeed, at one point during my fieldwork, when another anthropologist (working on a project that was unrelated to my own and who had been previously unknown to me) began her own fieldwork research in the clinic, Sheila snidely remarked to me, "They say that molecules change their behavior when they are observed under a microscope. So, can you imagine the changes that *two* anthropologists are going to make in this clinic?" On another occasion toward the end of my fieldwork, I had been asked by my direct supervisor in the clinic to present my findings in a meeting attended by staff and providers. During my brief talk, I remarked about the absence of explicit discussions of race by both clinic staff and the patients to whom they attended. I continued that this absence stood as a dramatic counterpoint and contradiction to the obvious racial geography of the clinic, "where patients who are predominately of color are attended to by providers who are, predominately, not of color." Sheila, who was present at the meeting, took to sarcastically referring to herself as a "provider not of color" in the days and weeks following my presentation. So, it was a pleasant surprise when she agreed to sit down for a formal interview. As it turned out, Sheila was the most politically radical of the staff that I had the opportunity to interview in depth, and her apparent disapproval of my research (and me) was a product of her focus on the inherent power differential between my research subjects and me; they had no choice, on a multiplicity of levels, but to be observed by me. I could only offer her reassurances that I considered my project as one engaged in a politics of liberation.

Sheila's resistance to racialist population discourse was evident when I asked her to compare her Alpha patients with those she had attended as a midwife in a hospital in California that accepted both private and public insurance. Upon attempting an answer, she found herself stymied, as she could not comfortably speak about her Alpha patients with generalities: "There's a whole—there's other populations of women here who are pregnant and . . . you know. But—so yeah, I don't know. There are so many women here, I'm not even sure how to categorize them." In Sheila's reference to *"other* populations of women," she indicates an awareness of the population discourse that stymied her and in which she hesitated to participate—wherein risk, disease, and pathology define a singular "Alpha patient population." What is also interesting about Sheila's response is that although I asked her a question about differences between her "patients," she answered using the discourse of "population," even while problematizing it.

Later in the interview, when I asked Sheila why she believed Medicaid mandated the treble testing of poor women for sexually transmitted diseases and infections, her response evidences her struggle with the fact that the dominant population discourse pathologized the "Alpha patient population," yet such pathologization was the condition of possibility for a regime that over-tested all in order to reach the few for whom the excess of technology was actually warranted.

KHIARA: What I found is that there's repeat [testing for gonorrhea and chlamydia]. It's not usually. . . . It's not part of ACOG standards or anything like that.

SHEILA: At thirty-six weeks. Actually I don't remember. . . . It could be [Center for Disease Control] guidelines for high risk populations.

KHIARA: That's my question. This "high risk population" thing: what makes them high risk?

SHEILA: [long pause] You're talking to somebody who just got back, like, five positive chlamydias at thirty-six weeks.

KHIARA: Really?

SHEILA: Oh, and I just did that. . . . I was doing the research and so I was kind of asking myself that: high risk? Low risk?. . . . You know, is it sexual partners, is it . . . ? I was doing that work just in this last week. Oh, that's an excellent, you know, it's an excellent question. What makes somebody likely to have chlamydia again, or for the first time, at thirty-six weeks? I don't know necessarily the answer right now, but we catch chlamydia; so that's interesting to me.

KHIARA: I'm glad you told me that because I wouldn't have known otherwise.

SHEILA: Well, it's just silly—I mean to say "high risk"—as you are so intimately familiar. . . . To say "the immigrant population" is kind of like putting everybody into one category.

In this exchange, Sheila wrestles with the construction of the "Alpha patient population" as a "high risk population." This is a construction she appears to want to reject outright as "silly"—that is, if she had not "just got back five positive chlamydias." However, instead of allowing the Medicaid program's success at identifying five women who contracted chlamydia during their pregnancies to justify the construction of the whole "Alpha patient population" as at risk, Sheila articulates her desire to identify the conditions that justify the treble testing of a woman: to do the "research," to identify more precise risk factors. If she could discover those factors, she (and the Medicaid prenatal care program more generally) could respect the nuances within the "Alpha patient population" and, in so doing, avoid pathologizing the whole group. Also fascinating about this exchange is the analogy Sheila draws toward the end: "high risk" is like saying "immigrant population." The argument she seems to imply is that discourses of "high risk" and "immigrant population" fabricate a homogeneity from incredible heterogeneity.

Sheila imagines a way out of racialist population discourse with the concept of the "culture of women." That is, when one must speak in generalities about the patients served within the WHC, she posits that indexing the commonality of their womanhood avoids doing violence to their multiplicity:

When people talk about the need for culturally competent care here, it's the culture of women. How do we treat women? Like, how do we treat me? How do we treat you?. . . . So, in that, I think we provide incredibly good culturally competent care. I just don't always know how we serve all of our patient populations well because there are so many cultures. Like: a thirty-seven-year-old Bengali woman is so different than a thirteen-year-old sixth grader who is pregnant, you know. It's just—those are two hugely different women.

One can recognize her use of the plural of population as an act of defiance against a logic that would deny her patients their overwhelming diversity. However, Sheila's most poignant rejection of racialist population discourse came when she spoke of the clinic in Bali for which, in the weeks following our interview, she would leave her job at Alpha: she referred to her patients there as "a population of people."

CONCLUSION

In his analysis of newly developed practices of administering populations of individuals with histories of psychiatric events in the United States and Britain, Castel (1991) writes of a "new mode of surveillance" to which the individuals within the populations are subjected. This is a surveillance that is justified and actualized under the banner of "prevention." He observes that the aim of the "new preventive policies"

> is not to confront a concrete dangerous situation, but to anticipate all the possible forms of irruption of danger. "Prevention" in effect promotes suspicion to the dignified scientific rank of a calculus of probabilities. To be suspected, it is no longer necessary to manifest symptoms of dangerousness or abnormality, it is enough to display whatever characteristics the specialists responsible for the definition of preventive policy have constituted as risk factors. (289)

It appears obvious that a similar process is in operation in the Alpha obstetrics clinic.

PCAP/Medicaid is designed to anticipate all possible forms of the irruption of danger—dangers posed by possibly failing maternal bodies, by possible external threats within the social environments of the woman, by a woman's possible lack of commitment to becoming a "responsible" mother. PCAP/Medicaid, essentially, polices possibilities. This is justified on the basis that the policed group displays "characteristics" that have been, as Castel notes, "constituted as risk factors." Pregnancy presents itself as the base risk factor; its intersection with the second risk factor, poverty, comes to justify all the immoderation and intemperance that the state ultimately brings to bear against the pregnant poor.

And so, in the absence of any apparent or exhibited danger or abnormality, yet in the presence of assumptions about the behavior, lives, and moral worth of the pregnant poor, a program of prevention *for* the pregnant poor becomes a program of suspicion *of* the pregnant poor. In light of her production as a suspect, as a persona who must be monitored because of the danger she poses to her own child, should there be any wonder that instead of the expected irruptions of danger, the clinic instead witnesses irruptions of contempt for the space and the people who must perform that suspicion? In the following chapter, I explore these irruptions of contempt more expansively.

SIX

Wily Patients, Welfare Queens, and the Reiteration of Race

AFTER FINALLY RECEIVING AUTHORIZATION TO begin my fieldwork from all relevant Institutional Review Boards (IRBs), well over a year after I began the approval process, I was eager to begin observation of the Alpha Women's Health Clinic (WHC). Dr. Christina Smith, my direct supervisor in the hospital, suggested that I introduce my research and myself to the clinic staff at the clinic's monthly interdisciplinary meeting. Accordingly, my fieldwork began with my describing my project (within the five minutes allotted to me) to a motley assemblage of nurses, doctors, midwives, and administrative assistants who drifted in and out of the classroom over the course of the meeting.

Subsequent to my brief talk, the executive director of Alpha Hospital gave a presentation titled "The Alpha Hospital Mission and Vision." She described "the unanimous sentiment" felt by Alpha employees that working at Alpha was a challenging endeavor. The presentation continued with a relatively grim portrait of the hospital. She depicted a hostile state of affairs in which the players in the clinic were positioned in oppositional relationships to one another: hospital and clinic administrators against providers (which include medical doctors, midwives, and nurse practitioners), providers against ancillary staff (which include patient care associates (PCAs), intake workers, and registered nurses), and ancillary staff against patients. After the director concluded, Dr. Smith commented that, with regard to the acrimonious relationship between ancillary staff and patients, her personal observations supported the director's description. She said that she received a substantial number of complaints from patients who were angered by the way they were treated by staff persons. Indeed, over the course of my fieldwork, my notes became filled with descriptions of outrageously hostile interactions between the ancillary staff and patients. These displays of antagonism became a banality—something I could observe on any given day I was in the clinic. It was the ordinariness of these contentious interactions that compelled me to inquire into their significance, their causes, and their effects.

I was led to conclude that belligerent confrontations between staff and patients result from patients being viewed by Alpha Hospital ancillary staff as uneducated and unintelligent, yet somehow incredibly shrewd manipulators of the Alpha "system." The intersection of these contradictions in the fantasy of the patient seeking health care from Alpha produces a figure I call the "wily patient." The wily patient, although stupid (simply put), nevertheless possesses the ability to craftily and astutely exploit the hospital for the purpose of attaining access to undeserved appointments, ultrasounds, and other gratuitous health care.

ON WILY PATIENTS

Within Alpha staff folklore exists the wily patient—a health care-seeking subject whose crushing stupidity is matched only by her formidable duplicity. Alpha staff tends to perceive as contemporaneous these contradictory characteristics. In the next section, I explore the first term within the wily patient equation—patient stupidity. An exploration of the second term, patient duplicity, follows.

Patient Stupidity

At Alpha, pregnant women with appointments to see their prenatal care providers are required to collect and submit urine so its glucose and protein levels can be measured. Subsequent to giving the staff persons working behind the front desk her clinic card (on which is stamped the patient's name, address, and insurance provider), appointment slip, and registration receipt,[1] the woman is instructed to take a paper cup and plastic tube and "do your urine." Indeed, one of the first Spanish colloquialisms I learned when I began conducting patient intake was "Haga la orina"—"Make urine." The woman is then allowed entrance behind a secured door that separates the waiting area from the internal labyrinth composed of doctors' and nurses' examination rooms. The pregnant patient is expected to use the internal restrooms to urinate into the cup, pour the urine into the tube, and seal the tube with a rubber stopper. She will usually keep the tube of urine with her until a PCA calls her to take the urine from her and record her blood pressure and weight.

After being told to "do your urine" at their first two or three prenatal care appointments, most patients realize that they must submit urine at every visit and, as a result, without prompting, take a paper cup and plastic tube for the purpose of collecting urine. However, there are always new patients. These women are often confused when the person conducting their intake points to the stack of cups and piles of tubes on the front desk and simply says, "Do your urine." Consequently, there is the occasional circumstance where a woman so instructed returns to the front desk after using the internal restroom and attempts to hand the person conducting intake an uncovered cup of urine. Instead of understanding such confusion as resulting from a lack of proper instruction, these incidents are largely explained in terms of patient "stupidity."

I witnessed such an attempt one day when I was behind the front desk observing the clinic. Sandra, a PCA who took great pride in her Jamaican heritage and who was sitting beside me, also observed the confused woman's attempt to give Minnie, a Puerto Rican intake worker who had worked in Alpha for over twenty-five years, the cup of urine. She laughed at Minnie, who was contorting her face in disgust, and said:

> These patients do the strangest things. When patients do that to me, I say to them, "What do you want me to do with that? Drink it?" They do the strangest things. You tell them to pee in the cup, they bring back [feces] in the cup. I used to work in the urology clinic and you tell them to pee in the cup, and they come back with semen in the cup. These patients are so stupid. So stupid.

Sandra's comments about the stupidity of Alpha patients are representative of a sentiment shared by many of the ancillary staff, who largely understand the patients seeking care at Alpha to be "stupid" people who frequently manifest their lack of intelligence in "strange" ways. The above example of the confusion generated by a poorly clarified directive to "do your urine," and the willingness of the staff to place it within a larger ideology of patient stupidity, is one of many.

A patient's failure to respond to her name when it is called by a PCA, nurse, provider, or other Alpha employee is usually an event also explained in terms of patient stupidity. The circumstance of a patient failing to respond to an Alpha employee who has summoned her (and subsequent explanatory attestations of patient "stupidity") is a ubiquity in the obstetrics clinic, largely due to the considerable size of the patient waiting area, the poor acoustics in the area, the absence of a microphone to amplify the speaker's voice, and the formidable lengths of most patients' waiting times. Instead of understanding the frequency of patient unresponsiveness as a function of just those very attributes of the clinic, the frustrated speaker and her observing colleagues unfortunately tend to look to the intelligence of the patients (or lack thereof) to explain the phenomenon. Indeed, most patient behavior of which the staff disapproves is perceived as a function of patient stupidity.

My observations led me to believe that many of the ancillary staff members subscribe to an ideology of Alpha patients as dim-witted and obtuse. This, I believe, partially explains the regularity of polemical interactions between patients and staff. Indeed, many of these confrontations can be described as attempts by the staff to reprimand "stupid" patients and castigate them for their imbecility.

Because of the frequency with which patients fail to respond to employees calling their names, I was able to witness numerous "reprimandings" of such unresponsive patients when they were ultimately located. On one occasion (which is descriptive of many), Sandra had called out a particular patient's name, Tameka Jones, several times. When no patient in the waiting area responded, Minnie also called the patient's name. When still no patient responded, Sandra called several other patients and escorted them into the nurses' triage room to take their vital signs. Ten minutes later, Sandra returned and called out "Tameka Jones" once again. This time, she responded. When the patient finally made her way over to Sandra, Sandra said, "You're Tameka? Then why didn't you respond when your name was called? I said, 'Tameka!' 'Tameka!' If you're Tameka, then why don't you put your hand in the air so that I can stop shouting?!" Sandra continued scolding the woman as she escorted her to the nurses' triage room. At the start of the harangue, the patient had offered an apology and the explanation that she had not heard Sandra. But, as the rant continued, the patient became angry and eventually spat back, "I'm not the only Tameka in the world! And it's your job to call the names. Do your job!"

Yet, the mythos of the Alpha patient as largely stupid is enacted alongside a competing, contradictory mythos of the Alpha patient as a fantastically shrewd manipulator of the Alpha system. Indeed, one might argue that in staff lore, the patients' stupidity is matched only by their artful cunning. Although these two characteristics may appear to contradict one another, they happily coexist in the mythology of the Alpha patient and are remarked on alongside one another in daily interactions in the Alpha clinic.

Patient Duplicity

According to the story articulated and accepted by most Alpha ancillary staff, when one finds oneself performing intake work behind the front desk of the WHC, one must be prepared to defend the clinic against the pilfering of its resources by patients. According to this mythology, although it is deplorable that patients tax the hospital of its resources by their sheer existence as patients—each one demanding expensive services the cost of which the hospital can only hope to recover from depleted state and federal coffers—the leeching of the hospital's assets by the patient does not end there. Indeed, patients are not satisfied to merely consume reasonable portions of the public-hospital-as-governmental-largesse. Through their cunning, the patients attempt to steal more time than that allotted to them, more resources than those allocated to them, and more services than those deserved by them. Thus, Alpha intake workers must always be primed to identify patient greed and deception, then act to protect the hospital from exploitation.

The fear of the swindling of clinic resources is manifest in the belief that many obstetrics patients "steal" Medicaid from the hospital. As previously noted, because Alpha, as a public hospital, is obliged to provide medical care to all patients without regard to their ability to pay, all obstetrics patients are encouraged to sign up for Medicaid if they do not already have it. Medicaid coverage means the hospital ultimately will be reimbursed by state and federal governments for the cost of the services it provides pregnant women, as opposed to absorbing the cost of the care itself. Thus, located within the WHC, among the examination rooms, ultrasound scanning rooms, and sites in which to dispose of biological waste, is the finance office, which assists patients in the Medicaid subscription process. The expectation is that once the hospital has successfully aided a woman in her pursuit of Medicaid coverage of her prenatal care expenses, the woman will continue receiving her care at Alpha, allowing the hospital to receive

Medicaid money from the government. However, many private hospitals in New York City will accept patients with Medicaid coverage, although (unlike Alpha) they will not assist patients in applying for it. Consequently, there is an articulated worry among Alpha staff that many patients begin prenatal care at Alpha for the sole purpose of enlisting the hospital to help them acquire Medicaid, after which they will take their business (and the government dollars associated with it) to another hospital.

This fear was exemplified one day when a man approached the front desk while I was sitting there chatting with a PCA, Carla, and another intake worker, Yolanda. Both Carla and Yolanda had been born and raised in Jamaica and had worked in Alpha for well over three decades; moreover, both had reputations among the ancillary staff, providers, and hospital administrators for the lack of tact, patience, and kindness with which they dealt with patients. Although I came to love spending time with Yolanda, whose excitability and consequent impatience with the women who approached her became strangely endearing to me, I was disgusted by the way Carla treated patients and avoided her at all costs for many months. However, by the end of my tenure in the clinic, Carla and I had reached a relative peace, and she even took to calling me her daughter.

On this day, the man introduced himself and said that he would like to apply for Medicaid for his wife, who was pregnant. After checking the wife's name in the computer system, it was revealed that she had had a PCAP appointment during the prior week and was scheduled to return to the clinic for her initial obstetric appointment during the following one. Yolanda informed the man that his wife had probably begun the Medicaid application process at her PCAP visit. If she had turned in all necessary paperwork on that day, then the man and his wife could expect confirmation of Medicaid coverage in the mail. Apparently satisfied with Yolanda's answer, the man left. Carla then turned to me and said, "What they want is to get Medicaid here and then go take it somewhere else. A lot of patients do that. They get the Medicaid here, and then they take it to another hospital." Yolanda then told me a story about a woman who came to her first prenatal appointment after applying for Medicaid, "and then we never saw her again. They say they live in the Bronx or in Staten Island. That's too far from here. Think about it. They're not going to deliver their babies here."

What was remarkable about this incident was that there was absolutely nothing to indicate that the man was interested in "stealing" Medicaid. To the lay observer, he seemed like an average expectant father; probably anxious that he and his wife would not be financially prepared for their child, he decided to pay a visit to the hospital to confirm that all requisites for Medicaid coverage had been satisfied. However, Carla and Yolanda saw something quite different in the figure of a man inquiring into the Medicaid application process. They saw a trickster conniving to exploit the hospital by consuming a valuable service while fully intending to deny the hospital the ability to reap the rewards of that same service. Indeed, during my tenure at the clinic, Yolanda was in the habit of asking every patient with a PCAP appointment if she expected to deliver her baby at Alpha. If a patient expressed even the slightest equivocation, Yolanda would chastise her, telling her to "come back when you've made up your mind." I came to learn that it was irrelevant whether a patient anticipated continuing prenatal care and giving birth at Alpha; the hospital, by legal fiat, was obligated to provide health care either way. Accordingly, Yolanda's endeavor to have prospective obstetrics patients verbally affirm their commitment to continuing their care at the hospital was a contrivance aimed at protecting the clinic and its resources from patient chicanery. Indeed, if Yolanda succeeded in dissuading these prospective obstetrics patients, her contrivance would have "protected" the clinic from duplicitous patients by obstructing women's entitlements to services.

Moreover, what becomes readily apparent after a short time of observation of the Alpha WHC is that the demand for gynecologic and obstetric services far outstrips the supply. For obstetric services, the incommensurate relationship between patient demand and provider supply results in the "next available appointment" being some weeks in the future. For instance, after confirming her pregnancy with a hospital-administered urine test, a pregnant woman could wait another two weeks before she receives a PCAP appointment—a prerequisite that all patients must satisfy before receiving an appointment for the "initial obstetric" evaluation ("Initial OB") with a prenatal care provider. Similarly, the Initial OB appointment, which a woman receives at the end of her PCAP appointment, may be yet another two weeks later. Thus, a new obstetric patient at Alpha can wait over a month before she finally receives a medical evaluation of her pregnancy. Unfortunately, for women seeking gynecologic care, the situation is far more acute: there are frequent, protracted stretches of time during which no new gynecology appointments are available. Although the providers attend to patients who have scheduled their appointments in past weeks and months, no future appointments can be scheduled. Hence, women seeking to make new gynecology appointments (or to reschedule an existing one) are met with the announcement, "There are no appointments in the computer. Try calling next week." Exacerbating the problem of the unavailability of future gynecology appointments is that when such appointments are inputted into the computer by administrators for dispensation to patients, the appointments are often for months in the future.

This circumstance makes the gynecology appointment a scarce commodity, viciously sought by prospective patients desiring gynecologic care and jealously guarded by the employees charged with the duty of dispensing them. Complicating the matter is that, although the large majority of scheduled gynecology appointments are reflected in the computer system (to which all intake workers have access), there are some categories omitted. Examples of these include urgent recalls (given to a woman when a laboratory test reveals a condition that must be treated in a timely manner), emergency room re-visits (given to a patient when a provider sees her in the emergency room and desires to follow up with her during normal clinic hours), and "reproductive choice" appointments (the two-week follow-up appointment given to women who have had surgical abortions, which are not inputted into the computer system for confidentiality reasons). The result is that there are many occasions where a woman presents herself to an intake worker with the claim that she has an appointment for that day and is subsequently rebuffed when the appointment is not found in the computer system. I cannot gauge the frequency with which women actually fabricate stories about having made or been given appointments, and, undoubtedly some women do tell lies to receive gynecologic care—especially in light of the paucity of available appointments. However, the intake workers have come to construct all Alpha patients (present and prospective) as mendacious by default. The patients are perceived as shrewd raconteurs, cunningly spinning calculated tales in order to extract undeserved resources and services from the clinic.

As an observer, I witnessed innumerable patient attestations of having made or been given appointments and staff rebuttals of such claims with the statement, "These patients will tell you anything," or more bluntly, "That's a lie." When I began conducting patient intake alongside the other intake workers, I occasionally found myself confronted by patients claiming to have appointments that I could not locate in the computer system. My intake colleagues would find amusing the lengths to which I would go to verify a patient's claim—by asking the head nurse if she had recalled the patient, checking with the resident who I knew had the habit of telling her patients to simply come in (without the benefit of a scheduled appointment), asking the surgical coordinator if she recognized the patient's name, or soliciting a PCA to search the patient's electronic medical records to find some indication why the woman would justifiably believe she should and would be seen on that day. Sometimes, my intake colleagues would simply remind me, "These patients lie all the time." At other times, they would impatiently reprimand me with, "Don't let these patients run you around. They'll say anything." On one occasion when my attempts to verify a patient's appointment were unsuccessful, I enlisted Minnie's help. Her search to find the provider or nurse who could have given the patient the claimed appointment was similarly unsuccessful. After the patient sat down to wait for the nurse who she maintained had called her to give her the appointment, Minnie reproached me by saying, "You've been here long enough to know: don't believe what these patients say. They'll tell you anything."

It should be noted that some staff members subscribe to the trope of patient mendacity while being simultaneously sympathetic to patients' efforts to obtain gynecological care. After a particularly nasty exchange during which Carla brusquely and repeatedly denied that a patient had an appointment on that day and which culminated with the patient calling Carla "estúpida," Minnie turned to me and said, "No wonder she [the patient] got angry. You have to see things from their point-of-view sometimes. I know they lie and tell stories and things, but you have to put that to the side. They want to get seen. Shoot, I'd make up stuff, too—tell them that so-and-so called me yesterday and told me to come in."

The mythology of the duplicitous, prevaricating patient has such prevalence among staff that it retains explanatory power even when patients do not seek the clinic's scarce resources. The image of the patient as fundamentally deceitful is available to explain all manner of patient–staff miscommunication. The following example is paradigmatic: I overheard a patient, in heavily accented English, inform Trisha, a Bahamas-born nurse who I thought had exceedingly poor interpersonal skills, that the patient had received a blood test from the clinic a couple of days ago and she wanted to find out the results. Trisha muttered that she would call the patient into her office in a second. After Trisha left, the patient turned to me and, in Spanish, said, "She wasn't happy that I asked for my results. But, they're mine! If she doesn't want to give them to me, I'll just ask someone above her." I replied that I did not know why the nurse would be reluctant to give the results to her, but I was confident that the patient would be assisted. The patient answered, "I hope so. But, she wasn't happy that I was asking for those results." A couple of minutes later, Trisha called the patient to her office, as promised. Shortly thereafter, the patient reappeared, visibly upset. She said to me in Spanish, "She showed me the results on the [computer] screen; it was negative—which is great. But, I need to take them with me. I need the results in my hand. I have to go on a trip and I need to show those results. It's fine. I'll just go to another hospital." After the patient left, I went to Trisha's office to ask her why she was not able to give the patient a printout of her results. Trisha looked bewildered and said, "All she said was, 'I want to show my boyfriend.'" When I returned to the front desk, Minnie, who had overheard all the exchanges between the patient and me, asked me why Trisha had been unable to give the patient a hard copy of her results. After relaying what Trisha told me, Minnie said, "I told you: don't listen to what these patients say. They never tell the truth. They tell you one thing and then tell someone else a completely different thing."

It is possible to reconcile Trisha's and the patient's versions of the event without recourse to a trope of patient duplicity. That is, it is possible that the patient needed a printout of her results because she was going on a trip *and* she wanted to show them to her boyfriend. Indeed, her boyfriend might have been the person to whom she needed to show the results in order to go on her trip. Or, she may have needed to make the trip in order to see her boyfriend and show him the results. Furthermore, after having heard the patient speak to Trisha in English, it seemed relatively obvious to me that the patient was not fully proficient; her English was functional, but labored. In the face of what she perceived as Trisha's reluctance to inform her of the results of the blood test, it is understandable that her imperfect grasp of the English language would fail her and she would be unable to fully explain why she needed a hard copy of her results.[2] Perhaps she believed the struggle to find the English words for her thoughts would be ultimately futile, given that those words would be heard by someone who did not appear committed to helping her. To the patient, Trisha was someone who expressed displeasure at a simple request, someone who appeared preemptively unsympathetic. Nevertheless, instead of attempting to resolve the patient's narrative in a manner coextensive with Trisha's narrative, Minnie relied on the mythos of the untruthful, duplicitous patient. This case of what could have been patient–staff miscommunication simply served to reiterate to Minnie the veracity of the trope of the mendacious patient.

The two characteristics outlined above, stupidity and duplicity, coexist within the mythology of the patient. Although they are contradictory—indeed, if patients are as stupid as staff believe them to be, they would lack the intelligence to decipher the cumbersome and abstruse Alpha bureaucracy well enough to manipulate and abuse it—the Alpha patient nevertheless embodies the paradox. The intersection of these contradictions in the fantasy of the patient produces the "wily patient." Interestingly, the figure of the wily patient bears a striking similarity to another ubiquitous character within political and popular discourse: the figure of the "welfare queen."

ON WILY PATIENTS AND WELFARE QUEENS

Much like the wily patient, the welfare queen is discursively constructed as a marriage of contradictions:[3] She is uneducated, yet informed enough to make lucrative her reproductive capabilities. She is stupid, yet smart enough to shift to the government the costs of maintaining her (luxurious, or at least undeservedly excessive) lifestyle to the tune of billions of dollars a year. Descriptions of the welfare queen abound: "If one takes a serious moment to envisage what the 'typical' welfare recipient looks like, perhaps the image is one of an urban, black teenage mother, who continually has children to increase her benefits and who just lies around all day in public housing waiting for her check to come" (Note 1994, 2019).[4] In other descriptions, the excessiveness of the welfare queen's enjoyment of governmental largesse in the form of cash assistance is underscored: "At worst, the conjured image is one of a gold-clad, cadillac-driving [sic], welfare queen who buys steak and beer with food stamps" (2019).

Former President Ronald Reagan should be credited with introducing the figure of the welfare queen to the nation and ensuring her popularity. Reagan insisted that she was made possible by "extreme" redistributive policies and social programs authored by liberal politicians; moreover, she exemplified everything that was wrong with "big government." The welfare queen was strategically deployed by Reagan. As Smith (2007) writes, the figure of the welfare queen—and the extramarital sex and blatant immorality she implies—enabled Reagan to enlist the support of the religious right in his efforts to reduce the size of social welfare programs. In so doing, he reiterated the perception that "out-of-wedlock births, rather than structural conditions, . . . cause impoverishment among single-mother-headed families" (104). But, what was key in Reagan's construction of the myth of the welfare queen was the sense that the single mother who received public assistance took more than what she needed; moreover, the structure of the programs allowed her to do so. The "typical welfare mother was bent on extracting every last penny from the poverty programs by fraudulently exaggerating the neediness of her household" (106). Hence, we arrive at Reagan's oft-cited, hyperbolic fantasy of the welfare queen: "One of Reagan's favorite anecdotes was the story of a Chicago welfare queen with '80 names, 30 addresses, 12 Social Security cards and tax-free income over $150,000'" (Edsall and Edsall 1991, 148).

In the figure of the welfare queen, not only do contradictions intersect, but they appear to exist in an imperfect dialectic. The prospective welfare queen's lack of education and intelligence compel her, in the face of certain death/poverty, to shrewdly capitalize upon her childbearing capabilities, or, rather, she shrewdly produces children, for which the government compensates her. She calculatingly produces more children to increase the size of government payments to her. Her scheme is successful, as she avoids the necessity of selling her labor (i.e., working) while simultaneously enjoying anything from a comfortable to a lavish standard of living. However, her cunning ultimately reveals her stupidity: although she receives a cash subsidy increase for an additional child, the newest child nevertheless effects a reduction in the per capita income of her individual family members.[5] Her stupidity prevents her from realizing the failure of her cunning. And the dialectic continues.

Implicit Racializations: A Genealogy of the Welfare Queen's Blackness

Although the figures of the wily patient and the welfare queen are analogous insofar as both are paradoxical unions of incongruous qualities, an important characteristic distinguishes them: the welfare queen is decidedly raced as Black. "By the 1990s, the image of the welfare queen had fully developed, and visual images in the media routinely displayed her as a black woman" (Onwuachi-Willig 2005, 1971). Meanwhile, the wily patient, capable of being recognized in any patient who presents herself (or himself) to the front desk of the Alpha Women's Health Clinic, appears to be un-raced. That is to say, all patients seeking care or services from Alpha may embody the wily patient without regard to a patient's ascribed race.

But, it is important to keep in mind that the figure of the welfare queen has never been explicitly raced as Black. Rather, the figure allows those who refer to it to gesture toward race—to speak about it—without expressly mentioning race at all. As noted by Marian Wright Edelman, "'[W]elfare' is not a direct signifier for race. Instead, it is but a 'code word' for race" (Note 1994, 2019). In fact, it is possible to conceive of the term "welfare" as a failed euphemism for race. It has failed insofar as euphemisms are generally polite methods of referencing topics perceived to be impolite; yet, there is very little polite in the signifier "welfare" as it is presently understood. I am reminded of my interview with eighteen-year-old Monica, who I initially met when she was pregnant with her first child. At the time of the interview, she was five months pregnant with her second child. After she had apprised me of the breathtakingly massive number of hardships she was experiencing—finishing high school, securing child care and housing, negotiating her own legal troubles, and coercing her intermittently unemployed and incarcerated boyfriend to provide financial assistance for their children—I suggested that her burdens might be reduced somewhat if she applied for and received welfare. She expressed profound disgust at the prospect:

MONICA: I really don't want to go there. Welfare is not . . . my
          mother never had welfare. My sister's on welfare, but she
          really needs the extra money. But, I don't want to do that.
          My mother doesn't, so why do I have to?
KHIARA: Why don't you like it so much?
MONICA: Welfare just sounds so bad. It does.
KHIARA: But it helps, though.
MONICA: [mouthing the words to herself] Welfare. Welfare. [To
          me] It don't even sound right. I don't like it. Old people in
          the projects maybe. I don't do that. It would make me go
          crazy.

For Monica, even the word "welfare" itself did not "sound right." That is, the things welfare signified were so noxious that they had managed to corrupt the signifier itself. Indeed, there is very little euphemistically polite about welfare. Irrespective of whether "welfare" was ever intended to be a courteous term of art, very few would disagree that when one speaks of the "welfare queen," one is speaking of a derided, debased, and *raced* figure.

Race and Deservingness   Yet, how did the welfare queen become Black? To begin an answer, welfare discourse itself is a form of nationalism, and it is figured within a capitalistic, moral economy of "deservingness."[6] That is, "the culture of capitalism measures persons, as well as everything else, by their ability to produce wealth and by their success in earning it; it therefore leads to the moral condemnation of those who, for whatever reason, fail to contribute or to prosper" (Katz 1989, 7). Yet, within the culture of capitalism, those individuals "who, for whatever reason, fail to contribute or to prosper," are not uniformly condemned. Rather, within the space of condemnation, one can distinguish those who are not to blame for their failure to prosper from those who are blameworthy. The former are the "deserving poor," whose status renders them capable of receiving pity, benevolence, and compassion (as well as the largesse of the people through the government). The latter, on the other hand, become the "undeserving poor."

In the early nineteenth century, the categories of "poor" versus "paupers" referred to the deserving and undeserving poor, respectively. Katz (1989) quotes the Reverend Charles Burroughs's articulation of the morality of poverty, in which acts of God produced the situations inhabited by the deserving poor. Conversely, God played no role in the predicaments inhabited by the undeserving poor; rather, the undeserving poor produced these (ungodly) situations themselves (13).

A tour through the history of the welfare state reveals the moral economy of deservingness has had its own history, marked by shifts in the boundary that partitions the deserving from the undeserving poor. Unemployed mothers without husbands, predecessors to the "welfare queen," once had a position on the "deserving" side of the binary. Within the 1935 legislation creating the Social Security system resided the Aid to Dependent Children (ADC) program (which would eventually become Aid to Families with Dependent Children (AFDC)), a program that was intended to provide grants to widows with children. It was believed that through no fault of their own, mothers whose husbands had died were unable to support themselves. They were worthy of government assistance, clearly distinguishable from those who were poor as a "willful result of indolence and vice" (Katz 1989, 14). However, by the 1960s, the line of demarcation within the moral economy of deservingness had shifted, and unemployed mothers without husbands, who were once the apotheosis of deservingness, became positioned within the category of the undeserving poor.

But what explains the shift? Most theories point toward the cause of the husband's absence. That is, the husbands of the originally intended recipients of ADC were gone because they had died. However, by the 1960s, recipients' husbands were absent because they had voluntarily abandoned the family (through divorce or desertion) or they were never "husbands" to begin with; the women had never married the fathers of their children. Although this may partially explain why the categories of deservingness had been redefined such that by the 1960s they excluded unemployed mothers without husbands, it is ultimately insufficient because it ignores the racial demographics of those who received government assistance in the form of ADC in the 1930s as compared to those who received AFDC in the 1960s. It is imperative to note that most women who received ADC at the program's inception were white—and most women who were making claims on AFDC by the 1960s were Black. Many scholars have observed that public support for government programs aiding single-parent families deteriorated as the beneficiaries of the programs shifted from the white widow to the never-married Black mother. Onwuachi-Willig's work is exemplary: "Racist assumptions have turned public opinion and policy against providing the American poor with welfare benefits as the image of its primary beneficiaries changed from deserving, chaste white widows to lazy, never-married black baby-makers. As welfare recipients became racialized as black, standard rhetoric changed to implicitly blame welfare mothers for the impoverished conditions in which they and their families live and, consequently, for societal problems that often stem from poverty" (2005, 1664).[7]

I propose that the shift within the moral economy of deservingness is informed by the shift in the racial demography of ADC/AFDC recipients. Essentially, within a hegemonic devaluation of Blackness and Black people, a behavior is more easily censurable and subject to moral opprobrium when it is performed by a Black person. In other words, divorce, desertion and never-marrying can be aligned with less difficulty with "immorality" when it is Black women who are divorcing, deserting and being deserted, and never-marrying. Moreover, the alignment of divorce, desertion, and failure to marry with immorality, and consequently underservingness, allows the category of the moral, deserving poor to retain its whiteness. Simultaneously, the category of the undeserving poor can be populated by people of color.

This is not to suggest that the category of the undeserving poor can never include white people. Indeed, in light of this country's history of racial oppression, it might be more accurate to say the category of the undeserving poor was originally populated *entirely* by white people. To explain: the moral economy of deservingness has always been articulated in terms of whose claims to (or pleas for) assistance by the state should be acknowledged and satisfied. Katz (1989) quotes Josiah Quincy who articulated in

1821 the principle on which rested the laws that provided relief to the poor: "'The impotent poor; in which denomination are included all, who are wholly incapable of work, through old age, infancy, sickness or corporeal debility.'" These are to be compared with "'[t]he able poor . . . who are capable of work, of some nature, or other; but differing in the degree of their capacity, and in the kind of work, of which they are capable.'" (12). No one disagreed about helping the impotent poor; but the able poor were another matter: "'[F]rom the difficulty of discriminating between this class and the former, and of apportioning the degree of public provision to the degree of actual impotency, arise all objections to the principle of the existing pauper system.'" (12). However, because Black persons were formally disenfranchised and could make *no* claims on the state, one could argue that they were positioned outside of the moral economy of deservingness altogether. Accordingly, the controversy concerned who among white persons—who, by legal fiat, were the only persons who had relationships to the state—should be heard. Thus, the category of the undeserving poor was originally only populated by white people. It was only subsequent to the enfranchisement of Black persons that a Black person could come to embody a member of the undeserving poor. Enfranchisement ironically raised the status of the Black person such that he or she could belong to the dregs of society.

Deservingness and Capitalism   However, the relationship between undeservingness and Blackness requires more illumination. That is, to claim Black people's performance of a behavior facilitates the behavior's alignment with undeservingness may inadequately describe the discursive forces at work. A more robust version of the argument may be to claim that Blackness is always already aligned with undeservingness. The elaboration of this argument begins by recognizing that what has historically determined an individual's location within the moral economy of deservingness has been the ability of that individual to be perceived as either accepting or rejecting capitalism's values. Those persons who have failed to "prosper or contribute" within the culture of capitalism, but who do so other than as a result of a conscious repudiation of the needs and requirements of capitalism, are accepted as the "deserving poor." Those suffering from disability of mind or body who have failed to sell their labor power cannot be said to have rejected the mandates of capitalism; their disability has simply rendered them incapable of entering the market as purveyors of labor power. The same can be argued about the widowed mothers for whom ADC was imagined; these women failed to sell their labor not because of a rejection of the demands of market capitalism, but because the existence of their children demanded the women labor in the home where they could care for them. Conversely, those categories of persons who have been perceived as knowingly and intentionally repudiating the mandates of capitalism are branded as undeserving poor. Indeed, the undeserving poor are all persons who consciously fail to enter into the labor market and willfully refuse to sell their labor, and who therefore threaten the foundation upon which market capital is built.

It becomes clear that those individuals who do not suffer some incapacity, but who nevertheless refuse to sell their labor, are guilty of more than laziness or apathy. Instead, they imperil the very base upon which market capitalism rests: the sale and purchase of labor power. The "pauper" who spends his days beneath a haze of intoxication, the "tramp" who earns his sustenance not through a wage but through his guile, the able-bodied woman who (negligently, recklessly, or intentionally) produces children (the care of which effectively precludes her labor market participation, etc.): these figures all have the potential to reverse the fortune of the formerly "lucky" money-owner who enters the market in search of that special commodity with transformative powers. The undeserving poor are those fortune-changers. As described by Marx (1867):

> He who was previously the money-owner now strides out in front as a capitalist; the possessor of labour-power follows as his worker. The one smirks self-importantly and is intent on business; the other is timid and holds back, like someone who has brought his own hide to market and now has nothing else to expect but a tanning. (196)

Repudiators of capitalism's mandates, the undeserving poor, invert this narrative. Having saved their own hide from the market, they are thought to smirk with the expectation of their eventual receipt of governmental charity.[8]

Capitalism and "American"-ness   To understand the undeserving poor as always already Black, one must acknowledge that the values of capitalism are in synchrony with the values of U.S. nationalism, which is to say that those ideals that are espoused as "American" or are associated with "American"-ness are readily identifiable as necessary to the successful operation of a capitalist economy. Hence, those characteristics of the ideal wage-laborer—a "good" work ethic, the ability and willingness to "work hard," as well as thriftiness, self-denial, frugality, and economic independence—are also those characteristics extolled as "American."[9] Accordingly, the rejection of this personality—in the form of a perceived "laziness" and an aversion to work, as well as through demonstrations of extravagance, indulgence, intemperance, and economic dependence—is denounced as "un-American."

Indeed, a person cannot even begin the process of becoming "American"—that is, a person cannot immigrate to the country and apply for inclusion in one of the various categories of immigrant "legality"—unless she avers that she will not become a "public charge" and depend upon public benefits for survival. This prerequisite to inclusion within the United States is codified at 8 U.S.C. § 1601. This section, titled "Statements of national policy concerning welfare and immigration," makes explicit the connection between "American"-ness and economic self-sufficiency:

> The Congress makes the following statements concerning national policy with respect to welfare and immigration:
>
> (1) Self-sufficiency has been a basic principle of United States immigration law since this country's earliest immigration statutes.
> (2) It continues to be the immigration policy of the United States that—
>   (A) aliens within the Nation's borders not depend on public resources to meet their needs, but rather rely on their own capabilities and the resources of their families, their sponsors, and private organizations. . . .
> (5) It is a compelling government interest to enact new rules for eligibility and sponsorship agreements in order to assure that aliens be self-reliant in accordance with national immigration policy.

This immigration policy, which equates "American"-ness with economic self-sufficiency, is reiterated on Form I-485, the document persons must file with the U.S. Citizenship and Immigration Services to become a permanent resident, a category of "legality" that might be understood as liminally "American." Petitioners are asked to indicate, by checking a box "yes" or "no," if ever they "have . . . received public assistance in the United States from any source, including the United States government or any state, county, city or municipality (other than emergency medical treatment), or are you likely to receive public assistance in the future?" A reasonable expectation might be that, in light of economic self-sufficiency being a "basic principle" of national immigration policy, a box checked "yes" might result in the denial of the application.

It is because of the discursive alignment of "American-ness" with "economic self-sufficiency" that the recipients of welfare are condemned in the court of popular opinion as "un-American"; they are perceived to represent par excellence the laziness, work aversion, extravagance, indulgence, intemperance, and economic dependence that threaten the future of "America" (Hancock 2004). In the compelling words of Lubiano (1992), the figure of the welfare queen, a "human debit," derives its problematic status because "responsibility for the destruction of the 'American way of life' is attributed to it" (338).

"American"-ness and Whiteness   Further complicating the analysis is the relationship between "American"-ness and racialized whiteness. That is, one could convincingly argue that "American"-ness has been historically (and is presently) identified with racialized whiteness. This is an argument eloquently made by W.E.B. Du Bois (1903) in *The Souls of Black Folk*. In his description of the double consciousness, he argues that Black persons in the United States are always aware of their "two-ness,—an American, a Negro; two souls, two thoughts, two unreconciled strivings; two warring ideals in one dark body, whose dogged strength alone keeps it from being torn asunder" (17). That the "Negro" identification of the "American Negro" is at war with the "American" portion of her identification is due to "American" and "American"-ness being associated with racialized whiteness. Thus, the "American Negro," whose U.S. citizenship is her birthright, is produced as the unity of antithetical poles—that is, "American"-ness, and a "Blackness" that negates it. In light of the simultaneity of "American"-ness and whiteness, "American Negro" reveals itself to be an oxymoron.

The axiomatic relationship between whiteness and "American"-ness is handsomely revealed through the use of ethnographic data in De Genova's and Ramos-Zayas's *Latino Crossings* (2003). The authors illustrate how the unequal sociopolitical status of Puerto Ricans and Mexicans (itself a result of the politics of citizenship) causes racialized distinctions between the two groups. As evidenced by the informants' candid opinions about themselves in relation to the other "ethnic" group with which they shared the urban space of Chicago and against which they tended to define themselves, there was a distinct sense that "American"-ness and "whiteness" were coincident. Indeed, "American"-ness had more to do with race than with citizenship. As such, "[N]either for African Americans nor for Puerto Ricans does birthright U.S. citizenship secure the status of 'American'-ness, which constitutes a national identity that is understood, in itself, to be intrinsically racialized—as White" (78). So powerful is the identification of "American"-ness with racialized whiteness that one Mexican informant articulated his sense that his proximity to "American"-ness, as demonstrated by his acceptance and enactment of putative "American" (read: capitalist) values, was linked to his ability to approximate an "Italian" phenotype (70).

The Always Already Blackness of the Undeserving Poor   We can now begin to see how the undeserving poor might be understood as always already Black. To the extent undeservingness is defined as the rejection of the values necessary to the functioning of a capitalist economy, and that capitalism's values define (and, consequently, are synchronous to) those values espoused as "American values," undeservingness describes an individual's distance from "American-ness." When one recognizes "American"-ness exists within discourse as "whiteness," the undeserving poor's distance from "American"-ness is their distance from "whiteness." Within the hegemonic bipolarity of white supremacy in the United States, a distance from "whiteness" results in an approximation to Blackness— hence, the always already Blackness of the undeserving poor.

This explains the racialization of the archetype of undeservingness, the welfare queen. The always already Blackness of the undeserving poor accounts for the persistence of the discursive construction of the welfare queen as Black—this in spite of the fact that Black women do not make up a majority of welfare recipients. No matter: the figure of the welfare queen continues to imply Black women. To borrow Lubiano's language again:

> [I]t does not matter that all such children needing state care are not black, or that poverty and unemployment are reasons that they need state care; what matters, what resonates in the national mind's eyes, is the constant media-reinforced picture of the welfare queen—always black. (1992, 340)

Although the figure of the welfare queen is very infrequently referred to in explicitly racial terms, its Blackness nevertheless remains, enduring and intractable.

Implicit Racializations: The Race-ing of the Wily Patient

It would appear that race represents a point of departure between the wily patient and the welfare queen; whereas the welfare queen is implicitly raced as Black, the wily patient is not similarly constructed. Insofar as the wily patient gets located in the thousands of patients attended to within Alpha Hospital, and insofar as Alpha patients are profoundly racially and ethnically diverse, the wily patient cannot be said to possess an exclusive racial ascription or identification. The wily patient is raced in accordance to the ascribed race of whoever happens to present herself within the hospital at any given moment. Or so it would appear.

In fact, a more critical "reading" of enactments of perceived patient wiliness intimates that the wily patient is, like the welfare queen, implicitly raced. To be precise, a close examination of the ethnographic data reveals that when patients are perceived as stupid, their supposed stupidity is often a function of their ascription as a racial Other. Similarly, professed patient duplicity is often a function of the ascription of "foreignness" to the alleged duplicitous party. The following example is illustrative.

A little background information: prior to receiving health care at Alpha Hospital, every patient must acquire an Alpha clinic card from the business office. On the card is printed the patient's name, address, the type of insurance a patient has (or if the patient pays out-of-pocket for medical services), and a medical record number (which is assigned to the patient by the business office when she first requests a clinic card). The only exception to this procedure is when a patient who has never received health care from Alpha seeks medical services in the Alpha emergency room (ER). Under such circumstances, the ER will assign the patient a medical record number, although the patient will later have to obtain a physical clinic card from the business office during regular business hours. The deceptively innocuous clinic card is an important item that a patient is reminded to bring with her to every visit as the raised characters on the card enable the patient's medical documents to be stamped with the patient's information. Additionally, appointments are tracked by entering the medical record number on the card into the computer.

One day when I was observing the clinic, a Spanish-speaking patient approached the desk and indicated to Yolanda that she had come for her initial obstetric ("Initial OB") appointment. (During the Initial OB appointment, which is scheduled for the woman at the end of her PCAP visit, the patient receives her first medical examination from a health care provider.) However, when Yolanda entered the patient's medical record number into the computer, no appointment was found. When Yolanda began telling the patient (in English) that she did not have an Initial OB appointment and asking her why she thought she had one (considering that the computer indicated that she had not even had a PCAP appointment), the patient gestured to me and asked me if I could translate for her. She told me that she had had a PCAP appointment the week before. However, at her PCAP appointment, she had used the name "Manuela Tenemaza"; consequently, all the prenatal care documents that would follow her throughout her entire pregnancy at Alpha had been stamped with "Manuela Tenemaza" and the medical record number assigned to that name. However, the patient told me her name was actually "Maria Galarza," and "Maria Galarza" (with a new, corresponding medical record number) was the name on the clinic card she had obtained from the business office after her PCAP appointment.

I asked Maria how it had come to pass that her actual name was entirely different from the name she had used on the day of her PCAP appointment. She answered that her first name is Maria, her middle name is Manuela, her maiden name is Tenemaza, and her husband's name is Galarza. She showed me her Ecuadorian passport, which verified that her name prior to her marriage was indeed Maria Manuela Tenemaza. She also showed me her husband's identification card, which indicated that his last name was indeed Galarza. She went on to explain that her PCAP appointment had been made by a nurse in the emergency room. She had sought medical attention from the ER after experiencing several days of persistent nausea and vomiting; it was at this ER visit that she discovered her pregnancy and the PCAP appointment was made. On that day, no one in the ER spoke Spanish. Moreover, when the nurse asked her for her name and how to spell it, Maria gave the nurse her passport. She said that she wanted to explain to the nurse that she was now married and her last name was now "Galarza," but she could not think of the English words with which to express herself. At any rate, the ER nurse had recorded her middle and maiden names as her name and assigned to this name a medical record number. When Maria went to the business office after her PCAP appointment to get a clinic card, she explained the error in Spanish to the person working there, and she was made a clinic card with her correct name and a new corresponding medical record number.

Maria's story seemed wholly truthful to me. Moreover, because Spanish is a second language for me, I can perfectly understand how the words of a relatively new language can fail to come to the non-native speaker, especially when she finds herself in a stress-inducing circumstance or environment. Moreover, the discovery of an unplanned pregnancy—particularly when that discovery occurs within the ER of a public hospital where no one, at the moment, speaks your first language—certainly qualifies as a stress-inducing circumstance and environment. Nevertheless, when I recounted Maria's explanation to Yolanda, she was unconvinced. She rhetorically and repeatedly asked, "She can't decide who she is?", and, "She doesn't know her own name?" In effect, Yolanda asked if Maria was deceitful or stupid, invoking both sides of the wily patient equation in one breath. Moreover, Maria had attempted to explain to the nurse who had attended to her during her PCAP appointment (a nurse who, significantly, spoke very little Spanish) that her name had been recorded erroneously. This nurse, who had frequently and good-naturedly teased me about the fact that I always carried with me a notebook in which I jotted down observations, approached me after hearing Yolanda's complaints and said, "I hope you write this down in your little book. I asked her [during her PCAP appointment] how she ended up with the wrong name. She said, 'I was in the emergency room and there were a lot of people around . . .' So many people that you forget your name? No. This is an example of a lie coming back to bite you in the butt." Maria Manuela Tenemaza Galarza's story could have been understood by the Alpha staff as an example of patient vulnerability and the ability of the space of the hospital to intimidate and, consequently, disempower the persons who seek health care there. Unfortunately, it instead served to reiterate to the Alpha staff the duplicity of the patients and the concomitant verisimilitude of the figure of the "wily patient."

Similarly, perceived patient stupidity, the other half of the "wily patient" calculus, is often attributable to some aspect of the patient's Otherness. This relationship was illustrated one day when an elderly Asian woman approached the front desk and said to Minnie, "Appointment." Minnie understood the statement as a request that she make a gynecology appointment for the woman. Because there were no available gynecology appointments showing in the computer system, Minnie responded, "You have to call next week to make an appointment." The woman's facial expression made it fairly obvious that she did not understand what Minnie had said to her. In situations like these, where the patient and the staff person do not speak the same language, the front desk workers are instructed to dial an extension on the telephone that will connect them with an interpreter service. The employee is then asked to designate the language for which interpretation services are requested. Once the desired interpreter is on the telephone, the staff person can communicate with the patient by having the interpreter translate the communications between staff person and patient. Accordingly, when the elderly patient did not appear to understand Minnie's direction to call the clinic at a later time, Minnie asked, "Do you speak Mandarin or Cantonese?" Again, the woman's facial expression indicated that she still did not understand what Minnie had asked her. In situations like these, where the patient does not understand the English word for the language she speaks, front desk workers are instructed to show the patient a slip on which "I speak . . ." is written in Spanish, French, Polish, Bengali, Mandarin, and Cantonese. The patient can then point to the language she speaks and the appropriate interpreter can be called. However, instead of showing the slip to the patient, Minnie picked up the telephone, dialed the extension for interpreter services, and asked to be connected to a Mandarin interpreter. She then asked the Mandarin interpreter to ask the patient, in Mandarin, if she spoke Mandarin. The patient did not understand. Minnie, deducing that the patient spoke Cantonese, proceeded to get a Cantonese interpreter on the telephone who was able to successfully broker communication between Minnie and the patient.

After the patient left, I told Minnie that she had solved the problem quite cleverly, but why had she not simply shown the patient the "I speak" slip and asked her to point to the language in which she wanted to communicate? Minnie responded, "Because they can't read." Puzzled, I responded, "Who can't read?" Minnie explained, "The patients. The patients can't read." Her blanket generalization perplexed me, and I could not hide my confusion. In response, Minnie said, "Trust me. These patients can't read." Minnie did not seem to realize that her interaction with the patient who had sparked this statement directly contradicted her assessment of patient literacy: this Cantonese-speaking patient had written on a piece of paper the clinic's phone number in Cantonese characters before she left.

Minnie's low opinion of the literacy of the patients seeking health care from Alpha was not confined to those she identified as Asian; comments she made over the course of my time in the hospital revealed that she generally considered the patients unlearned and uneducated. For example, on one occasion, a PCA named Linda was chatting with a group of bilingual, Spanish-speaking staff members about a Spanish language test she had recently failed. Linda, who had immigrated as a child to the United States from Jamaica, was taking the Spanish class as part of a course of study that would ultimately enable her to become licensed as a registered nurse. She was jokingly lamenting her poor Spanish language skills when Minnie remarked, "You are not going to use the Spanish you learn [in that Spanish class] because most of the people here haven't gone to school. They won't understand you. For example, if I say to them, 'Su prueba de embarazo salió positiva' ['Your pregnancy test was positive'], they won't understand what I'm saying. But, if I say, 'Está embarazada' ['You're pregnant'], they will understand." She continued, "These people didn't learn Spanish in school. They learned it from their parents. And they are going to teach it to their kids—just like they learned it." Remarkably, Minnie did not believe that the Spanish Linda was learning in school would, in the end, be usable as the patients with whom she would communicate would be unfamiliar with medical terminology or phrases as a product of an utter lack of familiarity with or incomprehension of biomedical discourse generally. Rather, Minnie believed that Linda's patients would find her school-acquired Spanish incomprehensible because they had not received a formal education and were, therefore, uneducated.

However, my experience directly contradicts the claim that Spanish speakers at Alpha would not understand a person whose Spanish was learned in school. I began studying Spanish in grade school, became fluent in college, and refreshed my fluency in graduate school. To my knowledge, none of the Spanish-speaking patients with whom I interacted at Alpha had trouble understanding my Spanish. Moreover, Minnie's assertion that patients would not comprehend the phrase "su prueba de embarazo salió positiva" was disproved almost daily, as patients constantly approached me and informed me that they needed to begin prenatal care because they took an at-home pregnancy test and "la prueba salió positiva." I found that although many patients exhibited a certain level of estrangement from biomedical discourse, most of those with whom I interacted were sufficiently fluent in biomedical terminology to understand those phrases that had become part of common parlance, such as "la prueba de embarazo salió positiva." Moreover, as their medical records revealed, most Spanish-speaking patients seeking health care from the WHC who were not born in the United States had received many years of formal education in the countries from which they emigrated. Now, it is possible that *some* patients had received no formal education in their countries of birth. However, Minnie had conceptualized the exception as the rule and declared all Spanish-speaking patients to be uneducated.

What deserves underscoring is that the wily patient, that simultaneously obtuse and duplicitous character, is a figure constructed by Alpha staff about patients who are largely racialized as something other than white. Thus, the wily patient is frequently and most often enacted by nonwhite individuals. What is revealed after some observation is that demonstrations of perceived patient stupidity time and again correspond with patients' ascription as migrant, immigrant, foreign, not "American," and otherwise undeservingly poor. Similarly, expressions of perceived patient duplicity regularly correlate with the patient's racialized Otherness. A reasonable interpretation is that patient wiliness—that is, the simultaneous duplicity and stupidity believed to be exhibited by those seeking gynecologic and obstetric care at Alpha Hospital—is a function of the patient's racialization as Other. One can say that the wily patient and the characteristics that define her are products of Alpha patients tending to be racial minorities. The wily patient, then, is an implicitly raced figure after all. In this way, the wily patient allows the Alpha staff to "speak race" and manipulate it within a political climate and particular social location that do not condone explicit discussions and manipulations of race.

The implicit racialization of the wily patient reveals that there is a closer affinity between it and the welfare queen than was previously imagined. As noted above, the welfare queen is itself a figure that, like the wily patient, is only implicitly racialized. As noted above, "welfare" is a "code word" for race, not a synonym. Smugly race-neutral on its face, references to "welfare" authorize debates about whether race is really what is under discussion. Harrison (1998) makes this point when she notes, "We find ourselves debating whether current political discourses on . . . welfare reform . . . encode race and reinforce racial domination. . . ." (610).[10] The figure of the welfare queen functions to disarticulate race, while ironically, simultaneously allowing those who conjure it to evoke race nonetheless. In this way, the welfare queen appears to be a not-so-distant relative of the tacitly raced wily patient whose racial Otherness is mostly unmentioned but constantly suggested. Hence, the wily patient is more like the welfare queen in racial terms than not, both for its dissimulation of race and its evocation of it nevertheless.

The similarities shared by the figures of the wily patient and the welfare queen, in terms of the contradictory characteristics that define them as well as their common implicit racialization, might not be understood as a mere fluke. That is, the welfare queen and the wily patient are parallel figures because the latter might be understood as a simple reflection of the former as she is imagined in the particular social context of a public obstetrics clinic where the "undeserving" poor are provided with Medicaid to finance their pregnancies. One might even argue that welfare legislation, which generates the welfare apparatus begrudgingly and with a contemporaneous problematization of those who benefit from it, produces the wily patient insofar as she is, by definition, a potential/possible/likely welfare queen. To take an argument made by Piccato (2001) in his incisive study of early twentieth-century criminology in Mexico and adapt it for my own purposes, Temporary Assistance for Needy Families (TANF) and its coercive, punitive, and reluctantly charitable state strategies have perpetuated the vilified figure of the welfare queen; moreover, it has created suspected welfare queens out of poor women. To the extent that the wily patient is marked as poor by her mere presence at a public hospital, she should be considered the embodiment of that suspicion. In other words, the wily patient might be understood as that which is engendered when suspicion of the welfare queen's presence is materialized within the WHC. The point is underscored if one considers that, at Alpha, the wily patient is frequently manifested precisely during her pregnancy. The wily patient's pregnant body is not read as a symbol of infinite possibility, joy, or self-fulfillment—a reading that may only be reserved for the non-poor. Rather, in light of TANF and the condemnation of welfare mothers in political and popular discourse, the (poor) wily patient's pregnancy is realized as the event that makes the welfare queen possible, the condition that makes the entire welfare apparatus necessary.

A caveat: although some may refer to any means-tested public assistance as "welfare," none of the Alpha patients with whom I spoke considered themselves to be "on welfare" or otherwise "collecting welfare" by virtue of their receipt of Medicaid. Rather, to most, "welfare" referred to cash assistance from the government and was understood as reserved for the most impoverished of the poor; Medicaid, on the other hand, represented for them a less stigmatized aid.[11] The distinction between "welfare" and "Medicaid" was vigorously defended by many of the women with whom I spoke.

THE BLACKENING/"ALIEN-ATION" OF THE WILY PATIENT

Although the figure of the wily patient is believed to be enacted by patients who tend to be persons of color, not all Alpha patients are such. That is, there are white persons, although a minority, among Alpha patients. That the wily patient is implicitly raced as a minority might be taken to suggest that those patients who are identified by staff as white would escape expectations of wiliness; the theory would be that when a staff member is confronted with a patient whose overt racialization directly contradicts the tacit racialization of the figure of the wily patient, the attribution of patient wiliness would fail. If true, white obstetric and gynecologic patients at Alpha would be perceived as less inclined to exhibit the supposed stupidity and cunning that define and characterize the wily patient. However, this expectation would prove to be unfounded.

The ethnographic data I have gathered does not support the claim that white patients at Alpha escape ascriptions of patient wiliness. The Alpha ancillary staff appeared to be equal opportunists insofar as any person who approached the Alpha reception desk was marked as suspicious. All persons who approached the OB/GYN desk were wily by default, by virtue of their physical location on the supplicant side of the desk that physically and metaphorically divided the staff from those seeking health care. The question that must then be posed is whether the implicit racialization of the figure of the wily patient is somehow mitigated by the fact of some Alpha patients' ostensible whiteness. Does the fact the wily patient is occasionally enacted by persons identified as white make the wily patient a race-neutral figure?

An examination of the figure of the welfare queen indicates that the question must be answered no. The welfare queen's racialization as Black is accomplished despite the demographics revealing that Black women do *not* comprise the majority of welfare recipients. According to statistics compiled by the Department of Health and Human Services and released in 2006, Black women accounted for only 35.7 percent of persons receiving welfare in the form of TANF; the majority is made up of white (33.4 percent), Latina (26.5 percent), Asian (1.8 percent), and Native American (1.4 percent). However, the statistics may be read as damning as Black women represent a preponderance of TANF recipients and disproportionately receive welfare-qua-TANF. However, these same numbers in no way demonstrate that the figure of the welfare queen ought to be racialized as Black. Instead, the data evidences that of every five TANF recipients, only two are Black. This hardly justifies conceptualizing the figure of the welfare queen as a Black woman. Nevertheless, it is so conceptualized. Expressed differently, the frequency of white and Latina recipients of welfare has not jeopardized the integrity of the construction of welfare as Black. Likewise, the (in)frequency of white wily patients does not jeopardize the durability of the construction of the wily patient as not-white.

The Wily Patient and the Black/White Binary

The figure of the wily patient is implicitly racialized as not-white, notwithstanding its intermittent enactment by patients who are racialized as white, because one may understand *all* Alpha patients to be racialized as not-white. This ostensible paradox may be unraveled by turning to legal scholar Cheryl Harris' review of *Whitewashing Race* (Brown, 2005). Harris begins with a defense of the "Black/White paradigm" of U.S. race relations, a lens which views "racial subordination as reflected by dichotomous constructions of Blackness and Whiteness." (2006, 915). She cites the authors' defense of their methodological choice to employ this paradigm in their endeavor to contest colorblind conceptions of race and racism:

> Whiteness in the United States has never been simply a matter of skin color. Being White is also a measure, as Lani Guinier and Gerald Torres put it, "of one's social distance from Blackness." In other words, Whiteness in America has been ideologically constructed mostly to mean "not Black." The increasing numbers of Asians and Latinos in the United States and the development of a Black middle class have not changed this ideological construction of Whiteness. . . . [The] dichotomy [is] not between Black and White, but between Black and non-Black. (916)

The Black/White paradigm is essential for understanding the bipolarity that characterizes U.S. racial dynamics. However, although Guinier and Torres conceptualize the racial dichotomy as Black/non-Black, this seems to conflict with ontologies of race throughout this country's history. History appears to show that Blackness was perceived to be self-evident; whiteness, alternatively, required demonstration. That is, the struggle has been for immigrant groups to demonstrate their whiteness, not their non-Blackness, within the hegemonic bipolarity of white supremacy. Indeed, Haney-Lopez's reading of the prerequisite cases illustrates that it was the petitioning immigrant's whiteness (as opposed to his non-Blackness) that was in dispute; it was the petitioner's burden to prove his whiteness, which would enable his naturalization as a U.S. citizen. Haney-Lopez verifies this reading, noting that courts have defined the white race "through a process of negation, systematically identifying who was non-White" (20). Accordingly, I find it more useful to dichotomize the Black/White binary in terms of white/not-white, in lieu of the Black/not-Black interpretation proposed by *Whitewashing Race*.

However, what is being described by the Black/White binary is not racialization per se; rather, the binary describes racial power and the racial privilege contemporaneous with it. On this point, Harris offers the following:

> Within the Black/White binary that undergirds prevailing social relations, "Black" and "White" signify ideological concepts and do not operate as phenotypic markers, nor even as racial categories in the sense of creating socially constructed communities. Rather, Black and White are relationally constructed. Whiteness is the position of relative privilege marked by distance from Blackness; Blackness, on the other hand, is a legal and social construction of disadvantage and subordination marked by the distance from White privilege. (917)

Yet, the racial politics present within the WHC demand at least some qualification of the Black–White binary. To read the degradation of the racial status of Alpha patients as, always, an approximation to Blackness, denies the work citizenship does to produce ambiguities, ambivalences, and incoherencies within the simple Black–White bifurcation.

In an insightful and compelling problematization of the Black–White binary, De Genova (2006) argues that it denies the work the figure of the Native American has performed in the history of the United States to make whiteness synchronous with the nation. Although African Americans were figured as the subjugated and subjugatable Other within the bosom of the nation, Native Americans were figured as the inassimilable, inexorable savage that lay just outside of the borders of the nation. De Genova contends that this category of the racialized outsider has persisted and has come to be occupied at various points in U.S. history (as well as at present) by Latinos and Asians. The perceived "foreignness" of Latino and Asian immigrants, which tends to appear as a simple question of citizenship, is that which excludes them from whiteness: "To be Latino and Asian within the space of the U.S. nation-state or its imperial projects has . . . nearly always meant having one's specific national origins as well as cultural, religious, and linguistic particularities—in short, the convoluted amalgam of one's foreign or alien status—rendered virtually indistinguishable from a conclusively racial condition of nonwhiteness" (12). De Genova does not claim that the experiences of Latinos and Asians within the United States are reducible to that of Native Americans; rather he endeavors to illuminate how the Black–White binary makes invisible the work that the enduring trope of the racialized outsider does to dia-critically produce whiteness as the position of racial privilege. "[T]he ra-cialized equation of Latinos and Asians with foreignness and their figura-tion as inassimilible aliens and permanent virtual immigrants" (3) is essential and must not be reduced to Blackness; instead, it is a distinctly Othered position from which the whiteness of the Self-as-Nation can be reiterated.

When considering the racial Othering of Alpha patients, one must bear in mind that the degradation of their racial status is frequently accom-plished through the reading of patients as not only undeserving (and, by implication, "Black"), but also as ineluctably "immigrant" and intractably "foreign." Which is to say, the racialization of patients is often produced by perceiving patients as the elided and sublimated third term of the Black–White binary. Further, the racialization accomplished by the reading of patients through the trope of the non-citizen immigrant outsider cannot properly be understood as an approximation to Blackness because—and this point bears underscoring—Blackness presupposes citizenship. Indeed, citizenship is the condition of possibility for the presumptively Black wel-fare queen; it is the welfare recipient's status as a U.S. citizen that enables her to make claims on the state. In its allowance of non-citizens to make claims on the state in the form of Medicaid during their pregnancies, New York State enables the non-citizen to reflect undeserving citizenship and, consequently, reflect Blackness. Yet, this approximation to Blackness does not make null or render insignificant perceived patient "foreignness."

Consequently, the heterogeneous racialized specificities of the individu-als within the WHC alternate between racial figurations. In one instance, they are "Blackened," as their undeservingness is figured through their re-ceipt of welfare-as-Medicaid. So Blackened, they are figured as "the despi-cable bottom of white 'American' society" (De Genova 2006, 3). Yet, their "Blackening" is not mutually exclusive to their racialization as (always al-ready non-white) "alien outsider," when their undeservingness is figured through their "foreign-ness," "immigrant-ness," "Third-World-liness"—their "U.S. Otherness." And so, at times, when the pendulum of Alpha patients' racial figuration has swung towards "Blackness," all patients—citizens and non-citizens, native-born and the undocumented—come to be racialized as such. At other times, when the pendulum has instead swung toward a racialized alien Otherness, all patients—including, ironically, African-American and white U.S. citizens—come to be racialized accord-ingly. So "alienated," they are not figured as the "despicable bottom" of the nation, but rather as outside the nation. They are the outside that has managed to come within. Importantly, within either racial figuration, Alpha patients remain disqualified from whiteness.

And so, the racial dynamics of the WHC reveal that the Black–White binary must be qualified to represent more appropriately the confusions, disjunctions, and irrationalities of race-thinking in the United States. Indeed, to persist as an organizing principle of U.S. society, race has had to be flexible enough to be manipulated in multiple and frequently contradictory ways, as required by the exigencies of the day. The dual racial figurations of Alpha patients ought to be understood as an example of the incoherencies produced when two distinct racial logics—deployed separately to accomplish different goals—intersect.

In sum, the patients seeking health care at Alpha Hospital are always disqualified from whiteness—whether they are racialized as Black or as alien, theirs is always a position far distanced from the privilege associated with whiteness. As I argued in Chapter 2, they are disadvantaged and subordinated insofar as their receipt of Medicaid ties them to a PCAP apparatus that enables state surveillance and regulation of their private lives. As I argued in Chapters 3 and 5, they are disadvantaged and subordinated insofar as they have very little control over the massive quantities of tests to which their pregnant bodies will be subjected as a result of their receipt of prenatal care with government assistance. Moreover, they are disadvantaged and subordinated insofar as the administrative apparatus at Alpha does not allow them the privilege of selecting the doctor(s) who will administer their prenatal care; thus, they cannot ensure that their provider's philosophy of pregnancy and childbirth aligns with their own. And importantly, as I argued in this chapter, they are disadvantaged and subordinated insofar as they are compelled to negotiate a clinic staffed by individuals who view them with contempt and treat them accordingly.

The positions of white privilege and Black/alien privation are physically manifested and spatially realized in Alpha's location as immediately adjacent to Omega Hospital, a private hospital that refuses to accept Medicaid. Omega's commitment to accepting only private insurance effectively creates mutually exclusive, class-divided patient "populations."[12] The result is that Omega attends to the wealthier, more privileged possessors of private insurance while Alpha attends to their poorer, less-privileged, publicly insured counterparts. Pursuant to this dichotomy, Omega's patients are "whiter" than that of Alpha, both in the sense that more Omega patients are racialized as white and that they are more privileged than Alpha patients. Furthermore, the segregation of patient "populations" into separate edifices has more than symbolic import: the unprivileged social positioning of the Alpha "population" is sensed by those whose duty it is to provide medical care and ancillary services to them. That is, the physical space of Alpha Hospital reflects this disadvantage and produces a feeling associated with it. A comparison made by Dr. Kramer, a second-year resident, is revealing in this regard. After I asked him to articulate the ways in which Alpha and Omega were different, he responded:

> Well, you know . . . [long pause] Almost everything. It just feels a lot different. You're still doing the same procedures. Treating the patients in the same way. Making the same medical decisions, for the most part. The attending [physicians] are a lot more involved at Omega. [At Omega,] there's a lot more supervision. It's not a negative or positive thing. It's just that that's their private patients. You're not just admitting someone. . . . For example, if I were doing an ultrasound on somebody at Omega, I know I have to have a little bit more. . . . For example, if something doesn't go well during an ultrasound at Alpha, she's probably not going to know that. Probably. So, it's an attitude thing. I mean, it's embarrassing a little bit; but, it's true. Sometimes, we'll take a phone call right in front of an Alpha patient. Sometimes it's important for patient care and [taking the phone call] is something that we should do. But, we wouldn't do the same thing if it were a private patient.

Interestingly, Dr. Kramer described the difference between Alpha and Omega viscerally, as something he could "feel." Although he asserted that he "treated the patients in the same way," an attestation that was averred by many of the residents I interviewed, he acknowledged that he allowed himself to indulge in admittedly inappropriate or unprofessional behavior while at Alpha. He is hopeful when he states that patients probably are not aware of those space-based indulgences.

However, my interviews with patients reveal that they are a bit more perceptive than Dr. Kramer permits; they, too, feel the relative disadvantage of Alpha as a place. Because of Omega's refusal to accept patients with Medicaid insurance, there is no blending of patient "populations" between Alpha and Omega, as there might be at private hospitals that accept Medicaid. The effect is that the space of Alpha (and the patients within it) becomes marked as not quite as consequential, not quite as worthy. Thus, these private and public hospitals adjacent to one another come to manifest the relative privilege associated with whiteness and the relative lack associated with non-whiteness.

One Alpha patient I interviewed, Rhonda, had given birth prematurely to twins at a well-known private hospital that accepted Medicaid insurance, Theta Medical Center. She described her experience there in wholly negative terms. In fact, a couple of weeks before I met her, she had just settled a lawsuit against the hospital alleging medical malpractice that resulted in cerebral palsy in one of her twins and the death of the other. When I asked her why she thought the physicians at the other hospital had given her unsatisfactory care, she—a self-identified Black Medicaid recipient who had been raised by her Puerto Rican mother after her African-American father abandoned the home—replied:

> I don't know. To this day, I still don't know. I don't want to say that it's a racist thing because you know what? Black, White, whatever, we all go through the same thing. Who knows? There was a White woman that was suing Theta, too. So, I can't say that it's a color thing. I think it was more of a Medicaid thing. Because they did have separate areas for us. There was a clinic for the Medicaid women. And then there was the pretty lounge over here. You know? And they were, you know, they call them perinatologists, you know? They had the "Perinatology Suite." Right here. And you had the little Jewish ladies with the wigs, White ladies, all that-upscale Black ladies. All up in there. And I'm like, "Well, damn! Let me go get on my mama's insurance or get on my daddy's insurance." You know? I'm like, "Damn!" They were looking good. They had beautiful, comfy chairs. The lighting was nice. It was beautiful. It was a suite. Meanwhile, "Y'all [Medicaid recipients are] over there. What they have is cute. But, y'all over there." After I had my son, for some reason, I don't know why, I went back on my job's [private] insurance. Which is crazy. I don't know if the hospital messed up, but I used it. I was a HIP patient. I was in the pretty area. Over here. All the Medicaid patients were in the crazy area over there. Yelling and screaming and carrying on. I was on this side.

Rhonda's experience illustrates Medicaid recipients can be marked as unprivileged and disadvantaged even in institutional spaces that purport to dissolve such markings. Instead of buildings that physically manifest white privilege and non-white disadvantage, as with Omega and Alpha, Theta Medical Center produced separate waiting areas that did that work.

Thus, the point is clearly about the stigmatization and neglect of Medicaid patients (an effect of their racialization as the undeserving poor). The end result is that Alpha, which is effectively an all-Medicaid hospital, achieves a special distinction as a racializing site.

And so, Alpha may also be understood to be a racializing institution. In the class-stratified, public-versus-private U.S. healthcare system, Alpha Hospital sits squarely on the subordinate, "non-white" public side as the prototypical beleaguered municipal hospital. Alpha's history of being chronically and severely underfunded (yet somehow miraculously remaining solvent enough to continue to serve the most indigent of the city's ill), is widely known and well-respected. Alpha is recognized as the site where "the most marginalized members of the society—the destitute, the homeless, the incurable, and the insane" are cared for (Opdycke 1999, 4). Indeed, Alpha has remained the consummate "poor person's hospital." As quoted in Opdycke's colorful and informative history of the institution, "'[Alpha] was where people went, a poor person's hospital,' recalls a neighborhood resident. 'If you had any money, you went somewhere else'" (105–06). Furthermore, the earlier discussion about undeservingness is relevant here inasmuch as Alpha has historically served the "undeserving poor," a category of persons private hospitals expressly refused.

> Like many charitable managers, trustees of private hospitals preferred patients who were clean, sober, and industrious—the group that contemporaries sometimes described as the "worthy" poor. The trustees were convinced that many people were poor simply because of their disorderly lives; giving free care to dissolute citizens, they reasoned, would only encourage their profligacy. . . . Solid citizens like disabled artisans and genteel widows were usually accepted [to private hospitals], while shady characters like tramps, prostitutes, and unwed mothers were passed on to the public hospitals. . . . Public hospitals nevertheless acquired a special responsibility for New Yorkers classed as unworthy. (21)

When one recalls the earlier discussion of the always already Blackness of the undeserving (or "unworthy") poor, one can better see how the institution of Alpha itself acquires racial characteristics; Alpha is itself racialized. Moreover, in a society where class and race are mutually constitutive, that Alpha's patients are the city's poorest also means its patients tend to be people of color. "Everyone knew that the public system treated far more than its share of the city's minority residents" (Opdycke 1999, 177).

Indeed, "even though non-whites represented only about 50 percent of the city's population by 1995, they accounted for about 80 percent of the public hospital's patient population" (185–86).

Further, the significance of a place that is renowned, indeed celebrated, for serving the racialized indigent refused by every other hospital does not escape the patients seeking health care there. Patients who were aware of Alpha's history understood that their status as an Alpha patient aligned them, to a certain extent, with the city's most dispossessed and detested. In this way, Alpha might be understood as a racializing institution insofar as it marks its patients as lacking power and privilege by virtue of their status as patients of the institution. Moreover, when that lack is read within a racializing logic, the patients are produced as lacking (racial) power and privilege—that is, the patients are produced as Black/alien.

Although the patients at Alpha Hospital experience a "non-whitening" because of their relatively disadvantaged and unprivileged social positioning, they are also "non-whitened" by their low socioeconomic status. Ong's insightful analysis of Asian immigrants' encounters negotiating the welfare state in the San Francisco Bay region is helpful. She notes that Cambodian immigrant groups were believed to be largely composed of peasants destined to become "human debits" through their petitions for welfare assistance from the state. As a result, "Khmers were socialized [in refugee-processing camps] to expect limited occupational options and taught subservient behaviors, as well as a flexible attitude towards frequent changes of jobs which would help them adapt to cycles of employment and unemployment" (Ong 1996, 742). Thus, their "minoritization" began prior to their setting foot on U.S. soil. Importantly, the "Blackening" of Cambodian refugees would have been less intelligible without the simultaneous "whitening" of other immigrant groups. Ong writes, "This positioning of Cambodians as black Asians is in sharp contrast to the model-minority image of Chinese, Koreans, and Vietnamese (including Sino-Vietnamese), who are celebrated for their 'Confucian values' and family businesses." (742). Ong explains the ideological positioning of Cambodian immigrants as "Black" within the bipolarity of the Black/White model of race in U.S. society as a consequence of the racialization of class. Looking to Roediger's historical analysis of Irish immigrants' struggle for the racial privilege that is produced by the acquisition of whiteness, she notes that the economic success of groups has been discursively constructed as being simultaneous with their "whitening." Exemplifying this construction are notions of the "model minority" and the "underclass," "both economic terms standing for racial ones" (739).

Although Roediger and Ong look to historical and present patterns of immigration to establish the fact of the racialization of class, by no means should their analyses be thought to apply solely to immigrant groups. That is, the "racializing logic of class attributes" is effected not only upon newly arriving categories of persons, but upon individuals and groups that presently reside in the United States. One can say the racialization of class "Blackens" the patients at Alpha, a group of individuals who are presumed to be poor by virtue of their receipt of public assistance in the form of "welfare." Although the Cambodian immigrants with whom Ong worked were "Blackened"/disqualified from whiteness by their low-wage employment, high rates of teenage pregnancy, and welfare-dependent families" (Ong 1996, 742), Alpha patients' identities as petitioners of subsidized health care from a public hospital analogously effect their Blackening/disqualification from whiteness. Insofar as whiteness is associated with the characteristic Medicaid recipients lack—economic self-sufficiency—their disqualification from whiteness is indisputable. Thus, the implicitly racialized figure of the "wily patient" can be imagined as enacted by every discursively racialized patient who turns to Alpha for health care, without regard to her overt racial ascription.

The Racial Sullying of White Alpha Patients

Interviews I conducted with racialized white Alpha patients support the proposed analysis: white patients seem to be aware of a "sullying" of their whiteness that is concomitant to their receipt of government assistance. They also seem to be aware that a racial privilege they possess in the United States "by birthright" has been somewhat corrupted by their present social positioning as a seeker of government-subsidized health care from a public hospital. Victoria, a graduate student who was studying sculpture, was pregnant with her first child when I met her in the Alpha waiting area. The fine arts program in which she was enrolled rendered her ineligible for insurance offered through the university. When she discovered her pregnancy, she signed up for Medicaid and came to Alpha on the recommendation of a friend. I asked about her first impressions of Alpha, and Victoria, a self-proclaimed "daughter of hippies," spoke about the general rudeness to which she had been subjected by hospital staff.

She described the midwives she had seen as "always kind, but the face of Alpha, the people who the patients interact with first, [is] not always kind." She continued: "When I came to the hospital, on two occasions, I was sent to the wrong floor. Now, in this country, I understand that I have a racial privilege. And with that privilege, I don't expect to be sent to the wrong floor. I don't expect to have to wait an hour and a half for the midwife to call me." When I responded that no one I had interviewed had ever explained the difficulties they experienced within the hospital in terms of racial privilege, she replied, "I realize that being conscious of my race privilege is unique, but, my having that experience of racial privilege is not unique at all."

White patients who were not as conscious of their racial privilege as was Victoria, or alternatively, who were not as willing or able to speak of it in those terms, also articulated the sense they had experienced a demotion in racial status by their receipt of health care from Alpha. Wendy, an unemployed writer who identified as "white" and who was pregnant with her second child when I met her, reminisced during our interview about her first pregnancy and the circumstances that found her unemployed and unexpectedly pregnant. She had been raised in the Bronx and the Morningside Heights area of Manhattan by her Puerto Rican father and white mother. After her parents divorced, her family had experienced intermittent bouts of poverty, during which her mother received welfare. Wendy stated she experienced "antepartum depression" when she discovered her pregnancy on the same day she had been fired from her waitressing job:

> WENDY: It was very hard. And I did a lot of research. And it took me a while to realize that I could come to Alpha without having insurance. And without having anything setup. That they would help me set it up.
>
> KHIARA: Did you look online?
>
> WENDY: Yeah. But, I was actually kind of late getting in here. I think part of that was the depression because it had me kind of, you know, isolated. I didn't want to go out and I didn't have the energy. And so tired. So tired. I couldn't get up. So, by the time that started fading, I was able to take care of some of the business and come in here and get the work done . . .
>
> KHIARA: So, when you arrived at Alpha, was it like a breath of fresh air?
>
> WENDY: No, I was really depressed.
>
> KHIARA: Why was it depressing?

WENDY: Well, it wasn't as nice as it is now.

KHIARA: You were in the other half? [The WHC was formerly located in
           the visibly older, more worn hospital building. However, the
           clinic was relocated to a newer, ambulatory care building
           approximately a year before I began my fieldwork.]

WENDY: Yeah. And, I was on . . . When I was little, my mom was on
           welfare for a while. And I think that [coming to Alpha] just
           kind of brought some of the . . . I think . . . It sucked. It felt very
           public. So, the idea of being on public assistance is not a
           cheerful thought. Um, but at the same time, my depression from
           the first trimester was starting to lighten up. So, it wasn't that
           bad. And I got a little part-time job—doing something where
           I was like in a mailroom or something. So, I mean, it wasn't
           bad. But, it wasn't . . . It was a relief. But, it wasn't a breath of
           fresh air.

Wendy could recall her and her mother's whiteness being sullied by the
necessity of receiving public assistance. When she had been a high school
English teacher with private insurance, she had escaped the depreciation
of her racial privilege and the enervation of her racial power that is usually
concomitant with the receipt of welfare. That she never took advantage of
the insurance by actually visiting a doctor or dentist does not negate the
protection of her racial privilege the insurance afforded; for Wendy, private insurance meant never needing to go to places that "felt very public."
However, the physical space of Alpha—which, at least prior to renova-
tion, was reminiscent of those "very public" places she had visited with
her mother—served to remind her of those times of vulnerability, of that
racial sullying. Later in the interview, which I was able to conduct because
Wendy had been waiting over an hour to see the midwife and was esti-
mated to have to wait another hour more, I asked her to elaborate on what
exactly "felt very public" about Alpha:

KHIARA: So, when you said that when you came to Alpha the first time,
           and it felt like public assistance, or it reminded you of those
           days of public assistance, is that a reference to waiting a long
           time?

WENDY: The waiting. Bureaucracy. The meetings with the social worker,
           and the dietician, HIV counselor. You know, like, all these
           services. And, it's obvious that they work a lot with people who
           don't have an education. Who are not citizens. Who are very,

very young. And sometimes I felt that they were relieved to work with me. Because I know what they're talking about. And I know a little bit about it. I speak English.

For Wendy, the "very public" feeling of Alpha was a by-product of the PCAP apparatus and the avalanche of requirements that accompany it. However, in the face of her forced submission to that apparatus, which would entail a repetition of the stripping of her racial power, she was able to hang on to some of her racial privilege by differentiating herself from what she imagined Alpha patients to be. Unlike the "other" Alpha patients, she was a citizen. She could speak English. She knew what the professionals were talking about, and she imagined their relief in the presence of a woman who was "like them" in terms of their power and privilege. Essentially, although Wendy could understand that her status as an Alpha patient signified a racial impoverishment, that she was "Blackened/"alienated" by her receipt of Medicaid, she seemed to argue that others were "Blacker"/more "alienated" than her: the ones who are not citizens, who speak no English, who have little education, and who do not know what the professionals are talking about—in short, who are still more disadvantaged and more likely to remain captive to their condition of dependency.

The initial response that one patient, Nancy, had when I introduced my study to her evidences an attempt to protect the racial privilege associated with racialized whiteness by differentiating oneself from "Blacker"/more "alienated" patients. I approached Nancy as she waited with her three-year-old daughter for an appointment with the midwife. I described my study to her as one that examines women's experiences with prenatal care in New York City and asked if she would be interested in participating. She replied in the affirmative, but with a caveat: "You should know that I am very different from all of the other women who come here." After I asked her to elaborate on what ways she was "different," she said, "Well, my situation is very different. This is just my second pregnancy. I have never been on welfare. The only reason why I have Medicaid is because my boyfriend's financial situation is very complicated right now and business has been very slow for him." Nancy's explanation of her "difference" revealed that she conceptualized Alpha patients as being women with multiple children (more than two) who collected welfare. Moreover, for Nancy, other Alpha patients' economic privation possessed a permanence and intransience. In contrast, her financial vulnerability was merely a provisional hardship, a phase she and her boyfriend would eventually overcome.

In this way, Nancy evinced her desire to distinguish herself from the persons who "truly" or "genuinely" belonged in Alpha and to whom I should direct my investigational inquiries. That is, she attempted to retain her racial privilege by arguing that the sullying of her whiteness was nothing more than an interim measure; thus, she was blissfully unaware that she shared significant similarities with the patients with whom she felt no cohesion.

Willa was pregnant with her second child when I met her in Alpha's waiting area. She had given birth to her first son at Kappa Medical Center, a private Catholic hospital in Manhattan that accepted Medicaid. She described her son's birth in overwhelmingly negative terms. After laboring for several hours without dilating, the obstetricians present ruptured her amniotic sac in an effort to accelerate her labor. (I refer to the physicians who delivered Willa's son as "the obstetricians present," as opposed to "her obstetricians," because she had never seen them before going to the labor and delivery ward to deliver her son. That is, Kappa was similar to Alpha insofar as the physicians who provided prenatal care to a publicly insured woman were not the same who would ultimately deliver the woman's baby.) However, instead of enabling her to dilate, the rupture of the sac caused her son's heart rate to fall precipitously. The physicians performed an emergency C-section to save her son's life. My interview with Willa and her Indo-Trinidadian husband, Anuj, was fascinating because I was able to bear witness to their attempts to understand how and why their son's birth had proceeded so differently from their desire for a "natural" birth. As they thought aloud to one another, their receipt of Medicaid figured prominently as an explanatory device. Willa wondered whether the physicians present at her son's birth were aware that they would ultimately deliver her son via C-section, yet had not informed her. Essentially, she wondered if her physicians' professed concern about her lack of dilation was in fact a charade inasmuch as they may have had every intention to deliver her son by C-section to expedite the delivery. Anuj answered her in the affirmative:

They know in advance. They can come in and determine in terms of your paperwork. There's some stuff that they do—like, third-worlders—like, "We're going to come in and do the sorcery. We're not going to tell you anything. You're going to have your baby. And there's all this background billing that we can do." That just happened. I'm like, "Dude, I'm college-educated. Don't tell me that. I know what's going on."

In Anuj's reading of their son's birth, he and his wife were treated as "third-worlders," a patently racialized figure. Their physicians' refusal or otherwise failure to inform them of the likelihood of a C-section delivery divested them of their choice and autonomy. In this manner, one can read Anuj's awareness of the "racializing logic of class attributes" and he and his wife's consequent positioning as non-white—this despite her manifest racialized whiteness and their attainment of high levels of education (which, pursuant to that same racializing logic of class attributes, would otherwise afford them a certain degree of "whitening"). However, Anuj is not white, neither in racial identity nor ascription. So, the combination of his phenotype and "foreign" name (despite educational attainments) with Willa's Medicaid-sullied whiteness arguably made them still more easily racially demoted. As the conversation continued, their lack of autonomy and "third-worlder"-ness was explicitly aligned with their receipt of Medicaid:

WILLA: You think they knew that when they broke the water that I was going to have a C-section?

ANUJ: It's like you know the building is going to fall down when you put it up. Of course they knew all that stuff. I just feel that we should have been told something ahead of time. And I felt that that was really, like, a clinic. [For Anuj and Willa, "clinic" was used to signify places that exclusively served Medicaid-receiving populations. Counterpoised to "clinics" were, presumably, "private offices."] At Kappa, is everybody on Medicaid or something?

WILLA: Nope—I went through the clinic. There was another part for people with private insurance.

ANUJ: Do they know ahead of time if you're going in for free? I don't know: I felt like if we were paying for health insurance. . . . We got worse care than them.

WILLA: That's true.

ANUJ: I just felt that they treated us like we were on Medicaid.

WILLA: Well, the weird thing is that after they broke the water, they watched his heart rate drop. And they didn't immediately go, "OK, C-section." [The attending] sort of played a quiz with the [resident]. He was like, "Look at what's happening." She's like, "Heart rate is dropping." He was like, "So, what does that mean?" And Anuj was, like, furious. [The resident] was like, "I think that maybe we should have a C-section." And [the attending] was like, "That is definitely what we should be doing." And she was like, "But, there's another woman scheduled to have a C-section." And he said, "But, this is an emergency. Take that one out and put her first." But, the whole question-answer . . . Like, they're playing a game. Like a school-game. . . .

ANUJ: And that's how you know that they knew this was going to happen—because they did that when it happened. Like, we don't need to be your test case. . . . He talked about how he was getting his kid a Benz—with one of the other doctors. [To Willa] You weren't there. It was when I was outside. And they talked about golf. Didn't pay attention to anyone. It was interesting—he didn't pay attention to any of the Filipino or Chinese nurses. And then, he came in and did his thing. I was like, "Dude, I can't believe you did all this crap-talking about how much money you're making, and then you waltz in and do a C-section." And then he didn't even look at us. He didn't even look at us. I'm like, that's ridiculous. I should have bugged out about that, but I had other stuff to bug out about.

While Anuj was present at his Medicaid-recipient wife's disempowering birth (most aspects of which Anuj was utterly impotent to eliminate or change), the physician who would perform invasive surgery on his wife converses with another presumably monied physician about his wealth and the luxury and leisure it affords him. Moreover, Anuj speaks of the physician's lofty class location as an issue of race; the physician's wealth and power were explicitly coupled with his disregard for the Filipino and Chinese nurses as well as Anuj. Thus, the physician's class position was counterpoised to a diverse array of persons not racialized as white, and this contrast implicitly racialized that wealth and power as white.

Willa and Anuj had decided to come to Alpha for their most recent pregnancy because they believed their identification as Medicaid recipients at Kappa had tagged them as available for poor treatment. They believed that at Alpha, where all patients received Medicaid, their class would no longer be an issue—that is, what I would call a "democratizing logic of class attributes" would trump Ong's "racializing logic of class attributes" with which they were faced at Kappa. They hoped that in a place with no class stratification, their status as Medicaid-recipients would not become a justification for the second-class treatment accorded to the poor/non-whites. Speaking again of Kappa, we had the following dialogue:

WILLA: That place is dirty, too. That clinic was dirty, too. That's what I'm saying—in New York, it's really hard to get good health care. There's a lot of great things about New York. But, I've had really bad experiences . . .

KHIARA: With doctors here?

WILLA: Yeah. You have to pay for it. If you pay for it, then you get care.

ANUJ: [inaudible]

WILLA: So, you think they have Medicaid?

ANUJ: I grew up knowing if someone was on welfare. I didn't know necessarily, but you feel it. Like, if you go to a poor school, you get a lunch ticket. You're broke, but everybody's broke. So, then, no one feels broke. But, if you go to a private hospital in Tribeca, you don't think everybody knows how you pay for your treatment there?

WILLA: Don't tell me that! He's been telling me that Medicaid's fine.

ANUJ: It is fine. I'm just saying: do people [providers] think that it's different? I don't know if they think that it's different. I do know that I've always had bad health care.

WILLA: Even when you're in a clinic where everybody has Medicaid? I don't feel like that here. Everybody has Medicaid here, right?

KHIARA: Yeah.

WILLA: I don't feel like that ["broke"] here. I felt like that at Kappa—even though you're at the clinic. When you're not supposed to feel like that [because everybody is "broke."] But, I really don't feel like that here.

Throughout the conversation, it was obvious that Anuj was much more aware of the "racializing logic of class attributes" than his wife. One exchange, following my prompting of the couple to speak more about the relationship they perceived between their status as Medicaid recipients and their experience during their son's birth, exemplifies this:

KHIARA: Now, you had Medicaid at Kappa, right?

WILLA: Yes.

KHIARA: And you were wondering if they knew that and maybe that's why you got treated . . .

WILLA: I don't think about these things.

ANUJ: I think about these things. Pull the race card! [laughs]

Anuj's response to my prompt indicates his awareness of the "racial-izing logic of class attributes." I had asked them a question about Medicaid, a question ostensibly about class. However, Anuj answered in racial terms—by "pulling the race card." It is interesting that Anuj, who would likely be phenotypically marked as non-white, claims to "think about these things" while his phenotypically white wife does not. This disparity in awareness of the relationship between class and race may illustrate the claim made by critical scholars that white privilege enables white people to never think of themselves in terms of race and to frequently discount the validity of race as an explanation for the predicaments, experiences, and disadvantages of others. It may also be attributable to Anuj being raised by a mother who received public assistance; consequently, he is aware of the multiple layers of subordination her gender, race, and class produced for her.

Nevertheless, during the interview Anuj and Willa made repeated attempts to differentiate themselves from the other "non-white" people with whom they shared a racialized class position. Like Wendy, they seemed to want to hold on to some of the racial power and privilege whiteness afforded them. To accomplish this, they argued that although their receipt of Medicaid might have positioned them as non-white, others were still more conclusively so. Anuj made such a distinction when he spoke about the difficulty he and his wife had experienced in their attempts to initiate prenatal care at Alpha. They had articulated the sense that the Alpha employees whose duty it was to assist patients were woefully undertrained to effectively serve those patients. Anuj said:

> The things that I complain about are actually because the people who are calling in the clinic situation are actually the people who work there. It's probably better for them. So, if, you know, I'm calling and I'm from Mexico and I don't speak English and have a high school education . . . If you called up and got somebody like that, you might actually get through [be able to communicate]. Instead of, "I'm broke, but I went to college; I read existentialism. Help me, I'm broke. Everything I took in college is useless! I went to art school and it's useless!" You can't call up and be like, "Yo . . ." I don't want to use too many expletives. [laughs] We're in the minority! We're educated, broke artists!

Anuj contrasts his wife and himself with the people who he imagines are served by "clinics": people from Mexico without college educations who do not speak English. Those people, he argues, are able to communicate with the clinic support staff, who he imagines are similarly situated to the clients they serve. Unlike "those people," he and his wife are "whiter": they have read existentialism; they have gone to college and graduate school. Thus, Anuj imagines that he and his wife were "in the minority" of the "non-white" population in which their "broke" status positioned them. They might have been "non-white," but they were "whiter" than some of their associates. Nevertheless, on the only occasion I explicitly asked the couple about race and the various experiences they had had during their pregnancies, they articulated a tension between their whitening and disqualification from whiteness; that is, they were torn between feeling the arrant success of the racializing logic of class attributes, yet feeling privileged due to Willa's racialized whiteness and their relatively high levels of education. I directed my question to Willa:

KHIARA: Do you guys feel that you were treated differently because you are ostensibly white?

WILLA: Right.

ANUJ: Do you think you were treated better? Worse? Different?

WILLA: No.

ANUJ: There's minorities in every . . .

WILLA: Well, I feel like maybe I get a little bit of preferential treatment here. But, then again, I go to my friends. [The midwife that attended to Willa was her friend.]

ANUJ: Here, it's fine.

WILLA: Anywhere. At Kappa—no, definitely, I got treated like shit. [laughs]

ANUJ: If you're a minority—in America, it's not a matter of "yeah, it's a White country and you're a Black person." It's like, you're a minority when you're not the same as the majority. It happens in hospitals—if [the hospital staff is poor, uneducated minorities] and most people are minorities, they're going to look at us . . . And it doesn't matter that I'm colored. They're going to look at us as privileged even though we're in there with Medicaid. We look a certain way, we speak a certain way; that's the minority when we go to a place where people are not like that.

WILLA: Sometimes I get worse treatment because I'm white.

KHIARA: Really?

ANUJ: Yeah.

KHIARA: Like where?

WILLA: At Kappa when I go. [Although Willa and Anuj opted not to return to Kappa for prenatal care, they continued to take their son to a pediatrician at the hospital.] It's just my sense—because a lot of it has to do with trusting the system. Because the thing is when you go to the hospital, basically—and doctors' offices—basically, things are set up. But, because I'm on Medicaid, which made me nervous, I'll be like, "So, what's the next step? [said anxiously]" They're just like, "Just chill out, relax. You're going to be fine." That's the difference. They're just like, "Oh my God, this lady is freaking out." I've been that lady.

ANUJ: You don't know the process. Most people don't know the process to go see a doctor. My mom went to the doctor. They churn her through the system and she comes out the other end. And she's still sick. When [their son] goes, I kinda want to see what's happening. And they're not used to that in Medicaid. I'll go and be like, "Hey, what's going to happen?" They're like, "I'm not sure I like what you're doing—because it's free."

WILLA: I used to get really stressed out because, you know . . . During the first pregnancy, especially, I didn't know if I was going to get my appointment. Am I going to have to pay the bill? How does this work? So, I was really kinda intense about it. No, I don't feel like even if I'm white—it doesn't matter; I don't have health insurance. If you don't have health insurance, you don't have health insurance. It doesn't matter. It's nerve-wracking.

Thus, Willa and Anuj articulate a tension between their sense that they were privileged by Willa's racialized whiteness and the whitening afforded to them by their higher education, yet disadvantaged by their receipt of Medicaid. Anuj believed their education allowed them to be recognized as "minorities" within a non-white population, thereby recouping some of their racial prestige. Willa, on the other hand, articulated the sense that the absence of health insurance coverage universally produced the uninsured as unprivileged without regard to the uninsured's racial ascriptions. Moreover, both articulated a sense that the privilege afforded to them by their educational attainment, insofar as it was coupled with their status as Medicaid recipients, effected a disempowerment when it manifested in posing inquiries to their healthcare providers. They both felt that they are treated poorly when they, as educated consumers, attempt to retain some autonomy by demanding from their physicians (who are accustomed to treating more disempowered Medicaid recipients) information regarding the course of treatment they could expect. Ultimately, Willa and Anuj seem to be very much aware of the contextuality of racial privilege and the tenuousness of their hold on it in the face of their status as Medicaid-recipients.

SOME CONCLUDING THOUGHTS

What the wily patient and the welfare queen underscore is that race and racism is not as easily apprehended in the United States as it once was. Explicit and egregious demonstrations of racism are not as enumerable as they were just half a century ago. Within public institutions, persons are no longer presumptively dehumanized on the basis of their racial ascription and reduced to a fraction of their racial Other. We have left behind the days where lawmakers and jurists can discuss the appropriateness of Black people's subjugation and repression in the United States as matter-of-factly as one would the weather. In essence, institutional oppression on the basis of race is no longer something one can readily point to and say, "There it is."

Moreover, we have left behind the days where racism was a unidirectional phenomenon practiced by white people on Black people—where "racism" was what happened when racist beliefs that white people held about Black people manifested themselves. Insofar as the most egregious demonstrations of race-based contempt I observed during my fieldwork were directed to people of color *by other people of color*, it suggests that non-white persons serve an important function in enacting contemporary forms of medical disenfranchisement as well as in reiterating and reproducing racial discourses. Simply put, racism is very much an aspect of racial minorities' social imaginaries as well. Ascription or identification as a racial minority does not immunize the person from participating in discourses that function to disenfranchise other racial minorities.

Nor does ascription or identification as a racial minority immunize the person from harboring ideas about racial biology or from believing that culture represents radical Otherness. As such, the "individual racism" discussed in Chapter 4 can be, and likely is, enacted by physicians of color— just as it is enacted by physicians racialized as white. When one considers this likelihood along with the observation that individual racism acts in concert with institutional racism to produce both racial disparities in health and the more discreet instances of medical disfranchisement that I observed in the Alpha WHC, it suggests that even if the physicians who worked in the WHC had not been predominately white, we may expect similar results.

Furthermore, Willa's and Anuj's story dramatizes that racial discourses that developed as ideas about racial minorities can and do function to disenfranchise white persons. Indeed, racism in the contemporary moment can no longer be described as "white people against people of color"—even though that description might have been accurate in earlier historical moments.

Moreover, the implicit racialization of the wily patient and the welfare queen serves to demonstrate that race, as an omnipresent social fact with potent material repercussions, need not be explicitly evoked in order for it to overdetermine the quality of persons' lives. This chapter illustrates that although race was only infrequently verbalized in its own terms by persons in the Alpha obstetrics clinic, it was always extant; it was always there. Although race undoubtedly worked in mysterious ways in the clinic, the operation of race produced an entire group of women as racially Other-ed bearers of despised fertility. The ethnography presented here should be understood as a description of race as it is remade, reaffirmed, reiterated, and reconsolidated on the bodies of pregnant women seeking prenatal care in the United States. As a study of race as a process, it is an invitation to future discussions of how we can intervene in the process in order to produce more equitable—more just—outcomes.

EPILOGUE

TWO YEARS AFTER I HAD concluded my research in Alpha Hospital, I received a voice mail from Rosa, a patient I met when I first began field-work there in the spring of 2005. Back then she had just turned forty and was about five months pregnant with her third child. Her oldest son, Victor, was twenty, and he, like Rosa, occupied the precarious status of being an undocumented immigrant in the United States; her sixteen-year-old daughter had remained in Ecuador. Rosa's third pregnancy had proceeded without complications, and she later gave birth to a healthy and beautiful baby girl. In that message I received from her in the fall of 2008—decades, it seemed, after I had last hugged her, congratulated her on her new baby, and wished her well—Rosa said to me in Spanish:

> Hi Khiara! It's Rosa. I'm pregnant again! Can you believe it? I have about three months left. I'm going to a hospital close to my house in the Bronx, but, I don't want to deliver there. Babies die in that hospital. The nurse told me. Can I get my prenatal care from this hospital, but then go to Alpha to deliver? Call me back and let me know!

I knew that if Rosa showed up at Alpha in active labor, the staff would allow her to deliver her baby at the hospital; they would not at-tempt to send her to her neighborhood hospital if the birth of the baby was imminent. But, if she showed up at Alpha with no record of prenatal care at the institution, and the physicians felt it was safe to send her to her neighborhood hospital, she would be transferred. I called Rosa back to inform her, in Spanish, that if she was certain she wanted to deliver at Alpha, her labor and delivery would go much more smoothly if she simply received her prenatal care there. She paused, then timidly said: "My English is not very good. And Victor is working at a restaurant now—he works during the day. And my husband also works. So, it would have to be just me. And my English is not very good. . . ." I interrupted her and told her that, yes, I would be happy to meet her at Alpha and, acting as her translator, help her sign up for prenatal care.

On the day I met Rosa in the obstetrics clinic, it had been two years since I had last set foot in the hospital. But, when I showed up that morning, the clinic appeared eerily unchanged from the days I had sat behind the reception desk and observed the comings and goings with a trusty notebook in my lap: the waiting room was bursting at the seams with pregnant women, most patiently (but a few impatiently) waiting for their names to be called, urine-filled test tubes clutched in some of their fists. Residents who appeared young enough to be college freshman hurried back and forth, white coats trailing in the wind. A midwife spoke to a patient in heavily accented Spanish. A health educator stood next to the secured doors, anxiously waiting to be buzzed in. A PCA chastised a patient about the importance of being on time for her appointments, informing her that the staff "can't wait all day for you to decide to show up."

The vast majority of faces working behind the front desk that morning were familiar to me, and most of my former colleagues greeted me with hugs; many chided me about leaving Alpha for "greener pastures," teasing me by claiming I left because I thought I "was too good for Alpha." As I waited for Rosa, I chitchatted with the staff about any and everything—including what happened to Yolanda. ["After you left, they moved her to a room where she can't talk to anyone! There are only filing cabinets in there. I don't know what you told them about her, but they put her in a room and told her not to talk to patients anymore!"] Eventually, Rosa arrived and I gave her the instructions and materials for the urine pregnancy test, explained that the intake worker had given her an appointment to return for her PCAP appointment (to meet with the health educator, social worker, financial officer, etc.), and translated the intake worker's admonishment that it was extremely important that Rosa bring with her the record of her prenatal care from her neighborhood hospital. (While I was helping Rosa, I overheard one of the women who answered the clinic's telephone tell a patient that the computer was showing that there were no available gynecology appointments and she ought to call back in a couple of weeks. The scarcity of gynecology appointments appeared to be an enduring feature of the WHC.) Scheduling the prenatal care appointment took very little time, and Rosa—who had traveled over an hour from her apartment in the Bronx for this requisite in-person visit to Alpha—was in and out of the hospital in less than fifteen minutes.

Rosa was not the only patient who kept in touch with me after I had completed my fieldwork at Alpha. Rhonda, who gave birth to a healthy girl at Alpha after her previous pregnancy had ended with the birth of premature twins, one of whom died, occasionally sent me random forwarded text messages about everything ranging from the importance of prayer to the beauty and strength of the Black woman. Monica, who had given birth to two children before her eighteenth birthday, called me periodically—inviting me to her children's birthday parties, sharing the news she had finally received her own apartment in a housing project in the East Village, complaining that her boyfriend had been arrested again (this time for destroying her furniture), etc. Wendy found me on a social networking Internet site and filled me in on the goings-on in her life—how she had moved to the South to live with her mother after New York City had proved too expensive a place in which to raise a family. I ran into Fiona on the Upper East Side where she was hurrying to her job at as a clerk at a grocery store.

And then there were the other women who I tried to find, but could not—like the woman whose name I would Google because her story of abuse, betrayal, and abandonment was so extreme and heartbreaking that I was certain her life would end tragically, perhaps as a headline in the *New York Post*.

Like Rosa, who could be required to travel hours in order to come to a hospital and make an appointment that more privileged, privately insured women could make over the phone—an appointment she thought necessary to make if she wanted to avoid giving birth in a hospital where "babies die"—the disparate grouping of women I encountered at Alpha could be described by their lack of privilege and by their marginalization. And therein lies the irony: I met these decidedly marginalized women in the most paradigmatic of state institutions, Alpha Hospital. Moreover, Alpha, as a state institution, functions as a hub of sorts of other state institutions, such as the Administration for Children's Services (ACS), the Department of Health and Human Services, the Office of Medicaid Management, the Health Resources and Services Administration, the U.S. Department of Agriculture, the Federal Nutrition Service, the Department of Corrections, etc. All of these bureaucratic departments function in close collaboration with Alpha such that an Alpha patient, with the smallest of effort, can be seamlessly swept up within the regulatory ambit of other state institutions. Indeed, this is precisely what happened to many Alpha patients with whom I worked—women who, subsequent to attempting to receive prenatal care at Alpha, found themselves with open and reopened cases with ACS, signed up for TANF, having applied for food stamps, and receiving WIC vouchers. With this in consideration, the irony is revealed: *the site of extreme marginalization in the U.S. is at the vortex of state institutions.*

A distinction should be made between the marginalized women at Alpha and their abandoned counterparts: the homeless men and women who are, for all intents and purposes, invisible to the state; the detainees at Guantanamo Bay who seem to be wholly without political, civil, or human rights; the embodiments of the figure of *homo sacer* in refugee camps, concentration camps, and all other manner of camps all over the globe. The profound vulnerability of these abandoned men and women results from their having been denied a relationship with the state. The patients at Alpha Hospital are different in a very important respect: the profound vulnerability of these marginalized women (and men) at Alpha, found within a maelstrom of state institutions, results from the tenacity and insistence of the state's relationship with them.

ON RESISTANCE, OR SOME FINAL CONCLUDING THOUGHTS

Many of the poor, pregnant women I have encountered do not passively accept state regulation of their bodies. Nor do they watch the vanishing of their privacy rights with disinterest. Nor do they submissively accept conscription into a biomedical model of pregnancy and the concurrent construction of their bodies as unruly. Nor are they always successfully interpellated as members of an "at risk population." As the figure of the wily patient makes clear, the poor, pregnant women I have encountered loudly, passionately, and eloquently articulate their anger and dissatisfaction with the order of things.

I was constantly made aware of discrete acts of resistance. Such acts may be as minor as a woman lying to the nutritionist about the (in)frequency of her cheese consumption, as did a clever patient who simply wanted to avoid being "hassled" about her vegan diet so as to shorten the length of her requisite nutritional assessment. Other acts of resistance are bolder, as when a patient refuses to answer the inquiries of the social worker, or avoids meeting with the social worker altogether by ignoring her when she calls out the patient's name in the waiting room. Additionally, a patient's refusal to be seen by a resident obstetrician and her demand for care from an attending physician might be interpreted as a bold act of resistance. This patient's mother, who had prompted the patient to insist upon an attending as her provider, told me, "I said to her [the patient, her daughter], 'You're not a guinea pig.' I know this is a teaching hospital; but, they need to find someone else to learn on." Indeed, the very selection of Alpha in lieu of another as the site of prenatal care should be understood as an act of resistance for many women who, like Rosa, do not blindly go to the nearest public hospital, but instead travel far to Alpha because they believe it has an excellent reputation and exceptional facilities.

I am also compelled to acknowledge that what is in operation within the Alpha obstetrics clinic should not be understood as a wholly repressive, entirely punitive bureaucratic and medical apparatus that successfully reiterates the racism, xenophobia, classism, and sexism that inform it. Indeed, Foucault cautioned that the repressive aspects of power were equally matched by its productive aspects:

> What makes power hold good, what makes it accepted, is simply the fact that it doesn't weigh on us as a force that says no, but that it traverses and produces things, it induces pleasure, forms knowledge, produces discourse. It needs to be considered as a productive network which runs through the whole social body, much more than a negative instance whose function is to repress. (1984, 61)

What I mean to underscore is the fundamental and inherent ambivalence of a power that is simultaneous in its productivity and repression.[1] Accordingly, although power may operate in the Alpha WHC as an entity that enables the problematization, surveillance, regulation, management, and punishment of the patients seeking prenatal health care there, all in the effort to produce "docile bodies," power concurrently operates to produce resistances.[2] Indeed, one of the most important pieces of evidence of resistance might be the legacy of social struggles that has compelled the state to provide prenatal care to women whose fertility has been otherwise ubiquitously condemned within prevailing discourses. One may, ironically, understand as a defiant act of resistance the ostensible submission of poor, pregnant women to a regime of prenatal care that purports to insure a healthy mother and child even as it disparages them and violates their autonomy. Writes Lupton, "[T]hose individuals who 'go along' with medical advice need not necessarily be viewed as passively accepting the orders of the doctor or the medical gaze, but rather could be seen as engaging in practices of the self that they consider are vital to their own well-being. . . ." (1997, 105). Thus, in the context of the discursive condemnation of poor mothers and their children, resistance may be seen in the poor mother who participates in a state-subsidized prenatal healthcare program; although an excess of technology may characterize the healthcare program, and although the woman must first be interpellated as a "high risk" vector of pathogens, the woman's participation in the program may nevertheless be understood as a resistant "practice of the self" that she considers vital to her own well-being as well as the well-being of her unborn child. These practices of resistance need not be understood as mutually exclusive: I could cite numerous examples of women who willingly and happily participated in one or more aspects of the regime of prenatal care set out for them by the state and their providers while vehemently rejecting another aspect. For example, one patient I interviewed early on in her pregnancy, Nancy, articulated her sense that pregnancy was a natural state of the body that did not demand the surveillance her providers sought to implement through a demand for frequent and numerous "routine examinations"; however, she also articulated that the pain of childbirth could be "too much" and might require medicinal analgesics and anesthesia. Her somewhat contradictory conceptualization of pregnancy and childbirth was realized: although she did, in fact, fail to keep many of her scheduled appointments over the course of her pregnancy, she was also the happy (and relieved) recipient of an epidural at the birth of her son. Nancy's experience accords with Lupton's observation that individuals may constitute themselves in varying and sometimes contradictory ways in their encounters with medicine: "[I]ndividuals may constitute themselves . . . as an autonomous, reflexive individual who refuses to take a passive, orthodox patient role [or] . . . as someone who 'follows doctor's orders,' who is a 'good patient'. . . . Sometimes they may pursue both types of subject position simultaneously or variously" (1997, 105).

In fact, I would like to imagine the very act of being pregnant as an act of resistance for many of the poor, expectant mothers who are served in the obstetrics clinic at Alpha Hospital. I was always moved whenever I saw in the waiting room a pregnant nanny with her white charge. I think of Ginsburg and Rapp's formulation of "stratified reproduction," a term used to "describe the power relations by which some categories of people are empowered to nurture and reproduce, while others are disempowered" (1995, 3). Ginsburg and Rapp explain:

> Low-income African American mothers . . . are stereotyped as undisciplined "breeders" who sap the resources of the state through incessant demands on welfare. But historically and in the present, they were good enough nurturers to work as childcare providers for other, more privileged class and ethnic groups. . . . The concept of stratified reproduction helps us see the arrangements by which some reproductive futures are valued while others are despised. (3)

Accordingly, I viewed resistance whenever I saw in the waiting area pregnant women of color employed as nannies, who not only value their own reproductive futures, but insist upon them—even while enacting an employment that recognizes their ability to nurture other women's children and simultaneously disregards or demeans their competency to nurture their own.

Indeed, resistance might be seen in the fact of many other of these poor, pregnant women's bodies. That is, in the face of the discursive problematization of their fertility, despite polemical attestations that their reliance on governmental aid is "un-American" and figures them outside of the deserving body politic, and notwithstanding that mythical and fantastical ideas of their children as the future scourges of society exist in the national imagination, the patients at Alpha Hospital embrace their fertility. They give birth to their babies and love them unconditionally. This, I believe, ought to be understood as a powerful, material act of resistance.

Finally, I offer this study as a conscious attempt to begin a resignification of the fertility of the poor. If it is true, as François Ewald has written, that "[s]ocial insurance is also an insurance against revolutions" (1991, 209), it is also true the most dispossessed of society—in this case, ironically, those with social insurance—are those most likely to imagine radical social change and bring it to fruition. And so, it is not just race that is reproduced in the Alpha WHC and the countless other locations across the United States in which can be found the nationally circulating discourses, politics, policies and practices that work to produce the Alpha WHC as the space it is. Also reproduced is the possibility—the hope—of a different, more just, society.

NOTES

INTRODUCTION

1. I have not used a pseudonym for Professor Rayna Rapp.

CHAPTER TWO

1. The New York City Health and Hospitals Corporation (NYCHHC) is a public benefit corporation, created in 1970 to oversee New York City's public health care system in all five boroughs. "The Corporation consists of 11 acute care hospitals, 6 Diagnostic and Treatment Centers, 4 long-term care facilities, a certified home health care agency, and more than 80 community health clinics. . . . Through its wholly owned subsidiary, MetroPlus, NYCHHC operates a Health Plan which enrolls members in Medicaid, Child Health Plus, and Family Health Plus." (New York City Health and Hospitals Corporation 2008).

2. "A PCAP provider is an Article 28 approved hospital outpatient department or freestanding diagnostic and treatment center (D&TC) that was approved by the NYSDOH to provide prenatal care in accordance with Part 85.40 of Public Health Law at 10 NYCRR." (Office of Medicaid Management 2007, 3). "If the application review process indicates the provider is qualified and the Department approves their enrollment, the provider is reimbursed at an enhanced Medicaid rate for the enriched package of services delivered" (4).

3. The statute provides: "Health and childbirth education services shall be given to each pregnant woman based on an assessment of her individual needs. . . . Such services shall be provided by professional staff, documented in the medical record and shall include but not be limited to the following: . . . rights and responsibilities of the pregnant woman; signs of complications of pregnancy; physical activity and exercise during pregnancy; avoidance of harmful practices and substances including alcohol, drugs, non-prescribed medications, and nicotine; sexuality during pregnancy; occupational concerns; risks of HIV infection and risk reduction behaviors; signs of labor; labor and delivery process; relaxation techniques in labor; obstetrical anesthesia and analgesia; preparation for parenting including infant development and care and options for feeding; . . . and family planning." 10 NYCRR § 85.40(g) (2009).

4. The statute provides: "The PCAP provider shall routinely provide the pregnant woman with HIV counseling and education[, and] routinely offer the pregnant woman confidential HIV testing. . . ." 10 NYCRR § 85.40(j) (2009).

5. The statute provides: "The PCAP provider shall establish and implement a program of nutrition screening and counseling which includes individual risk assessment including screening for specific nutritional risk conditions at the initial prenatal care visit and continuing reassessment as needed; . . . [and] documentation of nutrition assessment, risk status and nutrition care plan in the patient medical record. . . ." 10 NYCRR § 85.40 (f)(1), (f)(3) (2009).

6. The statute provides: "A psychosocial assessment shall be conducted and shall include: screening for social, economic, psychological and emotional problems; and referral, as appropriate to the needs of the woman or fetus, to the local Department of Social Services, community mental health resources, support groups or social/psychological specialists." 10 NYCCR § 85.40 (h) (2009).

7. The statute provides: "Following the determination of a pregnant woman's presumptive eligibility for Medicaid benefits, the PCAP provider shall act as a pregnant woman's authorized representative in the completion of the Medicaid application process if the woman provides consent for such action." 10 NYCRR § 85.40 (b)(2) (2009).

8. Although I never met a woman who had private insurance and elected to receive care from Alpha Hospital, one of the midwives informed me she had encountered some Alpha patients who were privately insured, yet chose to apply for and receive Medicaid because their private insurance required exorbitant co-payments.

9. Most germane to this project is the literature discussing the state's interest in reproduction. Treichler's work is illustrative. She notes, "The health of childbearing becomes a signal for the health of the state. Accordingly, deci-

sions about pregnancy, childbirth, and maternity have been concerns of the state as well as of the childbearing woman and her family" (1990, 120).

10. A Colorado court found that although a petition for neglect could not be "filed with respect to an unborn child because a fetus is not specifically included within the statutory definition of 'child,'" a pregnant woman who uses drugs can be found to have neglected her "child" if the infant tests positive at birth for controlled substances. See People ex. rel. T.T., 128 P.3d. 328, 329 (Colo. App. 2005). Compare the Colorado court's decision with a Maine statute, Me. Rev. Stat. Ann. tit. 22, § 4011-B (2007), requiring "a health care provider involved in the delivery or care of an infant who the provider knows or has reasonable cause to suspect has been born affected by illegal substance abuse . . . [to] notify the [Department of Human Services] of that condition in the infant," yet clarifying that the statute "may not be construed to require prosecution for any illegal action, including . . . the act of exposing a fetus to drugs."

In *Killing the Black Body*, Dorothy Roberts (1997) gives a history of the punitive response states have had toward women who use crack cocaine during their pregnancies. Instead of helping these women gain control over their addictions and lives, many states opted to punish pregnant drug users by prosecuting them for crimes against both their born and unborn children.

11. The disbelief of patients' prenatal care stories is part of a larger phenomenon whereby patients are largely viewed by Alpha employees as uneducated, yet somehow incredibly shrewd, manipulators of the "system." I explore the intersection of these contradictions in the fantasy of the patient—that is, the figure of the "wily patient"—in Chapter 6.

12. Gotbaum argued "[r]equiring a visit to conduct a pregnancy test prior to a prenatal care appointment is an unsound and unnecessary policy" (2007, 12). She recommended that "[i]nstead of requiring an additional visit, clinics should confirm pregnancy at the time of the first prenatal appointment. If the clinic-based pregnancy test produces a negative result, the appointment should be used to provide the woman with preconception or interconception care, or family planning and contraception counseling as appropriate" (Ibid., 3).

13. Legal theorist Austin Sarat has made a similar observation in his study of the "welfare poor." He writes: "The people I studied often spoke of an interminable waiting that they said marks the welfare experience. In the waiting they are frozen in time as if time itself were frozen; power defines whose time is valued and whose time is valueless" (1990, 347–48).

14. ACOG is a nonprofit organization comprised of physicians that report standards of health care in the OB/GYN specialty.

15. This language is taken from the "Alpha Hospital HIV Pre-Test Counseling" form, which is not a form prepared by NYSDOH.

16. The statute specifies that in order for a woman to be certified as eligible for WIC, she must be "determined to be at nutritional risk. . . . This

determination may be based on referral data submitted by a competent professional authority not on the staff of the local agency" (e.g., a nutritionist employed in the clinic where a woman receives her prenatal care). 7 C.F.R. § 246.7e (2006). A woman should be deemed eligible for WIC if she has, among other things, "[d]ietary deficiencies that impair or endanger health, such as inadequate dietary patterns assessed by a 24-hour dietary recall, dietary history, or food frequency checklist."

17. The overregulation and hyper-surveillance of poor women who rely on public assistance is well documented (Abramovitz 1996; Appell 1997; Dodson 1999; Mink 2001; Morgan and Maskovsky 2003; Piven and Cloward 1971; Roberts 1997; Smith 2007; Susser and Kreniske 1987).

CHAPTER THREE

1. In an interesting article, Mitchell and Georges (1998) compare Greek and Canadian women's experiences with ultrasound technology. Of Greek women, they write, "As the Greek pregnant women eagerly demand and consume ultrasound technology, they actively constitute themselves as modern pregnant subjects and, by implication, symbolically affiliate themselves with Europe and the West" (121). A similar process may be at work in the Alpha WHC. That is, poor women's demand for and consumption of ultrasound technology serves to affiliate them with the wealthier women who have always had access to fetal imaging technologies. Thus, ultrasound technology might be understood as a *technology of inclusion* for those who are disenfranchised from institutions that are accessible to those with class privilege.

2. On the fetishization of the fetus and the veneration of medical science as a part of "U.S. culture," Sharp (2006) has discussed Eleni Papagaroufali's study of perceptions about organ transfer in Greece, noting Papagaroufali was "struck especially by how readily U.S. Americans embrace biotechnological answers as solutions to human suffering" (238). Papagaroufali observed that "Greeks, in contrast, are far less committed to this paradigm, given that their nation remains peripheral to the scientific realm, one whose values are otherwise deeply entrenched in American society" (238).

3. Davis-Floyd (1987a) describes the "technocratic model of childbirth" as similarly disempowering. She argues standard procedures during medically managed childbirths "enact the view that the female body-machine is inherently defective and generally incapable of producing perfect babies without technological assistance from professionals" (292). This experience as described by Davis-Floyd might be understood as an unsurprising culmination—a concluding demonstration—of nine months of dependency and disempowerment during prenatal care within the biomedical, technocratic model of pregnancy.

CHAPTER FOUR

1. One example is the "Mortality and Morbidity Weekly Report" issued by the Centers for Disease Control, which notes that "[m]ultiple factors contribute to racial/ethnic health disparities, including socioeconomic factors . . . , lifestyle behaviors . . . , [and] social environment (e.g., educational and economic opportunities, *racial/ethnic discrimination*, and neighborhood and work conditions). . . ." (Centers for Disease Control 2005). Another example is a fact sheet released by the Centers for Disease Control Office of Minority Health Disparities, which notes that "[d]isparities occur for a variety of reasons, including unequal access to health care, *discriminations*, and language and cultural barriers." (Office of Minority Health Disparities 2007).

2. The Centers for Disease Control note that "sepsis, pneumonia (infection in the lungs), and meningitis (infection of the fluid and lining around the brain) are the most common problems" associated with Group B streptococcal infections in newborns. The CDC does not mention death or disability as expected results of Group B strep infection.

3. BiDil has its origins in the Veterans' Administrative Cooperative Vasodilator Heart Failure Trials (V-HeFT I and II), which were intended to test the efficacy of the combination of hydralazine and isosorbide dinitrate in the general population (Ellison et al. 2008). The FDA failed to approve the drug subsequent to V-HeFT I and II. "The FDA found the data produced by the V-HeFT trials to be too muddled to meet the regulatory criteria of statistical significance to establish efficacy for the new drug. The data could support no conclusion as to whether BiDil worked or not" (Kahn 2008: 738). It was at this point that post hoc subgroup analyses of the trials were conducted. These post hoc analyses were used to argue that, while the drug was ineffective in the general population, it had had greater efficacy on the 49 African-Americans who had received the drug combination in the V-HeFT I and II. (Kahn 2008: 738 –39). The African American Heart Failure Trial (A-HeFT), which only enrolled self-identified African American people, was conducted in order to prove the efficacy of the drug combination in African Americans. The FDA approved BiDil as a race-specific drug based on the data provided by A-HeFT. But, as Kahn (2008) notes, "One of the great ironies of the BiDil approval is that the results of the A-HeFT trial say nothing about whether BiDil works differently or better with African Americans than with other groups, because the trial enrolled *only* African Americans. . . . Without a comparison population there can be no scientific basis for a claim of differential efficacy based on race" (739).

4. There are numerous examples of the persistence of biological notions of race. (Bolnick, et al. 2007; Braun 2005; Duster 2006; Fausto-Sterling 2008; Hammonds 2006; Kahn 2008; Obasogie 2007).

CHAPTER FIVE

1. For example, when an ostensibly white person was found to have been suffering from sickle cell anemia, a thorough genealogy of the patient's family revealed, conveniently, the possibility of the presence of "negro blood" in the patient: "The father was a healthy white man. . . . The mother, although considered a white person by her neighbors, had dark skin and the features of a Cuban, and was of Cuban descent. It is well known that Cuba is a violent melting pot, with the negro the predominant type" (quoted in Tapper 1995, 87). Essentially, the data revealed the ostensibly white person suffering from the "black-related disease" was, in fact, a Black person. Not satisfied with having protected the status of sickle cell anemia as a "black-related disease" in this instance, two concerned physicians went so far as to insulate from future attacks the integrity of this instantiation of medico-racial knowledge:

> [S]ince it is known that the sickling trait is a dominant character in its hereditary transmission, and since interbreeding between the colored and white races is more or less consistently taking place in many regions, including this country, we may in future generations expect the presence of this peculiar blood trait in an increasing number of apparently white descendants. Because of the tendency to deny such descent by those who are free of all negro features, no history will be obtained of such racial origin in affected individuals, thereby increasing the number of apparently pure white cases of sickle cell anemia (quoted in Tapper 1995, 88).

2. For example, when "a woman of Spanish and Scotch [sic]-Irish descent" sought help from two U.S. American physicians after losing her ability to walk (a common symptom of sickle cell anemia), the physicians advised "[t]here must be caution in calling this sickle cell anemia because no evidence of negro blood could be found" (quoted in Tapper 1995, 83). The mutual exclusivity of whiteness and sickle cell anemia was so entrenched that when one physician, Castana, rather radically went on record as having discovered a case of the disease in a white person, succeeding physicians sought to preserve the integrity of their medico-racial schema with the explanation, "[T]he semi-lunar or sickle-like gigantocytes [described by Castana] . . . represent degenerative erythrocytes and are not *true* sickle cells" (87).

3. Procacci (1991) writes that the promiscuity that is thought to describe the poor is part of a larger discourse of the poor's mobility—their refusal or inability to be sedentary: "Mobility also means *promiscuity*: indecipherable couplings, difficult to use as cohesive supports for the social fabric; spontaneous solidarities which elude 'legal' or 'contractual' definition, evading any attempt to orient them towards the goal of the social project" (1991, 161). And so, promiscuity appears as symptomatic of a more encompassing antisocial malaise.

4. Rose (1994) cogently articulates the important role medical practice and discourse has played historically in the construction of "populations": "[M]edical thought and medical activity, through the rationalities that unified the inhabitants of geographical space as a social body, though the compilation of statistics of birth, death, rates, and types of morbidity, through the charting of social and moral topographies of bodies and their relations with one another, played a key role in 'making up' the social body and in locating individuals in relation to this dense field of relations bearing upon the individual" (55). Although Rose emphasizes the work medicine has done in the creation of "populations" out of nations-qua-geographical bodies, the same rationalities, compilations, and chartings have worked to create "populations" out of subordinate groups within "the nation."

5. In a similar vein, Ian Hacking (1991) notes that statistics have been called a "'moral science': the science of deviancy, of criminals, of court convictions, suicides, prostitution, divorce. . . . It was above all the science that studied, empirically and *en masse*, immoral behavior" (182).

6. Writes Nye, "In Britain . . . biology served class and anti-urban perspectives; with the exception of racist portrayals of east European Jews, the underclass was not black, Italian or Slavic as in America, but simply poor" (1993, 688–89).

7. As Nye (1993) states, "[T]he momentous events of 1848–51, which encouraged revolutionaries like Marx to think about the common people as a disenfranchised and oppressed class, made bourgeois intellectuals think about them as a biological subspecies horrible to contemplate and malign in intent. Biology suddenly became useful for thinking about politics, and a medical model of diagnosis and cure became a fashionable way of analyzing problems of poverty, education and labour" (688). In the case of PCAP and the "Alpha patient population," the intellectuals have been replaced with physicians, epidemiologists, and legislators, and the quasi-biological subspecies is now a behavioral and environmental subpopulation. The medical model of diagnosis and cure is no longer a "fashionable way of analyzing problems of poverty," but rather a technique with which to manage the effects of poverty.

8. There appears to be a division among Foucauldian theorists about the relationship between the "individual" and the "population," and how much singularity the individual manages to retain when he or she becomes part of a population. In his ruminations on "biopower" in *The History of Sexuality, Vol. 1,* Foucault speaks about the biopolitical state's interest in both an "anatomo-politics of the human body," which takes as its focus the individual and his or her bodily capacities, and a "biopolitics of the population" that focuses on the "species body" (1978, 139). Foucault's focus on sex was due to the biopolitical state's use of it as a single technique that accomplished the dual aim of regulating both the individual and the larger population. He writes, "Sex was a means

to access both the life of the body and the life of the species" (146). And again, he notes, "Broadly speaking, at the junction of the 'body' and the 'population,' sex became a crucial target of a power organized around the management of life rather than the menace of death" (147).

Foucault's theorization of a biopolitical state with interests both at the individual level and at the population level seems to have produced a split among Foucauldian theorists over the question of whether the modern state's "power over life" in the form of an "anatomo-politics of the human body" means the state acts on the individual in his or her uniqueness, or whether the modern state's "power over life" in the form of a "biopolitics of the population" means the state acts on the individual as a crumb of the population—without specific regard to his or her uniqueness. Rose (1994) for one, interprets Foucault as concerned with individuality. Describing Foucault's work in *Birth of the Clinic*, Rose writes:

> As the medical record meticulously inscribes the details of the individual history of the patient in a stable, transferrable, comparable form, it renders the sufferings of the sick person knowable in a new way, in relation to the population of patients of which he or she forms an element. . . . Further, one could now, for the first time, observe the similarities and differences between symptoms in different individuals at any one time and over time. This provided the conditions for a statisticalization and normalization of diseases. . . ." (60)

In Rose's reading of Foucault, the individual in his or her uniqueness retains a primacy. Although the "sick person" is part of a "population of patients," he or she preserves an individual history that does not become effaced by the "statisticalization" of disease. However, other Foucauldian theorists have written about the effacement of the individual (and his or her individual history) by population. For example, Castel (1991) writes about the movement "from dangerousness to risk"—that is, a movement from a "subject or a concrete individual" who embodied or represented a danger to "a combinatory of factors, the factors of risk" (281). The movement from dangerousness to risk was one from acting on individuals with individual histories to acting on history-less individuals as the cell of a population: "The essential component of intervention no longer takes the form of the direct face-to-face relationship between the . . . professional and the client. It comes instead to reside in the establishing of flows of population based on the collation of a range of abstract factors deemed liable to produce risk in general" (281).

However, the conflict about the level of individuality the individual retains when governed by the modern state may be a question of which mode the state assumes at any given time. That is, individual histories may be more relevant when the state seeks to acquire knowledge about the population and less relevant when the state acts on the individual "through large-scale campaigns" designed to achieve some aim for the population, such as "the improvement of its condition, the increase of its wealth, longevity, health, etc." (Foucault 1991, 100). At any rate, it is evident that Foucault did theorize that, at least at some times, the individuality of the persons who compose populations is relevant to the biopolitical state; but, more important to the argument I make in this chapter, it is evident that Foucault also theorized that, at other times, the individuality of the persons who compose populations is wholly irrelevant to that same state:

> [T]he population is the subject of needs, of aspirations, but it is also the object in the hands of the government, aware, vis-à-vis the government, or what it wants, but ignorant of what is being done to it. Interest at the level of the consciousness of each individual who goes to make up the population, *and interest considered as the interest of the population regardless of what the particular interests and aspirations may be of the individuals who compose it,* this is the new target and the fundamental instrument of the government of population. (1991, 100) (emphasis added)

Accordingly, when I write that Alpha is a statistical institution that forces its individual patients to part with their unique histories and motivations, I am referring to the line of Foucauldian theory that tracks the mode of governmentality that effaces the particularity of individuals.

9. Indeed, the banality of the statement "I am high risk" bears witness to the process of "making up people"—that is, the "tendency to embrace the terms used to count us as part of our subjective understanding of ourselves" (Haggerty 2002, 101).

10. Haggerty (2002) makes a similar point when he notes "statistical categories and surveys brought new entities into the world" (98).

11. This phenomenon may be understood as an element of a larger phenomenon in which statistical norms are constructed, and any and all departures from the norm are understood as failures. "The mathematical norm is a measure of central tendency in a set of numbers; the mean, median or mode. The second approach to norms refers to proscribed behavior, with behaviors that fall outside of 'the norm' being deviant by definition. In this latter tradition, the terms 'normal' and 'abnormal' are often synonymous with 'good' and 'bad'" (Haggerty 2002, 100). Moreover, "Although these mathematical and proscriptive understandings of the norm are often seen to be quite distinct, their separation is not absolute" (100).

12. François Ewald writes about a certain Janus-faced quality possessed by "risk": as a neologism of insurance, "risk" evokes "the objective probability of an accident, regardless of the action of will"; however, within judicial reasoning, as well as within common parlance, "risk" evokes fault and blameworthiness. "Judicial reasoning springs from a moral vision of the world: the judge

supposes that if a certain individual had not behaved as he or she actually did, the accident would not have happened" (Ewald 1991, 202). And so, every invocation of risk conjures its staid, objective sense simultaneous with its morally culpable sense. The bodies of Alpha patients, interpellated and read as signs of risk, reflect that ambivalence.

13. On the relationship between "statistics," "demographics," and "population," Fogel (1996) offers "statistics" and "demographics" as that which results when one "see[s] the world as populational groups" (16).

14. "The actual Enumeration shall be made within three years after the first meeting of the Congress of the United States, and within every subsequent term of ten years, in such manner as they shall by law direct."

15. "Representatives and direct taxes shall be apportioned among the several states which may be included within this union, according to their respective numbers, which shall be determined by adding to the whole number of free persons, including those bound to service for a term of years, and excluding Indians not taxed, three fifths of all other Persons."

16. "[T]he emergence of modern forms of management, discipline and government . . . is the principal context for governmentality, as a regime which link self-subjection with societal regulation" (Turner 1997, xv).

17. One of the more lamentable characteristics of the Alpha obstetrics clinic was the inability to have a physician, nurse practitioner, or midwife speak to the patients who called the clinic telephone with their concerns. Accordingly, when a patient phoned with a medical question of any kind, the medically untrained staff who answered had been instructed, through an (appropriate) abundance of caution, to encourage the woman to go to the labor and delivery emergency room to be examined by an on-staff physician. (The alternative was for the person who answered the phone to attempt to flag down a registered nurse and pose the patient's question to her. Such attempts, however, were impractical due to the high volume of incoming telephone calls and the already overburdened workdays of the registered nurses.) The resultant increased number of visits to the hyper-medicalized and –medicalizing Alpha Hospital, and the consequent elevated number of screenings of a woman's pregnant body, served to reinscribe patients' body as unruly ones and reiterate the technocratic model of pregnancy, which assumes the inherent instability and danger of the pregnant body.

CHAPTER SIX

1. A registration receipt is given to the woman after she "opens her visit" at the financial services desk. By "opening the visit," the hospital documents that the woman was present on that day to receive an indicated service (i.e., initial obstetric visit, prenatal care revisit, ultrasound, postpartum care, gynecologic

care, etc.). This documentation enables the hospital to bill the insurance company (which, in the case of prenatal care patients, is Medicaid) for the proffered service.

2. Dorian (1982) provides an analogous example of the tenuous language skills of a speaker failing that speaker in stress-inducing circumstances. Her research on speech communities in Scotland led her to a community that had some members whose grasp upon Gaelic was fragile at best. Although these "low proficiency semi-speakers" were far from fluent in Gaelic, they were able to fully participate in community life because they understood social norms of speech and speaking. Relevant to the discussion at hand, Dorian tested the command of Gaelic possessed by a "low proficiency semi-speaker." She notes, "[I]t proved extremely difficult, almost impossible even, to interview this semi-speaker in Gaelic, since the presence of the tape-recorder produced a nervousness which compounded her difficulties with Gaelic" (30).

3. In her scathing critique of the Anita Hill/Clarence Thomas public spectacle and debacle, Wahneema Lubiano (1992) takes note of another fascinating marriage of contradictions. She argues Senators Orrin Hatch and Strom Thurmond defended Thomas (and his claim that the confirmation hearings functioned as a "high-tech lynching") by disparagingly describing Hill as a "lesbian, spurned woman." She writes:

> The logic of narratives that demonized Hill didn't seem to require rational defense whether or not such narratives were vulnerable to rational critique. . . . It doesn't matter that no one was ever lynched on behalf of a lesbian, or that being a woman spurned by a man implies heterosexuality (342–43).

And then, instructively:

> That lesbian and spurned woman cannot be rationally linked together simply means that a debased discourse doesn't care whether the terms of "othering" are logical or not. Any demonic narrative will do in a pinch. . . . [I]t simply depends upon what demon is most effective in making the sense of the world that power requires (343).

In this way, the paradoxical assertion that the wily patient and welfare queen are stupid, while simultaneously duplicitous, reveals itself as an example of a "debased discourse" whose work is to "other" the figure about which it speaks. Lubiano's analysis demonstrates it is not so much that power requires the wily patient/welfare queen be the possessors of this specific set of contradictory traits; rather, power simply requires the wily patient/welfare queen be "othered" in order that the speakers can define themselves and their values in contradistinction to the figure.

4. As early as the 1960s, articulations of the welfare queen—remarkably similar to descriptions made within the last decades—were present in public

discourse. Onwuachi-Willig (2005) cites a speech made in 1958 by Mississippi State Representative David Glass, who had proposed the mandatory sterilization of unmarried mothers. She quotes the Congressman as saying, "The Negro woman . . . because of child welfare assistance, [is] making it a business, in some cases of giving birth to illegitimate children. . . . The purpose of my bill was to try and stop, or slow down, such traffic at its source" (1670).

5. In the state of New York, the monthly grant for a family of two is $179, whereas the grant for a family of three is $238 and the grant for a family of four is $307. In effect, the state gives each individual in a two-person household $89.50, each individual in a three-person household $79.33, and each individual in a four-person household $76.75. Thus, each additional member in a family effects a reduction in the amount of money the state allocates to an individual member of the family. In essence, bearing a child for the purpose of increasing the size of a welfare grant does not make economic sense. Accordingly, it should come as no surprise that evidence supports the conclusion that the size of a welfare grant does not inform welfare recipients' decisions as to whether or not to have additional children (Kominos 2007; Note 1994; Smith 2002).

6. I use the term "moral economy of deservingness" to refer to a system of ideas in which some people are thought to be poor for "good" reasons while others are thought to be poor for "bad" reasons. Those in the former category are justified in making demands on the state; however, those in the latter category do not "deserve" assistance, and the state is justified in refusing to assist them.

7. Onwuachi-Willig (2005) notes that white women comprised 96 percent of the recipients of state pension programs, which provided economic assistance to "worthy" women and their children. President Roosevelt federalized these programs by creating ADC, which would eventually become AFDC as part of the New Deal. At its inception, "white women accounted for 85% of the AFDC rolls while black women, many more of whom were poor, accounted for a mere 13%" (1668). However, contemporaneous with the federalization of state pension programs and the establishment of ADC was the creation of the Survivor's Insurance Program, which provided cash assistance to the families of workers who qualified for retirement benefits; in essence, Survivor's Insurance provided monetary aid to the families of white workers. Hence, the (white) widows who would have otherwise been beneficiaries of ADC/AFDC were shifted to the Survivor's Insurance programs, which resulted in Black women comprising a greater percentage of those who were ADC/AFDC beneficiaries. Moreover, "[b]y the late 1960s, a string of cases had made welfare a statutory right in the United States, which enabled the number of black women on welfare rolls to continue to increase" (1669). Black women began to preponderate on the lists of welfare beneficiaries, and "welfare" began to become racialized as Black.

8. Such arguments, which equate undeservingness with a rejection of capitalism's demand that potential laborers do, in fact, labor, continue to be articulated in the present. Lawrence Mead, one of the "architects" of the work requirements that are built into TANF, is one of these articulators. The doggedness with which he insists welfare recipients work is based upon his equation of morality with work, and, conversely, immorality with not working. Thus, he argues there "are 'moral distinctions the public insists on drawing among claimants at the public trough.' In Mead's view, 'the public wants to hear . . . a moral language that links benefits and obligations'" (Koons 2004, 21–22).

9. De Genova and Ramos-Zayas (2003) have observed this sentiment in their study of the racialization of persons from Puerto Rico and Mexico in Chicago, noting "the quiet and routine exploitation of seemingly docile 'immigrants' can be conveniently reinterpreted by employers as 'hard work,' the stuff that perpetually animates the 'American Dream'" (78).

10. Cahn's (1997) argument reaches a similar conclusion. She writes: "Thus, regardless of the actual impact of Aid to Families with Dependent Children ('AFDC') regulations, their implementation is perceived as affecting blacks, even though this perception does not reflect reality. Indeed, welfare reform can be seen as an attempt to control poor black women. Thus, although welfare is not explicitly raced, it is implicitly a raced issue" (966).

11. Persons who qualify for TANF tend to be much needier than those who qualify for Medicaid. As a consequence, although persons who are eligible for Medicaid are not always eligible for cash assistance under TANF, those who are eligible for cash assistance under TANF are likely eligible for Medicaid. In fact, prior to the welfare reform of 1996, families that received assistance under the AFDC program were automatically enrolled in Medicaid (House Ways and Means Committee 2000). The law now requires that states provide Medicaid coverage to families who would have qualified for AFDC if the program still existed.

In New York, a pregnant woman whose income is at or below 200 percent of the federal poverty line is eligible for Medicaid assistance. Further, there is no resource limit—meaning the woman can own a house, car, and other assets without it affecting her eligibility. However, eligibility for TANF is much stricter: to qualify, the income of a family that includes a pregnant woman cannot exceed 100 percent of the federal poverty line, nor can it exceed 185 percent of the "Public Assistance Standard of Need" which "consists of six separate items whose value must be added together to arrive at a needs level for a particular applicant/recipient" (Health Resources and Services Administration 2008).

12. I use quotation marks around the word "population" in order to invoke the meaning usually signified by the concept while simultaneously problematizing it. See Chapter 5.

1. Consider Clarke et al. (2003) in this light: "[W]e refuse interpretations that cast biomedicalizations as a technoscientific tsunami that will obliterate prior practices and cultures. Instead we see new forms of agency, empowerment, confusion, resistance, responsibility, docility, subjugation, citizenship, subjectivity, and morality. There are infinite new sites of negotiations of power, alleviations as well as instigations of suffering, and the emergence of heretofore subjugated knowledges and new social and cultural forms" (185).

2. Lupton (1997) argues that there is a contradiction within Foucault's theorization of power, insofar as he posited the possibility of "docile bodies" within a theory that understands power as that which generates resistances to it. "There is somewhat of a disjunction, therefore, between Foucault's notion of the 'docile body' and his recognition of resistance at the local sites at which power operates and the inevitability of the failure of disciplinary and surveillance strategies directed at the patient" (102). If resistance to power is simultaneous to the repression it effects, the docility of bodies would never be complete. That is, the "docile body" is a limit to (a productive) power that would be impossible to reach. Essentially, the realization of complete docility would be foiled by "the local techniques and strategies of power, or the micro-powers that are exercised at the level of everyday life, and the ways that resistance may be generated at those levels by people refusing to engage in those techniques and strategies." (103).

Abramovitz, Mimi. 1996. *Regulating the lives of women: Social welfare policy from colonial times to the present.* Boston: South End Press.

Abu-Lughod, Lila. 1991. Writing against culture. In *Recapturing anthropology: Working in the present,* ed. Richard G. Fox, 137–62. Santa Fe: School of American Research Press.

Ackerman, Bruce. 1991. *We the people, vol. 1: Foundations.* Cambridge, MA: Harvard University Press.

Alan Guttmacher Institute. 1993. *The cost implications of including abortion coverage under Medicaid.*

American Anthropological Association. 1998. American Anthropological Association statement on "race". http://www.aaanet.org/stmts/racepp.htm.

American Congress of Obstetricians and Gynecologists. 2007. Bleeding during pregnancy. http://www.acog.org/publications/patient_education/bp038 .cfm.

Appell, Annette R. 1997. Protecting children or punishing mothers: Gender, race, and class in the child protection system. *South Carolina Law Review* 48: 577– 613.

Armstrong, Elizabeth M. 2000. Lessons in control: Prenatal education in the hospital. *Social Problems* 47(4): 583–605.

Athanasiou, Athena. 2006. Bloodlines: Performing the body of the "demos," reckoning the time of the "ethnos". *Journal of Modern Greek Studies* 24: 229–56.

Becker, Cinda. 2002. We have survived, and we're stronger; during the year since America's trauma of Sept. 11, New York hospitals—and healthcare organizations nationwide—have taken the painful lessons to heart. *Modern Healthcare* Sept. 2, 2002: 22.

Benjamin, Walter. 1996. Critique of violence. In *Selected writings, vol. 1: 1913–26*, eds. Marcus Bullock and Michael W. Jennings. Cambridge, MA: Harvard University Press.

Birke, Lynda. 2000. *Feminism and the biological body.* New Brunswick, NJ: Rutgers University Press.

Blanchet, Therese. 1984. *Meanings and rituals of birth in rural Bangladesh.* Dhaka, Bangladesh: University Press Ltd.

Boone, Margaret. 1988. Social support for pregnancy and childbearing among disadvantaged blacks in an American inner city. In *Childbirth in America: Anthropological perspectives*, ed. Karen Michaelson, 66–79. South Hadley, MA: Bergin and Garvey.

Bowers v. Hardwick, 478 U.S. 186 (1986),

Bridges, Khiara M. 2002. On the commodification of the black female body: The implications of the alienability of fetal tissue. *Columbia Law Review* 102: 123–56.

———2006. An anthropological meditation on *ex parte anonymous*. *California Law Review* 94: 215–42.

Brown, Michael K., Martin Carnoy, Elliott Currie, Troy Duster, David B. Oppenheimer, Marjorie M. Schultz, and David Wellman. 2005. *Whitewashing race: The myth of the colorblind society.* Berkeley: University of California Press.

Browner, Carole. 1985. Traditional techniques for diagnosis, treatment, and control of pregnancy in Cali, Colombia. In *Women's medicine: A crosscultural study of fertility regulation*, ed. Lucille F. Newman, 99–124. New Brunswick, NJ: Rutgers University Press.

———1986. The politics of reproduction in a Mexican village. *Signs* 11: 710–24.

Browner, Carole H. and Nancy A. Press. 1995. The normalization of prenatal diagnostic testing. In *Conceiving the new world order: The global politics of reproduction*, eds. Faye Ginsburg and Rayna Rapp, 307–22. Berkeley: University of California Press.

———1996. The production of authoritative knowledge in American prenatal care. In *Medical anthropology: Contemporary theory and method*, eds. Carolyn F. Sargent and Thomas M. Johnson. Westport, CT: Praeger.

Browner, Carole and Carolyn Sargent. 1990. Anthropology and studies of human reproduction. In *Medical anthropology: Contemporary theory and method*, eds. Thomas M. Johnson and Carolyn F. Sargent, 215–29, Westport, CT: Praeger.

Braun, Lundy. 2005. Spirometry, measurement, and race in the 19th century. *Journal of the History of Medicine and Allied Sciences* 60(2): 135–69.

Cahn, Naomi R. 1997. Representing race outside of explicitly racialized contexts. *Michigan Law Review* 95: 965–1004.

Campbell, Deborah. 2007. Impact of perinatal health issues on infant mortality and morbidity in the Bronx. www.aecom.yu.edu/uploadedFiles/Bronx CREED/D.Campbell%20present.ppt.

Carey v. Population Services, International, 431 U.S. 678 (1977).

Castel, Robert. 1991. From dangerousness to risk. In *The Foucault effect: Studies in governmentality*, eds. Graham Burchell, Colin Gordon, and Peter Miller, 281–90. Chicago: University of Chicago Press.

Centers for Disease Control. 2005. Health disparities experienced by black or African Americans—United States. *Mortality and Morbidity Weekly Report* 54(01): 1–3.

Chalmers, Beverley. 1990. *African birth: Childbirth in cultural transition*. River Club, South Africa: Berev.

Chang, Robert S. 2002. Critiquing "race" and its uses: Critical race theory's uncompleted argument. In *Crossroads, directions, and a new critical race theory*, eds. Franciso Valdez, Jerome M. Culp and Angela P. Harris, 87–96. Philadelphia: Temple University Press.

Christie, Sally K. 2002. Foster care reform in New York City: Justice for all. *Columbia Journal of Law and Social Problems* 36: 1–34.

Clarke, Adele. 2003. Biomedicalization: Technoscientific transformations of health, illness, and U.S. biomedicine. In *American Sociological Review* 68(2): 161–94.

Cohen, Jean L. 2002. *Regulating intimacy: A new legal paradigm*. Princeton, NJ: Princeton University Press.

Cooper, T. 2003. The jungle out there. *The New York Times*, July 30, 2003.

Crenshaw, Kimberlé, Neil Gotanda, Gary Peller and Kendall Thomas, eds. 1995. Critical race theory: The key writings that formed the movement. New York: New Press.

Dailey, Anne C. 1993. Constitutional privacy and the just family. *Tulane Law Review*. 67: 955–1031.

Davis-Floyd, Robbie E. 1987a. Obstetric training as a rite of passage. *Medical Anthropology Quarterly* 1(3):288–318.

———1987b. The technological model of birth. *Journal of American Folklore* 100(398): 93–109.

———1992. *Birth as an American rite of passage*. Berkeley: University of California Press.

———1994. The technocratic body: American childbirth as cultural expression. *Social Science and Medicine* 38(8): 1125–40.

De Genova, Nicholas. 2002. Migrant "illegality" and deportability in everyday life. *Annual Review of Anthropology* 31:419–47.

———2004. The legal production of Mexican/migrant "illegality." *Latino Studies* 2(2):160–85.

———2006. Introduction: Latino and Asian racial formations at the frontiers of U.S. nationalism. In *Racial transformations: Latinos and Asians remaking the U.S.*, ed. Nicholas De Genova, 1–22. Durham, NC: Duke Unversity Press.

———2007. The stakes of an anthropology of the United States. In *The New Centennial Review* 7(2): 231–77.

De Genova, Nicholas and Ana Yolanda Ramos-Zayas. 2003. *Latino crossings: Mexicans, Puerto Ricans, and the politics of race and citizenship.* New York: Routledge.

Dodson, Lisa. 1999. *Don't call us out of name: The untold lives of women and girls in poor America.* Boston: Beacon Press.

Dolgin, Janet L. 1994. The family in transition: From *Griswold* to *Eisenstadt* and beyond. *Georgetown Law Journal* 82:1516–71.

Dorian, Nancy C. 1982. Defining the speech community to include its working margins. In *Sociolinguistic Variation in Speech Communities*, ed. Suzanne Romaine, 25–33. London: Arnold.

Dorr, Gregory Michael and David S. Jones. 2008. Introduction: Fact and fictions: BiDil and the resurgence of racial medicine. *The Journal of Law, Medicine & Ethics* 36(3):443–48.

Douglas, Mary. 1966. *Purity and danger: An analysis of concepts of pollution and taboo.* London: Routledge and Kegan Paul.

Dubois, W.E.B. 1903. *The souls of black folk.* New York: Fawcett, 1961.

Duden, Barbara. 1991. *The woman beneath the skin: A doctor's patients in eighteenth-century Germany*, trans. Thomas Dunlop. Cambridge, MA: Harvard University Press.

———1993. *Disembodying women: Perspectives on pregnancy and the unborn*, trans. Lee Hoinacki. Cambridge, MA: Harvard University Press.

Duster, Troy. 2003. Buried alive: The concept of race in science. In *Genetic nature/culture*, eds. Alan H. Goodman, Deborah Heath, and M. Susan Lindee. Berkeley: University of California Press.

———2006. Lessons from history: Why race and ethnicity have played a major role in biomedical research. *The Journal of Law, Medicine & Ethics* 34(3):487–96.

Dvorchak, Robert. 1990. All the trappings of war-zone medicine, in the middle of a city, *Los Angeles Times*, Nov. 4, 1990, A40.

Eakins, Pamela, ed. 1986. *The American way of birth.* Philadelphia: Temple University Press.

Edsall, Thomas Byrne and Mary D. Edsall. 1991. *Chain reaction: The impact of race, rights and taxes on American politics.* New York: W.W. Norton.

Eisenstadt v. Baird, 405 U.S. 438 (1972).

Ellison, George T.H., Jay S. Kaufman, Rosemary F. Head, Paul A. Martin, and Jonathan D. Kahn, 2008. Flaws in the U.S. Food and Drug Administration's rationale for supporting the development and approval of BiDil as a treatment for heart failure only in black patients. *The Journal of Law, Medicine & Ethics* 36(3):449–57.

Ewald, François. 1991. Insurance and risk. In *The Foucault effect: Studies in governmentality*, eds. Graham Burchell, Colin Gordon, and Peter Miller, 197–210. Chicago: University of Chicago Press.

Fang, Jing, Shantha Madhavan and Michael H. Alderman. 2000. Maternal mortality in New York City: Excess mortality of black women. *Journal of Urban Health* 77(4):735–44.

Fausto-Sterling, Anne. 2008. The bare bones of race. *Social Studies of Science* 38:657–94.

Fein, Esther B. 1998. At ["Alpha"], luring back new mothers with luxury. *The New York Times*, Feb. 1998, 33.

Fineman, Martha. 1995. *The neutered mother, the sexual family, and other twentieth century tragedies.* New York: Routledge Press.

Fisher, Julia M. 2005. Book review: Marriage promotion policies and the working poor: A match made in heaven? In *Boston College Third World Law Journal* 25:475–97.

Fogel, Aaron. 1996. Bruegel's *The Census at Bethelehem* and the visual anticensus. *Representations* 54:1–26.

Foucault, Michel. 1973. *The birth of the clinic: An archaeology of clinical perception,* trans. A.M. Sheridan-Smith. New York: Pantheon.

————1977. *Discipline and punish: The birth of the prison*, trans. Alan Sheridan. New York: Random House.

————1978. *History of sexuality. vol. 1.* Translated by R. Hurley. New York: Pantheon.

————1991. Governmentality. In *The Foucault effect: Studies on governmentality*, eds. Graham Burchell, Colin Gordon, and Peter Miller: 87–104. Chicago: University of Chicago Press.

Fraser, Gertrude. 1995. Modern bodies, modern minds: Midwifery and reproductive change in an African American community." In *Conceiving the new world order: The global politics of reproduction*, eds. Faye Ginsburg and Rayna Rapp, 42–58. Berkeley: University of California Press.

————1998. *Afro-American midwives, biomedicine, and the state.* Cambridge, MA: Harvard University Press.1995.

Gálvez, Alyshia. 2007. Para Superarse. Unpublished manuscript.

Georges, Eugenia. 1996a. Abortion politics and practice in Greece. *Social Science and Medicine* 42(4):509–10.

———1996b. Fetal ultrasound imaging and the production of authoritative knowledge in Greece. In *Medical anthropology: Contemporary theory and method*, eds. Carolyn F. Sargent and Thomas M. Johnson. Westport, CT: Praeger.

Ginsburg, Faye and Rayna Rapp, eds. 1995. *Conceiving the new world order: The global politics of reproduction*. Berkeley: University of California Press.

Glendon, Mary Ann. 1991. *Rights talk: The impoverishment of political discourse*. New York: Free Press.

Goldberg v. Kelly, 397 U.S. 254 (1970).

Goode, Judith. 2002. From the New Deal to bad deal: Racial and political implications of US welfare reform. In *Western welfare in decline: Globalization and women's poverty*, 65–89. Philadelphia: University of Pennsylvania Press.

Gotbaum, Betsy. 2007. Hurdles to a healthy baby: Pregnant women face barriers to prenatal care at city health centers. http://pubadvocate.nyc.gov/policy/documents/Hurdlestoa HealthyBaby.pdf.

Griswold v. Connecticut, 381 U.S. 479 (1965).

Grutter v. Bollinger, 539 U.S. 306 (2003).

Haberman, Jürgen. 1962. *The structural transformation of the public sphere*, trans. Thomas Burger. Cambridge, MA: MIT Press, 1989.

Hacking, Ian. 1982. Biopower and the avalance of printed numbers. *Humanities in Society* 5:279–95.

———1982. "Biopower and the avalanche of printed numbers." In *Humanities and Society* 2:279 – 95.

———1986. Making up people. In *Reconstructing individualism: Autonomy, individuality, and the self in Western thought*, eds. Thomas C. Heller, Morton Sosna, Arnold I. Davidson, Ann Swidler, and Ian Watt. Stanford, CA: Stanford University Press.

Haggerty, Kevin D. 2002. Review: The politics of statistics: Variations on a theme. In *Canadian Journal of Sociology* 27(1):89–105.

Halm, Robert A. and Marjorie A. Mueke. 1987. The anthropology of birth in five U.S. ethnic populations: Implications for obstetrical practice. *Current Problems in Obstetrics, Gynecology, and Fertility* 4:134–71.

Hammonds, Evelynn M. 2006. Straw men and their followers: The return of biological race. *Social Science Reserach Council*, June 7, 2006, raceandgenomics.ssrc.org/Hammonds.

Hancock, Ange-Marie. 2004. *The poltiics of disgust: The public identity of the welfare queen*. New York: New York University Press.

Haney-López, Ian F. *White by law: The legal construction of race*. New York: New York University Press.

Harper, Margaret, Elizabeth Dugan, Mark Espeland, Anibal Martinez-Borges, and Cynthia McQuellon. 2007. Why African American women are at greater risk for pregnancy-related death. *Annals of Epidemiology* 17(3): 180–85.

Harris v. McRae, 448 U.S. 297 (1980).

Harris, Cheryl I. 2005. Review essay: Whitewashing race: Scapeboating culture. *California Law Review* 94: 907–43.

Harris, Mark. 2008. Checkout time at the asylum. *New York Magazine*, Nov. 24, 2008.

Harrison, Faye V. 1998. Introduction: Expanding the discourse on "race". *American Anthropologist* 100:609–31.

Health Resources and Services Administration. 2008. *New York Medicaid & S-Chip eligibility.* http://www.hrsa.gov/reimbursement/.

Hoberman, John. 2005. The primitive pelvis: The role of racial folklore in obstetrics and gynecology during the twentieth century. In *Body parts: Critical explorations in corporeality*, eds. Christopher E. Forth and Ivan Crozier. 85–104. Lanham, MD: Lexington Books.

———2007. Medical racism and the rhetoric of exculpation: How do physicians think about race? *New Literary History* 38(3): 505–25.

Hodgson v. Minnesota, 497 U.S. 417 (1990).

Horn, David G. 1988. Welfare, the social, and the individual in interwar Italy. *Cultural Anthropology* 3(4):395–407.

———1994. *Social bodies: Science, reproduction, and Italian modernity.* Princeton, NJ: Princeton University Press.

House Ways and Means Committee. 2000. Washington, D.C.: Green Book.

Huntington, Samuel. 1993. The clash of civilizations? *Foreign Affairs* 72(3): 22–49.

———1996. *The clash of civilizations and the remaking of world order.* New York: Simon & Schuster.

Institute of Medicine. 2005. *Addressing racial and ethnic health care disparities: Where do we go from here?* http://www.iom.edu/Object.File/Master/33/249/BROCHURE_disparities.pdf.

Jordan, Brigette. 1978. *Birth in four cultures: A cross-cultural investigation of childbirth in Yucatan, Holland, Sweden and the United States*, 4th ed. Prospect Heights, IL: Waveland Press.

———1997. Authoritative knowledge and its construction. In *Childbirth and authoritative knowledge: Cross-cultural perspectives*, eds. Robbie E. Davis-Floyd and Carolyn F. Sargent. Berkeley: University of California Press.

Kahn, Johnathan. 2008. Exploiting race in drug development: BiDil's interim model of pharmacogenomics. *Social Studies of Science* 38(5):737–58.

Kay, Margarita, ed. 1982. *Anthropology of human birth.* Philadelphia: F.A. Davis.

Katz, Michael. 1989. *The undeserving poor: From the war on poverty to the war on welfare*. New York: Pantheon Books.

Kominos, Teresa. 2007. What do marriage and welfare reform really have in common? A look into TANF marriage promotion programs. *St. John's Journal of Legal Commentary* 21:915–49.

Koons, Judith E. 2004. Motherhood, marriage, and morality: The pro-marriage moral discourse of American welfare policy. *Wisconsin Women's Law Journal* 19:1–45.

Landes, Joan B. 1998. Introduction. In *Feminism, the public and the private*, ed. Joan B. Landes, 1–20. Oxford and New York: Oxford University Press.

Lazarus, Ellen. 1988. Poor women, poor outcomes: Social class and reproductive health. In *Childbirth in America: Anthropological perspectives*, ed. Karen Michaelson, 39–54. South Hadley, MA: Bergin and Garvey.

———1990. Falling through the cracks: Contradictions and barriers to care in a prenatal clinic. *Medical Anthropology* 12(3):269–88.

Lazarus, Ellen and Elliott H. Phillipson. 1990. A longitudinal study comparing the prenatal care of Puerto Rican and white women. *Birth* 17(1): 6–11.

Lefebvre, Henri. 1947. *Critique of everyday life, vol. 1*, trans. John Moore. London: Verso.

Lindsey v. Normet, 405 U.S. 56 (1972).

Lock, Margaret. 1993. Cultivating the body: Anthropology and epistemologies of bodily practice and knowledge. *Annual Review of Anthropology* 22:133–55.

Lochner v. New York, 198 U.S. 45 (1905).

Lock, Margaret and Nancy Scheper-Hughes. 1996. A critical-interpretive approach in medical anthropology: Rituals and routines of discipline and dissent. In *Medical anthropology: Contemporary theory and method*, eds. Carolyn F. Sargent and Thomas M. Johnson. Westport, CT: Praeger.

Lubiano, Wahneema. 1992. Black ladies, welfare queens, and state minstrels: Ideological war by narrative means. In *Race-ing justice, engendering power: Essays on Anita Hill, Clarence Thomas, and the construction of social reality*, ed. Toni Morrison, 323–63. New York: Pantheon.

Lupton, Deborah. 1997. Foucault and the medicalisation critique. In *Foucault, health and medicine*, eds. Alan Petersen and Robin Bunton, 94–110. (London: Routledge).

MacKinnon, Catherine A. 1991. Reflections on sex equality under law. *Yale Law Journal* 100:1281–28.

Maher v. Roe, 432 U.S. 464 (1977),

Malthus, Thomas Robert. 1826. *An essay on the principle of population*. London: John Murray.

Mangold, Susan Vivian. 2001. Transgressing the border between protection and empowerment for domestic violence victims and other children: Empowerment as protection in the foster care system. *New England Law Review* 36:69–127.

Martin, Emily. 1987. *The woman in the body: A cultural analysis of reproduction*. Boston: Beacon Press.

Marx, Karl. 1867. *Capital: A critique of political economy*, trans. Ben Fowkes. New York: Random House, 1976.

Michael H. v. Gerald D., 491 U.S. 110 (1989).

Michaelson, Karen. 1986. *Childbirth in America: Anthropological perspectives*. South Hadley, MA: Bergin and Garvey.

Mink, Gwendolyn. 2002. 1998. *Welfare's end*. Ithaca, NY: Cornell University Press.

———— Violating women: Rights abuses in the welfare police state. In *Lost ground: Welfare reform, poverty and beyond*: 95–112. Cambridge, MA: South End Press.

Mitchell, Lisa M. and Eugenia Georges. 1998. Baby's first picture: The cyborg fetus of ultrasound imaging. In *Cyborg babies: From techno-sex to techno-tots*, eds. Robbie Davis-Floyd and Joseph Dumit. New York: Routledge.

Morgan, Sandra and Jeff Maskovsky. 2003. The anthropology of welfare "reform". In *Annual Review of Anthropology*, 32:315–38.

Morrison, Toni. 1992. *Playing in the dark: Whiteness and the literary imagination*. Cambridge, MA: Harvard University Press.

Mullings, Leith. 1995. Households headed by women: The politics of race, class, and gender. In *Conceiving the new world order: The global politics of reproduction*, eds. Faye Ginsburg and Rayna Rapp, 122–39. Berkeley: University of California Press.

National Center for Health Statistics. 2007. Health, United States, 2007, with chartbook on trends in the health of Americans. Hyattsville, MD: Table 52.

New York City Health and Hospitals Corporation. 2008. Frequently asked questions. http://www.nyc.gov/html/hhc/html/about/faq.shtml.

————2009. Hospitals, medical centers, home care services: ["Alpha"] Hospital Center. http://www.nyc.gov/html/hhc/html/facilities/alpha.shtml.

New York City Human Resources Administration. 2009. Pregnant women: Prenatal Care Assistance Program for Women. http://www.nyc.gov/html/hia/html/public_insurance/pregnant.shtml.

New York State Department of Health. 2005. Safe motherhood: Triennial report 2003–2005. http://mail.ny.acog.org/website/SafeMotherhoodrev.pdf.

————2009. Medicaid in New York State. http://www.health.state.ny.us/health_care/medicaid.

Note. 1994. Dethroning the welfare queen. *Harvard Law Review* 107:2013–30.

NYC.gov. 2010. http://www.nyc.gov.

Nye, Robert A. 1993. "The rise and fall of the eugenics empire: recent perspectives on the impact of biomedical thought in modern society." *The Historical Journal* 36: 697 – 700.

Obasogie, Osagie. 2007. Oprah's unhealthy mistake. *Los Angeles Times*, May 17, 2007.

Office of Medicaid Management. 2007. Prenatal Care Assistance Program (PCAP): Medicaid policy guidelines manual. New York: New York State Department of Health Press.

Office of Minority Health and Health Disparities. 2009. Eliminating racial and ethnic health disparities. http://www.cdc.gov/omhd/About/disparities .htm.

Olsen, Frances E. 1982. The family and the market: A study of ideology and legal reform. *Harvard Law Review* 96:1497–1578.

Omi, Michael and Howard Winant. 1994. *Racial formations in the United States: From the 1960s to the 1990s*. New York: Routledge and Kegan Paul.

Ong, Aihwa. 1996. Cultural citizenship as subject-making: Immigrants negotiate racial and cultural boundaries in the U.S. *Current Anthropology* 37:737–62.

Onwuachi-Willig, Angela. 2005. The return of the ring: Welfare reform's marriage cure as the revival of post-bellum control. *California Law Review* 93:1648–96.

Opdycke, Sandra. 1999. *No one was turned away: The role of public hospitals in New York City since 1900*. New York: Oxford University Press.

Orr, Cara C. 2005. Married to a myth: How welfare reform violates the constitutional rights of poor single mothers. *Capitol University Law Review* 34:211–49.

Osborne, Thomas. 1997. Of health and statecraft. In *Foucault, health, and medicine*, eds. Alan Petersen and Robin Bunton, 173–88. London: Routledge.

Parker, Willie J. 2003. Black-white infant mortality disparity in the United States: A societal litmus test. Commentary on A partnership to reduce African American infant mortality in Genesee County, Michigan. *Public Health Reports* 118(4):336–37.

Pashukanis, Evgeny Bronislavovich. 2002 [1924]. *The general theory of law & Marxism*. New Brunswick, NY: Transaction.

Pateman, Carole. 1998. The patriarchal welfare state. In *Feminism, the public and the private*, ed. Joan B. Landes, 241–76. Oxford and New York: Oxford University Press.

People. 2004. Courtney implodes, Scoop, July 26, 2004, 20.

Petchesky, Rosalind. 1987. Foetal images: The power of visual culture in the politics of reproduction. In *Reproductive technologies: Gender, motherhood, and medicine*, ed. M. Stanworth, 57–80. Minneapolis: University of Minnesota Press.

Piccato, Pablo. 2001. *City of suspects: Crime in Mexico City, 1900–31*. Durham, NC: Duke University Press.

Piven, Francis F. and Richard A. Cloward. 1971. *Regulating the poor: The functions of public welfare*. New York: Random House.

Planned Parenthood v. Casey, 505 U.S. 833 (1992).

Procacci, Giovanna. 1991. Social economy and the government of poverty. In *The Foucault effect: Studies in governmentality*, eds. Graham Burchell, Colin Gordon, and Peter Miller, 151–68. Chicago: University of Chicago Press.

Rabinow, Paul. 1992. Artificiality and enlightenment: From sociobiology to biosociality. In *Zone 6: Incorporations*, eds. Jonathan Crary and Sanford Kwiner, 234–52. Cambridge, MA: MIT Press.

Ramos-Zayas, Ana Y. 2007. Becoming American, becoming black: Urban competency, racialized spaces, and the politics of citizenship among Brazilian and Puerto Rican youth in Newark. *Identities: Global studies in culture and power* 14: 85–109.

Rapp, Rayna. 2000. *Testing women, testing the fetus: The social impact of amniocentesis in America*. New York: Routledge.

Reverby, Susan M. 2008. Special treatment: BiDil, Tuskegee, and the logic of race. *The Journal of Law, Medicine & Ethics* 36(3):478–84.

Roberts, Dorothy E. 1995. In the context of welfare and reproductive rights: The only good poor woman: Unconstitutional conditions and welfare. *Denver University Law Review* 72:931–48.

———1997. *Killing the black body: Race, reproduction, and the meaning of liberty*. New York: Vintage.

———2008, Race, pharmaceuticals, and medical technology: Is race-based medicine good for us?: African American approaches to race, biomedicine, and equality. *Journal of Law, Medicine & Ethics* 36:537.

Roe v. Wade, 410 U.S. 113 (1973).

Roediger, David R. 1999. *Wages of whiteness: Race and the making of the American working class*. New York: Verso.

Rose, Nikolas. 1994. Medicine, history, and the present. In *Reassessing Foucault: Power, medicine, and the body*, eds. Colin Jones and Roy Porter, 25–47. New York: Routledge.

Roth, Louise Marie. 1999. The right to privacy is political: Power, the boundary between public and private, and sexual harassment. *Law and Social Inquiry* 24:45–71.

Rylko-Bauer, Barbara. 1996. Abortion from a cross-cultural perspective: An introduction. *Social Science and Medicine* 42(4):479–82.

Sandel, Michael J. 1989. Moral argument and liberal toleration: Abortion and homosexuality. *California Law Review* 77:521–38.

Sanger, Carol. 2005. Regulating teenage abortion in the United States: Politics and policy. *International Journal of Law, Policy, and the Family* 18:305–18.

Sarat, Austin. 1990, ". . . . The law is all over": Power, resistance, and the legal consciousness of the welfare poor. *Yale Journal of Law and Humanities* 2: 343–80.

Sargent, Carolyn. 1989. *Maternity, medicine, and power: Reproductive decisions in urban Benin*. Berkeley: University of California Press.

Sault, Nicole. 1994. How the body shapes parenthood: "Surrogate" mothers in the U.S. and godmothers in Mexico. In *Many mirrors: Body image and social relations in anthropological perspective*, ed. Nicole Sault, 292–318. New Brunswick, NJ: Rutgers University Press.

Scheper-Hughes, Nancy and Margaret M. Lock. 1987. The mindful body: A prolegomenon to future work in medical anthropology. *Medical Anthropology Quarterly* 1(1):6–41.

Scheininger, Pamela. 1998. Legal separateness, private connectedness: An impediment to gender equality in the family. *Columbia Journal of Law and Social Problems* 31:283–319.

Schiebinger, Londa. 1993. *Nature's body: Gender in the making of modern science*. Boston: Beacon Press.

Scott, Gale. 2006. Maternal deaths plague NY. *Crain's New York Business*, June 26, 2006, 3.

Scott v. Sanford, 60 U.S. 393 (1856).

Segal, Sheldon. 1997. Contraceptive update. *New York University Review of Law and Social Change* 23:457–69.

Sharp, Lesley A. 2006. *Strange harvest: Organ transplants, denatured bodies, and the transformed self.* Berkeley: University of California Press.

Shaw, Nancy Stoller. 1974. Forced labor: Maternity care in the United States. New York: Pergamon Press.

Shonick, William and Walter Price. 1977. Reorganizations of health agencies by local government in urban American centers: What do they portend for "public health?" *Health and Society* 55(2):233–71.

Silag, Phoebe G. 2003. To have, to hold, to receive public assistance: TANF marriage-promotion policies. *Journal of Gender, Race and Justice* 7:413–38.

Smith, Anna Marie. 2002. The sexual regulation dimension of contemporary welfare law: A fifty state overview. *Michigan Journal of General and Law* 8:121–218.

———2007. *Welfare reform and sexual regulation*. New York: Cambridge University Press.

Stark, Shelley and Jodie Levin-Epstein. 1999. *Excluded children: Family cap in a new era*. Washington D.C.: Center for Law and Social Policy, http://www.clasp.org/publications/excluded_children.pdf.

State v. Luster, 204 Ga.App. 156, 419 S.E.2d 32 (1992).

Steinhauer, Jennifer. 2000. In a competitive market, city runs ads for its hospitals. *The New York Times*, March 28, 2000, B7.

Stewart, Kathleen. 1996. *A space on the side of the road: Cultural poetics in an "other" America*. Princeton, NJ: Princeton University Press.

Sullivan, Ryan. 1985. "AIDS: ["Alpha"] tries to cope with disease it cannot cure. *The New York Times*, Dec. 23, 1985, A1.

Sundaram, V., KL Liu, and F. Laraque. 2005. Disparity in maternal mortality in New York City. *Journal of the American Medical Women's Association* 60(1):52–57.

Susser, Ida and John Kreniske. 1987. The welfare trap: A public policy for deprivation. In *Cities of the United States*, ed. Leith Mullings, 51–68. New York: Columbia University Press.

Swift, Kelley P. 1995. *Hope v. Perales*: Abortion rights under the New York state constitution. *Brooklyn Law Review* 61:1473–1546.

Tapper, Melbourne. 1995. Interrogating bodies: Medico-racial knowledge, politics, and the study of a disease. *Comparative Studies in Society and History* 37(1):76–93.

Teitelbaum, Lee. 2006. Family history and family law. *Utah Law Review* 2006:197–240.

Thomas, Kendall. 1992. Beyond the privacy principle. *Columbia Law Review* 92:1431–1516.

Thomas, Susan L. 1998. Race, gender, and welfare reform: The antinatalist response. *Journal of Black Studies* 28:419–47.

Treichler, Paula. 1990. Feminism, medicine, and the meaning of childbirth. In *Body/politics: Women and the discourses of science*, eds. M. Jacobus, Evelyn Fox Keller, and Sally Shuttleworth, 132–56. New York: Routledge.

Tucker, Myra J. et al. 2007. Black–white disparity in pregnancy-related mortality from five conditions. *American Journal of Public Health* 97(2): 247–51.

Turner, Bryan S. 1992. Regulating bodies: Essays in medical sociology. London: Routledge.

———1995. From governmentality to risk: Some reflections on Foucault's contribution to medical sociology. In *Foucault, health and medicine*, eds. Alan Petersen and Robin Bunton, ix–xxi. London: Routledge.

Tutton, Richard, Andrew Smart, Paul A. Martin, Richard Ashcroft, and 2008. Genotyping the future: Scientists' expectations about race/ethnicity after BiDil. *The Journal of Law, Medicine & Ethics* 36(3):464–70.

United States Congress. 1987. Omnibus Budget Reconciliation Act of 1987, Pub. L. No. 100-203.

———1996. Personal Responsibility and Work Opportunity Reconciliation Act of 1996, Pub. L. No. 104-193, § 101.

United States Department of Agriculture. 2006. WIC Fact Sheet. http://www
.fns.usda.gov/wic/WIC-Fact-Sheet.pdf.
———2008. Women, infants, and children program for pregnant, breastfeeding, and postpartum women, About WIC. http://www.fns.usda.gov/wic/
aboutwic/default.htm.
United States Department of Health and Human Services Administration for
Children and Families. 2006. Table 8: Temporary Assistance for Needy
Families –Active cases, percent distribution of TANF families by ethnicity/
race October 2005–September 2006. http://www.acf.hhs.gov/programs/ofa/
character/FY2006/tab08.htm.
U.S. News & World Report. 1975. When the doctor says "take him to a hospi-
tal"; A close-up look at 4 institutions. June 16, 1975, 56.
Van Wolputte, Steven. 2004. Hang on to your self: Of bodies, embodiment,
and selves. *Annual Review of Anthropology* 33:251–69.
Visweswaran, Kamala. 1998. Race and the culture of anthropology. *American
Anthropologist* 100(1):70–83.
Ward, Martha C. 1989. The politics of adolescent pregnancy: Turf and teens in
Louisiana. In *Births and power: Social change and the politics of reproduction*,
ed. W. Penn Handwerker, 101–13. Boulder, CO: Westview Press.
Washington, Harriet A. 2007. *Medical apartheid: The dark history of medical
experimentation on Black Americans from colonial times to the present.* New
York: Doubleday Press.
Werbner, Richard. 1998. Beyond oblivion: Confronting memory crisis. In
Memory and the post-colony: African anthropology and the critique of power,
ed. Richard Werbner, 1–17. London: Zed.
West Coast Hotel v. Parrish, 300 U.S. 379 (1935).
Wiegman, Robyn. 1993. *American anatomies: Theorizing race and gender.* Dur-
ham, N.C.: Duke University Press.
White House (The). 2002. Working towards independence. http://www.white
house.gov/news/releases/2002/02/welfare-book-01.html.
Williams, Patricia J. 1991. The alchemy of race and rights: Diary of a law pro-
fessor. Cambridge, MA: Harvard University Press.
Youngberg v. Romeo, 457 U.S. 307 (1982).
Zuger, Abigail. 2001. They had everything they needed, except survivors to
treat. *The New York Times*, Sept. 18, 2001, F3.

INDEX

Abu-Lughod, Lila, 132
ACOG Antepartum Record, 52, 53
Administration for Children's Services
    (ACS), 253–54
Aid to Dependent Children (ADC) pro-
    gram, 214–15, 270n7
Aid to Families with Dependent Children
    (AFDC) program, 214–15, 270n7,
    271n10
Alpha Hospital, 2–9, 15; affiliation
    with Omega Hospital of, 25,
    28–30; as bureaucratic vortex,
    253–54; emergency room of, 2,
    7–8, 29, 221; impact of Medicaid/
    Medicare on, 26–28; legal custody of
    infants at, 48–49, 72–73; Medicaid
    PCAP program at, 12–13, 15–16,
    30, 48–49, 205–7; new birth-
    ing center at, 23, 28, 87–88, 239;
    pseudonym for, 11–13; as public
    hospital, 23, 24–25, 42; rate of
    C-sections at, 184–85; reputation of,
    5–8, 21–24; as site of racialization,
    24–26, 29; teaching role of, 16, 29,
    78–79

"The Alpha Hospital Mission and Vision,"
    201–2
Alpha Hospital Psychosocial Screening
    Form, 57
Alpha Women's Health Clinic, 1–9, 11,
    15–17, 30–40; acrimony towards
    patients at, 17–18, 201–2, 248–49,
    261n11; demand for services at, 207–
    9, 253; high risk services at, 103–6,
    121–22; language barriers in, 51, 210,
    223–24, 269n2; leadership in prenatal
    health care of, 23–24; racial and cul-
    tural stereotypes in, 16–17, 130–42;
    research methodology at, 13–15; staff
    hierarchies at, 10–11, 32–39, 85–89,
    180. See also ancillary staff at WHC;
    medical providers at Alpha's WHC;
    patient population at the WHC;
    Prenatal Care Assistance Program
alterity. See cultural difference
alternative/demedicalized care, 89–90, 92–96
American Anthropological Association, 8
American Congress of Obstetricians and
    Gynecologists, 52, 79–81, 160,
    261n14

American-ness, 217–20
amputations, 119
ancillary staff at WHC, 32–39; acrimony
    towards patients of, 17–18, 201–2,
    261n11; in clinic's racial hierarchy,
    10–11, 85–86; perceived incompe-
    tence of, 35–36; socioeconomic level
    of, 36–39
antenatal steroids, 113
at risk populations. *See* risk
attending physicians, 31–32, 85

Bangladeshi patients, 128–30
Benedict, Ruth, 131–32
BiDil, 123–26, 263n3
biological racism, 10, 114, 123–27,
    263n3; cultural determinist contexts
    of, 132–42; in genetic screening,
    132–34; in pathology and risk of
    WHC's patients, 151–67, 198, 256,
    265n7; *vs.* Boas's value-neutral con-
    ception of race, 131–32
biopower, 45–49, 147; docile bodies of,
    254–57, 272nn1–2; governmentality
    of risk in, 174–79, 199–200, 256,
    268nn14–16; immigration status in,
    47, 98–99; numerical objectification
    of, 148, 175, 268nn13–14; power
    over life in, 45, 265–67n8; prison
    metaphors of, 68–71; quality of the
    labor force in, 177; of reproduction,
    45–46, 260n9; state regulation of, 46,
    48–49, 60–72, 261n10, 262n17.
    See also populations
biosociality, 169–74; creation of identity
    in, 167, 170–71, 256, 265–67nn8–
    10, 268n17; moral control in, 46–48,
    171–73, 265n5, 267nn11–12; race
    and class in, 173–74
birth control, 77, 98, 156, 158–59
Birth of the Clinic (Foucault), 265–67n8
blackness, 220
black-related diseases, 153, 264nn1–2.
    See also sickle-cell disease
black/white binary, 229–36
Boas, Franz, 131–32
Burroughs, Charles, 214

Cahn, Naomi R., 271n10
capitalism: American-ness of, 217–20;
    desirability of poverty under,
    99–100, 178; moral economy of
    deservingness under, 213–20, 270–
    71nn6–10
Castel, Robert, 199, 265–67n8
census-taking, 175, 268n14
Chang, Robert S., 134–35
Chinese patients, 138–39, 184–85
chronic pelvic pain, 156–57, 183
citizen/non-citizen binaries, 231–32
Clarke, Adele, 169–70, 177, 272n1
*The Clash of Civilizations and the Remak-
    ing of the World Order* (Huntington),
    134
class. *See* socioeconomic class
clinic. *See* Alpha Women's Health Clinic
contempt, 127–30
contraception, 77, 98, 156, 158–59
C-sections, 184–85, 241–43
cultural difference, 130–42, 185; Boas's
    view of, 131–32; as deterministic,
    132–42; genetic screening in, 138–
    39; in post-racial America, 134–35.
    See also Otherness

Davis-Floyd, Robbie, 83, 93–94, 262n3
De Genova, Nicholas, 219–20, 230–31,
    271n9
Delta Hospital, 8–9, 104–5
demography, 148
Depo-Provera injections, 98
deservingness, 213–20, 270–71nn6–10
diabetes, 152, 156–57, 161–63, 172
Discipline and Punish (Foucault), 68–70
disempowerment by the fetus: at Alpha's
    WHC, 92–98; docility resulting
    from, 272nn1–2; Duden's analysis
    of, 90–93
docile bodies, 272n68, 255
doctors. *See* medical providers at Alpha's
    WHC
Dorian, Nancy C., 269n2
drug and alcohol use, 46, 77, 261n10
Du Bois, W. E. B., 219
Duden, Barbara, 90–93

Edelman, Marian Wright, 213
education of patients, 52–53
endometriosis, 118, 128–29, 140
ethnicity. *See* race/ethnicity
eugenics movement, 164–65, 265n7
Ewald, François, 257, 267n12
Expected Date of Confinement letter, 65
experimentation, 117

Federal Nutrition Service, 254
fetus. *See* disempowerment by the fetus
Figlio, Karl, 158
financial officers, 42–43, 64–66
Fogel, Aaron, 163–64, 268n13
folklore of black women's strength, 16–17,
    113, 117–18, 122
Foucault, Michel: on biopower, 45,
    68–71, 147; on the individual,
    265–67n8; on populations, 146–50,
    265–67n8; on power, 255, 272n2.
    See also biopower
Fraser, Gertrude, 93–94

Gálvez, Alyshia, 141
Gamma Medical Center, 181
genetic screening, 132–34, 138–39, 144–45
Georges, Eugenia, 262n1
gestational diabetes, 161–63
Ginsberg, Faye, 256–57
glucose challenge test, 77–78, 161–63
Gotbaum, Betsy, 261n12
governmentality of risk, 174–79, 199–200,
    256, 268nn13–16
Group B streptococcal infection, 115–16,
    263n2
Guinier, Lani, 229

Hacking, Ian, 148, 170–71, 265n5
Haggerty, Kevin D., 167, 267nn10–11
Haney-López, Ian F., 229
Harper, Margaret, et al., 112–14
Harris, Cheryl, 229–30
Harrison, Faye V., 134, 226
Hatch, Orrin, 269n3
health care: correlations with poverty of,
    164–67, 181–84, 265n7; racialized
    status of, 109–10

Health Resources and Services Administra-
    tion, 253
heart disease, 172
hepatitis, 119–21, 156–57
Hepatitis B vaccination, 77–78
high blood pressure, 60, 108, 152, 156–57
high risk pregnancy services, 103–6, 121–
    22, 177–79, 181–83. *See also* risk
Hill, Anita, 269n3
The History of Sexuality, Vol. I (Foucault),
    147–50, 265n8
HIV/AIDS, 172; counseling and testing
    for, 42–43, 53–54, 77, 160–61,
    260n4, 261n15; treatment in public
    hospitals of, 26, 78–79
Hoberman, John: on physician racism,
    111–12, 135; on racial contempt,
    127–29; on racial hardiness, 117–19
Horn, David, 149
Human Chorionic Gonadotropic (HCG)
    hormone, 91
Huntington, Samuel, 134
hyperfertility, 117, 123, 136, 156–57
hypertension, 152, 156–57
hysterectomy, 117, 119

immigrants/immigration: biopolitics of,
    47, 98–99; citizen/non-citizen bina-
    ries for, 231–32; Medicaid funding
    of, 65; stereotypes of, 185–96, 271n9
individual racism, 110–11, 248–49
infant mortality rates, 107–14, 263n1
Institute of Medicine (IOM) report, 109–
    10, 112, 136
institutional racism, 110–11
intake procedures, 16, 34, 41–45, 49–73,
    239–40; biopolitical analysis of, 45–
    49, 68–73; confirmation of preg-
    nancy in, 49–50, 91, 202–3, 261n12;
    documentation of, 67–68, 202,
    268n1; financial officer meetings
    in, 42–43, 64–66, 205–6, 260n7;
    HIV counselor meetings in, 42–43,
    53–54, 160–61, 260n4, 261n15;
    language barriers in, 51, 210, 223–
    24, 269n2; nurse/health educator
    meetings in, 42–43, 51–53, 260n3,

intake procedures, *(continued)*
261n14; nutritionist meetings in,
42–43, 54–57, 260n5, 261n16; risk
assessment in, 154–57; social worker
meetings in, 42–43, 57–64, 260n6;
state surveillance in, 66–68, 262n17;
waiting periods for, 51, 261n13
interpreters, 51, 223–24

Kappa Medical Center, 241–47
Katz, Michael, 214
Killing the Black Body (Roberts), 261n10

Latina patients: racialized distinctions
among, 219–20; stereotypes of,
128–29, 130, 139–42, 192–96
Latino Crossings (De Genova and Ramos-
Zayas), 219–20
lower-limb amputations, 119
Lubiano, Wahneema, 219, 220, 269n3
Lupton, Deborah, 75, 169, 256, 272n2

Marx, Karl, 217
maternal mortality rates, 107–14, 263n1
Mead, Lawrence, 271n8
Medicaid/Medicare in NY, 9, 23, 26–28,
30; application process for, 65–66,
260n7, 271n11; creation of, 44;
excessive medicalization of patients
under, 79–81, 151–52; health education requirements of, 155–56; intake
intrusions of, 16, 39–40, 42–44; as
less stigmatizing than welfare, 227;
marked Otherness of patients with,
232–36; pregnancy-related services
of, 44, 48, 64–66, 150–51, 205–7,
260n8; psychosocial risk in, 57–58;
technocratic model of pregnancy of,
83–90, 262n3. *See also* Prenatal Care
Assistance Program
medical folklore. *See* folklore of black
women's strength
medicalization of poor pregnant bodies,
16–17, 74–81; antiseptic sites of, 85–
86; comparisons with midwife care
of, 81–83; disempowerment by the
fetus in, 90–98, 272nn1–2; racialized

contexts of, 119–22; technocratic approach of, 83–90, 262n3; ultrasound
imaging in, 84–85, 104, 262n1
medical providers at Alpha's WHC, 31–32,
86–89; in clinic's racial hierarchy, 10–
11, 85–86, 180; racism of, 16–17,
110–16, 142–43, 248–49. *See also*
physician racism
MetroPlus, 259n1(ch.2)
Mexican patients, 139–42, 194–95
midwifery, 31–32, 82–83, 85–89; birthing
center deliveries of, 87–88; racial contexts of, 94; technocratic constraints
upon, 88–89
Mitchell, Lisa M., 262n1
morbidity and mortality rates, 107–14,
263n1

nation, 179. *See also* populations
natural childbirth, 94. *See also* midwifery
neglect, 46, 261n10
New Deal, 270n7
New York City Health and Hospitals
Corporation (NYCHHC), 24, 42,
259n1(ch.2)
New York Department of Corrections, 254
New York State Department of Health
(NYSDOH), 52–53, 259n2, 261n15
New York State Medicaid program. *See*
Medicaid/Medicare of NY
Nissen, Steven, 125
nurse/health educators, 42–43, 51–53,
260n3
nutritional risk, 154–57, 261n16
nutritionists, 54–57, 260n5, 261n16
Nye, Robert A., 164–65, 265nn6–7

obstetrical hardiness, 117–19
Office of Medicaid Management, 253
Omega Hospital, 25, 28–30; health
insurance policies of, 28, 232–34;
medical providers at, 31–32; rate of
C-sections at, 184–85
Omega University School of Medicine
(OUSOM), 28–29, 31–32, 119–20
Omnibus Reconciliation Act of 1987, 44
Ong, Aihwa, 236–37

Onwuachi-Willig, Angela, 215, 269n4, 270n7
Opdycke, Sandra, 235
orchidectomies, 119
Otherness, 226; black-white binary of, 229–36; racialized poverty of, 236–48. *See also* cultural difference

Papagaroufali, Eleni, 262n2
Parker, Willie J., 114
pathology, 152–54, 184–85; risk assessments for, 154–57; social constructions of, 157–63
Patient Education Flow Sheets, 53
patient population at the WHC, 17, 30–31, 144–46, 150–67; attribution of risk to, 154–57, 167–79, 181–83, 198, 256; classifications of, 41; deracialized discourse of, 196–99; Medicaid-required intrusions of, 16, 39–40; presumed homogeneity of, 155–57, 168–69; presumed pathology of, 151–67, 184–85, 198, 264–65nn3–4; racialist discourse of, 179–96; stereotypes of duplicity of, 205–11, 222–23, 269n2; stereotypes of stupidity of, 185–96, 202–5, 221–25; theoretical understandings of, 146–50, 265nn4–8. *See also* populations; wily patients
pauperism. *See* poverty
PCAP. *See* Prenatal Care Assistance Program
PCAs (Patient Care Associates), 1, 32, 85–86. *See also* ancillary staff at WHC
pelvic inflammatory disease, 118, 129
Petchesky, Rosalind, 84–85
pharmacogenomics, 124–25
physician racism, 16–17, 110–16, 142–43, 248–49; in acceptance of biological race, 114; in acceptance of cultural determinism, 128–29, 132–42; in folklore of black women's strength, 116–22; objects of contempt in, 127–30
physicians, 31–32, 85–89. *See also* medical providers at Alpha's WHC

Piccato, Pablo, 227
placenta previa, 96–97
populations, 146–50; ambiguous boundaries of, 148–50, 265nn4–7; attributions of risk to, 168–69; biosociality of, 169–74; governmentality of risk in, 174–79, 199–200, 268n16; individual identity in, 167, 170–71, 265–67nn8–9; logic of difference in, 179–96; numerical objectification of, 148, 175, 268nn13–14. *See also* patient population at the WHC
poverty: correlations with health of, 164–67, 181–84, 265nn6–7; creation under capitalism of, 99–100, 178; moral economy of deservingness in, 213–20, 270–71nn6–8; presumed homogeneity of, 168–69; racialized Otherness of, 226–27, 236–48
pregnancy-related hemorrhage, 112–13
Prenatal Care Assistance Program (PCAP), 12–13; creation of, 44; excessive medicalization of, 16, 74–81, 151–52; health education protocol of, 52–53, 155–56; immigration status in, 44; intake apparatus of, 16, 34, 41–73, 154–55, 239–40; Medicaid funding of, 44, 48, 64–66, 205–7; pregnancy protocols of, 76–81, 88–89; providers of, 42, 259n2; science of poverty in, 164–67
preterm birth, 113
primitive pelvis, 117–18, 140–41
prison (carceral) nets, 68–71
private hospitals. *See* Omega Hospital
Procacci, Giovanna, 164, 165, 168, 178, 264n3
promiscuity, 161, 166, 264n3
prostitution, 159–61
pseudonyms, 11–13
Psychosocial Screening Form, 57
Public Advocate for the City of New York, 50–51, 261n12
public hospitals, 24–26; AIDS treatment at, 26, 78–79; funding of, 23, 24–25, 42; impact of Medicaid/Medicare on, 26–28, 232–36; marginalization

public hospitals, *(continued)*
  of, 25–26, 253–54; private hospital affiliations of, 28–29. *See also* Alpha Hospital

Quincy, Josiah, 215–16

Rabinow, Paul, 165, 169; on biosociality, 171, 172–73; on new genetics, 173–74
"Race and the Culture of Anthropology" (Visweswaran), 131–32
race/ethnicity: biologized notions of, 10, 114, 123–27, 263n3; logic of difference in, 179–96; in normative assumptions of body types, 57; salience during pregnancy of, 10–11; scholarly definitions of, 8, 9; *vs.* culture, 130–42
racialized contexts, 24–26, 179–96, 264–65nn3–4; of alienated white patients, 236–49; of American-ness, 219–20; black/white binary in, 229–36; of deservingness, 213–20, 270–71nn6–10; of excessively medicalized care, 29, 93–94, 118–22, 151–52; of folkloric discourses on black women, 16–17, 113, 117–22; of health and health care, 109–10; of historic exploitation, 116–22; of ignorant patients, 185–96; of immigrant patients, 231–32, 271n9; impact of Medicaid on, 28; of infant and maternal mortality rates, 107–13, 263n1; of objects of contempt, 127–30; in pathology and risk analysis, 151–67, 256; of physician practice, 110–16, 135, 263n2; radical Otherness in, 130–42; of sexual stereotypes, 128–29; of sickle cell disease, 153–54, 157, 264nn1–2; of welfare queens, 17–18, 130, 195, 211–20, 228, 269n4; of wily patients, 221–27
radical Otherness. *See* Otherness
Ramos-Zaya, Ana Yolanda, 219–20, 271n9
Rapp, Rayna, 9, 256–57

Reagan, Ronald, 18, 211–12
registered nurses, 31–32, 85
regulatory apparatus. *See* Medicaid/Medicare of NY
research methodology, 13–15
resident physicians, 31–32, 85, 195
risk, 12–13, 167–79, 254; assessments of, 154–57; creation of biosocial identities of, 169–74, 198, 256, 265–67nn8–12, 268n17; governmentality of, 53, 174–79, 199–200, 256, 268nn14–16; high risk patients, 103–6, 121–22, 177–79, 181–83; nutritional risk, 54–56, 98, 261n16; procreative risk, 77, 98, 156, 158–59; of STDs, 80, 159–61; unruly pregnant bodies of, 16–17, 96–100, 268n17
Roberts, Dorothy E., 10, 128–29, 261n10
Roediger, David R., 236–37
Roosevelt, Franklin D., 270n7
Rose, Nikolas, 163, 265–67n8, 265n4

Sarat, Austin, 261n13
scientific racism. *See* biological racism
self-regulation, 175–77, 268n16
self-sufficiency, 218–19
sexuality: of poor unruly bodies, 80, 160–61, 211–12, 264n3; racial stereotypes of, 128–29
sexually transmitted diseases (STDs), 77–78, 80, 159–61
Sharp, Lesley A., 262n2
sickle-cell disease, 119–21, 133, 152–54, 157, 163, 264nn1–2
Smith, Anna Marie, 69–71, 211–12
social workers, 42–43, 260n6; discharge interviews with, 59; intake interviews with, 57–64
socioeconomic class, 9; of ancillary clinic staff, 36–39; correlations with health of, 164–67; medicalization of poverty in, 74–100, 151–52; in morbidity and motality rates, 99, 108–9; racialized poverty in, 226–27, 236–48; state regulation of poverty in, 42–44, 68–73; structure under capitalism of, 99–100, 178

The Souls of Black Folks (Du Bois), 219
staff of Alpha's WHC. *See* ancillary staff at WHC; medical providers at Alpha's WHC
state regulatory apparatus. *See* Medicaid/ Medicare in NY
state-sanctioned violence, 72
statistical institutions. *See* risk
sterilization, 119, 129
Stewart, Kathleen, 166
stratified reproduction, 257
structural racism, 110–11
"Study of Syphilis in the Untreated Negro Male," 126
substance abuse, 46, 77, 261n10
syphilis, 118, 126

Tapper, Melbourne, 153, 157, 163
technocratic model of pregnancy, 83–90; desirability of, 93–96, 262n1; disempowered bodies in, 90–98, 254–57, 262n3, 272nn1–2; seeing too much in, 96–97
technoscientific identities, 169–74, 265–67nn8–10
Temporary Assistance for Needy Families (TANF), 69–71, 227, 228, 254, 271n8, 271n11
Testing Women, Testing the Fetus (Rapp), 9
Thomas, Clarence, 269n3
Thurmond, Strom, 269n3
Torres, Gerald, 229
Treichler, Paula, 260n9
tuberculosis, 77–78, 153
Turner, Bryan S., 171–72, 268n16
Tuskegee syphilis experiments, 126
two-tier health care system, 24, 26–28, 232–33

ultrasound imaging, 84–85, 104, 262n1
undocumented immigrants. *See* immigrants/immigration
universal health care, 12–13

unruly pregnant bodies, 16–17, 96–100, 268n17; antiseptic sites of examination for, 85–86; disempowerment by the fetus of, 90–98, 254–57, 262n3, 272nn1–2; sexual stereotypes of, 80, 160–61, 211–12, 264n3; as sites for medical education, 78–80; technocratic model of, 83–90. *See also* medicalization of poor pregnant bodies
urine tests, 49–50, 91, 202–3, 261n12
U.S. Constitution, 175, 268nn14–15
U.S. Department of Agriculture, 254
U.S. Department of Health and Human Services, 253

vasa previa, 76, 145, 186–87
Visweswaran, Kamala, 123, 131–32, 134

Washington, Harriet, 117–18
welfare queens, 130, 195, 211–27, 269n4; financial allocations for, 270n5; racialized undeservingness of, 17–18, 212–20, 226–27, 228, 270–71nn6–10; Reagan on, 18, 211–12; stereotypes of, 211–12, 269nn3–4
whiteness, 219–20; in black/white binary constructs, 229–36; poverty-based demotions of, 236–49
Whitewashing Race (Brown), 229–30
wily patients, 17–18, 201–49, 261n11; acts of resistance by, 254–57, 271nn1–2; as welfare queens, 17–18, 130, 195, 211–27, 269n4; duplicity of, 205–11, 222–23, 269n2; implicit racialized Other ness of, 221–27; racialized poverty of, 236–49; racialized white patients as, 227–36; stupidity of, 202–5, 221–25
Women, Infants, and Children Program (WIC), 52, 254; food provided by, 83; nutritional risk in, 154–55; referrals to, 54–56, 77, 261n16

Text:	11.25/13.5 Garamond
Display:	Garamond
Compositor:	Westchester Book Group
Indexer:	Jan Williams